GENETICS IN HUMAN REPRODUCTION

Genetics in Human Reproduction

Edited by
ELISABETH HILDT and SIGRID GRAUMANN

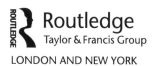

Routledge
Taylor & Francis Group

LONDON AND NEW YORK

First published 1999 by Ashgate Publishing

Reissued 2018 by Routledge
2 Park Square, Milton Park, Abingdon, Oxon, OX14 4RN
711 Third Avenue, New York, NY 10017

Routledge is an imprint of the Taylor & Francis Group, an informa business

Publisher's Note
The publisher has gone to great lengths to ensure the quality of this reprint but points out that some imperfections in the original copies may be apparent.

Disclaimer
The publisher has made every effort to trace copyright holders and welcomes correspondence from those they have been unable to contact.

A Library of Congress record exists under LC control number: 98074633

ISBN 13: 978-1-138-31497-9 (hbk)
ISBN 13: 978-1-138-31498-6 (pbk)
ISBN 13: 978-0-429-45661-9 (ebk)

Contents

VI

Part Five: Choices and decision making

Part Six: Health care, justice and regulation

List of Contributors

Matthew D. Bacchetta is Managing Director at the Cornell Medical Center, New York Hospital, Department of General Surgery.

Deryck Beyleveld is Professor of Jurisprudence at the University of Sheffield and Founding Director of the Sheffield Institute of Biotechnological Law and Ethics (SIBLE).

Dieter Birnbacher is Professor of Philosophy at the University of Düsseldorf.

Ruth Chadwick is Head of the Centre for Professional Ethics and Professor for Moral Philosophy at the University of Lancashire.

Sarah Franklin is Senior Lecturer in Anthropology at Lancaster University.

Sigrid Graumann is Scientific Coordinator of the Network for Biomedical Ethics together with Hille Haker.

Jennifer Gunning is Research Associate in Medical Law and Ethics at Cardiff Law School.

Hille Haker is Research Assistant at the Department of Ethics and Social Sciences (University of Tübingen) and Scientific Coordinator of the European Network for Biomedical Ethics together with Sigrid Graumann.

Elisabeth Hildt was the Scientific Coordinator of the European Network for Biomedical Ethics from 1996 until March 1998.

Jürgen Horst is Chairman of the Department of Human Genetics at the University of Münster.

Maureen Junker-Kenny is Head of the School of Hebrew, Biblical and Theological Studies at Trinity College, Dublin.

Lene Koch is Senior Research Fellow at the University of Copenhagen, Institute of Social Medicine.

Walter Lesch is Research Assistant at the Interdisciplinary Institute for Ethics and Human Rights at the University of Fribourg.

Ingeborg Liebaers is Professor of Clinical and Experimental Genetics and Head of Clinic of the Academic Hospital at the Dutch-speaking Brussels Free University.

Brian A. Lieberman is Professor of Gynaecology at the Manchester Fertility Services.

Barbara Maier is gynaecologist at the Salzburg Frauenklinik and teaches medical ethics at Vienna University.

Ulrike A. Mau is Clinical Geneticist at the Department of Anthropology and Human Genetics at the University of Tübingen.

Alexandre Mauron is Associate Professor of Bioethics at the University of Geneva Medical School.

Tony McGleenan is Lecturer in Jurisprudence at the School of Law at the Queen's University of Belfast and legal adviser to the European Commission Euroscreen Project.

Emma McIntosh is working on her PhD in the area of benefit assessment in health economics with particular attention to the technique of conjoint analysis.

Dieter Meschede is Research Assistant at the Institute of Human Genetics at the University of Münster.

Hansjakob Müller is Professor of Human Genetics and Head of the Department of Medical Genetics of the University Children's Hospital Basel and of the Laboratory of Human Genetics of the Basel University Clinics.

Ingmar Persson is Professor at the Department of Philosophy at Lund University.

Ysbrand Poortman is Vice President of the European Alliance of Genetic Support (European Alliance of Muscular Dystrophy Associations).

Alexandre Quintanilha is Director of the Centre for Experimental Cytology, University of Porto, Portugal, and President of the Scientific Board of the Institute of Biomedical Sciences Abel Salazar.

Stella Reiter-Theil is Research Coordinator at the Centre for Ethics and Law in Medicine, University Hospital Freiburg i. Br.

Gerd Richter is Internist and Gastroenterologist at the Department of Internal Medicine of the Philipps-University of Marburg.

Mandy Ryan is MRC Senior Fellow, Health Economics Research Unit, at the Department of Public Health, Aberdeen.

Paul Schotsmans is Professor of Medical Ethics and Director of the Centre for Biomedical Ethics and Law at the School of Medicine, K.U. Leuven.

Bernard Sèle is Geneticist and Professor of Reproductive and Developmental Biology at the Grenoble University Medical School (France) and Director of the IVF Laboratory.

Jacques Testart is Professor at the Institut de Physiologie et Psychologie de la repoduction humaine, Centre de recherche de l'INSERM.

Paul J.M. van Tongeren is Professor of Philosophical Ethics at the Catholic University of Nijmegen and Chairman of the Center for Ethics of the Catholic University of Nijmegen.

Guido de Wert is a Senior Research Fellow at the Institute for Bioethics, Maastricht, and Associate Professor in Medical Ethics at the Erasmus University Rotterdam.

Joke de Witte is biologist and philosopher and a staff member of the Center for Ethics in Nijmegen.

Reiner Wimmer is Professor of Philosophy at the University of Tübingen.

Preface

Since the birth of the first child conceived by in vitro fertilisation almost two decades ago the field of assisted reproduction is expanding continuously. Though, in the beginning of this development there has been an intensive discussion about the moral permittance of artificial intervention in human procreation and many aspects are still controversial in the public, today assisted reproduction is widely established as infertility treatment in medical practice.

In the 70s and 80s the ethical discussion was dominated by the problems related with artificial procreation as such, poor success rates of IVF, surrogate motherhood, split in social, biologic and genetic parenthood, cryoconservation and spare embryos, male domination of women's bodies, research with human embryos to improve the methods and similar topics. In spite of the fact that most of the stressed problems are still prevalent there is a change in the concentration on points of emphasis perceptible during the last years. The background for this alteration of the ethical discussion forms the experience of the establishment of the clinical practice of assisted reproduction and in vitro fertilisation as well as the presence of results of empirical follow-up studies on the one hand and the technological innovations in this field on the other hand. The new techniques pre-implantation diagnosis (PID), intracytoplasmic sperm injection (ICSI), in vitro ovum nuclear transplantation (IVONT), and in the future possibly germline gene therapy are bringing human genetics and assisted reproduction together.

Though, the theoretical possibility to check up the embryo in vitro for genetic "abnormalities" may have been from the beginning of in vitro fertilisation an idea of great influence on the part of the involved scientists, the expected benefits and the feared dangerous consequences of pre-implantation genetic diagnosis are rather new topics of public interest. Although not being feasible in human beings at the moment, also germline gene therapy – for which IVF is the presupposition – is a matter of intensive medical and ethical discussion.

Medical, social and ethical issues relating to the latest developments in IVF are discussed in the first book of the *European Network for Biomedical Ethics* with the title "In Vitro Fertilisation in the 1990s – Towards a Medical, Social and Ethical Evaluation" which has been issued 1998 at Ashgate with Elisabeth Hildt and Dietmar Mieth being the editors.

The present volume concentrates on the issues related to the current as well as to the possibly future technological progress in genetic technologies linked to IVF, i.e. preimplantation diagnosis and germline gene therapy, from a scientific and medical as well as from a social, juridical and ethical point of view.

This book contents the contributions of the second symposium of the *European Network for Biomedical Ethics* 'Genetics in Human Reproduction' which took place from February 26th to March 1st, 1998 in Maastricht, Netherlands. It provides a multidimensional view on the moral questions raised by PID and related technologies by collecting contributions from researchers coming from various European countries, working in different disciplines and arguing on various theoretical backgrounds.

The basic scientific data concerning preimplantation diagnosis and other micromanipulative procedures, as well as considerations concerning the chances and risks going along with these technologies from a scientific and medical point of view are discussed in Part One of this volume. These contributors are all physicians and scientists which does not mean that they leave out the ethical questions. The individual interests playing a role in PID and other micromanipulative procedures and their moral implications, e.g. concerning the responsibilities of prospective parents, the scientists involved, and society as a whole, are further examined in Part Two. Part Three concentrates on moral rights and duties regarding the possibilities of the new techniques on the one hand and the moral status of the embryo on the other. Part Four collects contributions with controversial moral views on the social implications of PID and related technologies. The contributors to Part Five are stressing the moral significance of desires, moral implications of reproductive choices and the role of counselling in the decision making process in the context of PID and related technologies.

The book is completed by Part Six with questions of justice in health care systems and legal regulation of PID and other micromanipulative technologies in the European context.

Acknowledgements

This volume is a collection of the lectures given at the symposium "Genetics in Human Reproduction" (Maastricht, February 1998) which was organised by the *European Network for Biomedical Ethics* in co-operation with the Instituut voor Gezondheitsethiek, Maastricht.

We want to heartily thank Ruud ter Meulen for making this Maastricht conference possible. We are especially indebted to the local organisers Guido de Wert and Angelique Heijnen.

Without the co-operation of a great number of persons, the symposium could not have been held and this book could not have been prepared. In particular, we would like to thank Katja Ruppel and Christof Mandry for invaluable help with the organisation of the symposium. Katja Ruppel and Annika Thiem carried out a great deal of the editorial work on this book, Glenn Patten and Hille Haker gave us support with proof-reading. We also want to thank the Center for Ethics in the Sciences and Humanities, University of Tübingen, for technical support, and Michael von Doering for organisational help.

In particular, this volume owes its existence to the enormous co-operation of all contributors and to the great support of the members of the *European Network for Biomedical Ethics*. We want to take the opportunity to express our thanks for their personal engagement.

We are grateful to the European Commission, Dr. Christiane Bardoux, DG XII, Science, Research and Development, for the generous funding of the *European Network for Biomedical Ethics*, the symposium "Genetics in Human Reproduction", and the publication of its results.

Elisabeth Hildt
Sigrid Graumann

These lectures were also the contributions at the Second Symposium of ENBE in Maastricht/NL in April 1998. The first symposium resulted in the publication of *In Vitro Fertilisation in the 1990s* edited by Elisabeth Hildt and Dietmar Mieth, which concentrated on interdisciplinary approach and dialogue about IVF in a general meaning and in assisted procreation. This second volume focuses on PGD-techniques, scientific, social, legal and ethical aspects. It will be followed by a third volume (from the symposium in Sheffield in January 1999), the purpose of which is the social and ethical debate on Human Procreation, promoting the controversy but also common 'points to consider'.

As the Director of the Network I would like to thank the editors of this book but also say thank you for the teamwork in the co-ordination of the whole project, including management, newsletters and research activities.

Dietmar Mieth

List of Abbreviations

AC	Amniocentesis
ACGT	Advisory Committee on Genetic Testing
AID	Artificial insemination with donor sperm
ART	Assisted reproductive technology
bp	Base pairs
BRCA 1	(Breast cancer predisposition gene)
BRCA 2	(Breast cancer predisposition gene)
CA	Conjoint analysis
CBA	Cost-benefit analysis
CBAVD	Congenital bilateral absence of the vas deferens
CEA	Cost-effectiveness analysis
CF	Cystic fibrosis
CFTR	(Cystic fibrosis gene)
CHA	Catholic Health Assosiation of America
CUA	Cost-utility analysis
CVS	Chorionic villus sampling
DMD	Duchenne's muscular dystrophy
DNA	Deoxyribonucleic acid
EAGS	European Alliance of Genetic Support Groups
ECJ	European Court of Justice
ESHG	European Society of Human Genetics
ET	Embryo transfer
FAP	Familial adenomatose polyposis
FISH	Fluorescence in situ hybridisation
GLGT	Germline gene therapy

HBOC	Hereditary breast/ovarian cancer
HD	Huntington's disease
HEXAA	Beta-N-acetylhexoaminidase A
HFE (Act)	Human Fertilisation and Embryology (Act)
HFEA	Human Fertilisation and Embryology Authority
HIV	Human immunodeficiency virus
ICSI	Intracytoplasmic sperm injection
IRB	Institutional Review Board
IVF	In vitro fertilisation
IVM	In vitro maturation
IVONT	In vitro ovum nuclear transplantation
MELAS	Mitochondrial encephalomyopathy, lactic acidosis, and stroke-like episodes
MESA	Microsurgical sperm aspiration
mtDNA	Mitochondrial DNA
NABER	National Advisory Board on Ethics in Reproduction
nDNA	Nuclear DNA
NF 1	Neurofibromatosis type 1
NHS	National Health Service
PCR	Polymerase chain reaction
PEP	Primer extension preamplification
PGC	Principle of generic consistency
PGD	Preimplantation genetic diagnosis
PGS	Preimplantation genetic screening
PID	Preimplantation diagnosis
PKU	Phenylketonuria
PND	Prenatal diagnosis
PPA	Prospective purposive agents
TBHR	Take baby home rate
TESE	Testicular sperm extraction
TNT	Therapeutic nuclear transfer
WHO	World health organisation
WTP	Willingness-to-pay

Part One
MEDICAL AND SCIENTIFIC VIEW

1 Clinical experience with PID and ICSI[*]

Ingeborg Liebaers[1,3], K. Sermon[1], C. Staessen[2], H. Joris[2], W. Lissens[1], E. Van Assche[1], P. Nagy[2], M. Bonduelle[1], M. Vandervorst[2], P. Devroey[2], A. Van Steirteghem[2]

[*]This article was reproduced with kind permission of Human Reproduction.

[1]Centre for Medical Genetics and [2] Centre for Reproductive Medicine, Dutch speaking Brussels Free University, Laarbeeklaan 101, 1090 Brussels, Belgium.
[3]To whom correspondence should be addressed.

Abstract

Preimplantation genetic diagnosis (PID) is a novel procedure which may be considered as a very early prenatal diagnosis for couples at risk for transmitting genetic diseases. Using the polymerase chain reaction (PCR) or fluorescence in situ hybridisation (FISH) the genotype or the sex of biopsied cleavage stage embryos obtained after in vitro fertilisation can be determined and selected embryos are then transferred. In vitro fertilisation with intracytoplasmic sperminjection is the method of choice to obtain embryos analysed through PCR to reduce contamination by residual sperm DNA. In our series of 61 PID cycles for 29 couples at risk since a period of 4 years the ongoing pregnancy rate per cycle was 15 %, per transfer 19 % and per patient 31 %. Of the 6 morphologically normal children born, one who is still alive and doing well, weighed 850 gr. because it was born at 25 weeks after a complicated triplet pregnancy. More experience is needed to correctly evaluate the efficiency and safety of this novel technique as well as its place in the prevention of genetic disease.

Introduction

Preimplantation genetic diagnosis (PID) is a novel technique which permits determination of the genotype of an oocyte before fertilisation or of an embryo before implantation. On the one hand, this procedure became possible because of the almost simultaneous development of IVF, micromanipulation, PCR and fluorescence in-situ hybridisation (FISH). On the other hand, patients or couples with a recurrence risk for genetic diseases were asking such a procedure so as to avoid the need for pregnancy termination after conventional prenatal diagnosis. The first clinical PID was reported by Handyside and Winston in 1990 (Handyside et al. 1990). Preclinical studies had convinced them that their was apparently no harm in biopsying a cleavage-stage embryo at the 6- to 8-cell stage (Hardy et al. 1990). Since then several groups have performed PID successfully using either PCR or FISH to analyse blastomeres from 3-day-old embryos (Harper 1996, Lissens et al.1996) or to analyse polar bodies from oocytes before fertilisation (Verlinsky et al. 1996).

Intracytoplasmic sperm injection (ICSI) certainly has its use in PID. In the first place it has an advantage over conventional in vitro fertilisation (IVF) in that it avoids contamination by sperm in PID of a cleavage-stage embryo, using the polymerase chain reaction (PCR). Moreover, for some couples with a concurrent genetic risk such as cystic fibrosis (CF) in cases of congenital bilateral absence of the vas deferens (CBAVD), pregnancy will be obtained more often after ICSI with spermatozoa retrieved from the epidydimis than after regular IVF (Silber et al. 1994). Klinefelter patients who on rare occasions may produce a very low number of spermatozoa may try to father a child through IVF and ICSI with spermatozoa extracted from an ejaculate or more often from a testicular biopsy and in this experimental setting the number of sex chromosomes in the embryos will have to be evaluated before transfer. The outcome of these treatment cycles in Klinefelter patients have partially been published and will be updated separately (Staessen et al. 1996, Tournaye et al. 1996). In this article our clinical PID experience in case of a recurrence risk for monogenic diseases will be reported and the place of ICSI will briefly be discussed.

Materials and methods

Twenty-nine couples were counselled at the Centre for Medical Genetics between February 1993 and February 1997 prior to PID. Except for 3 of them with a lower risk (see appendix) they had a 25% or 50% risk of having children with CF (with or without CBAVD in the male) (n=8), with non-fragile X mental retardation (n=3), with hemophilia A (n=2), with Duchenne's muscular dystrophy (DMD) (n=4), with retinitis pigmentosa (n=1) or with myotonic dystrophy (n=11). The reason why these couples chose PID rather than regular prenatal diagnosis were in general (A) infertility or subfertility necessitating IVF as well as the genetic risk (n=15), (B) one or several pregnancy terminations after chorionic villus sampling (CVS) or amniocentesis (AC) (n=8) and (C) moral, emotional or religious objections against abortion in itself (n=6) or in combination with another indication (n=4). Table 1 summarises the indications and the outcome of PID in Brussels over a period of 4 years. Couples were prepared for IVF (4 cycles) or for IVF with ICSI (57 cycles) according to standard protocols (Staessen et al. 1993, Van Steirteghem et al. 1993, 1995). A brief history of each couple is given in the appendix.

Blastomere biopsy

Embryos were biopsied in the morning of day 3 after insemination or microinjection. From the 7-cell stage on, two blastomeres per embryo were removed, while from 4-cell to 6-cell embryos only one blastomere was taken. A micropipette was used with an inner diameter of 40 to 45 µm while the embryos were immobilised by means of a holding pipette. These biopsies were performed in HEPES-buffered Earle's medium. First, a hole was made in the zona pellucida. This was done by blowing a stream of Acidic Tyrode's solution until the zona pellucida ruptured. Two different procedures to obtain blastomeres have been used. In the first cycles, the hole in the zona was turned to the 12 o'clock position. One or 2 blastomeres were pushed through the hole by pushing with a bevelled pipette with an inner diameter of 40 µm. Later, a blunt pipette with an inner diameter of 40 µm to 45 µm and a smoothened opening was passed through the hole. The hole was placed at the equatorial plane of a blastomere containing a nucleus before aspiration (Ao et al. 1996).

Diagnosis by the PCR method

Under continuous microscopical supervision, blastomeres were washed three times in Ca^{2+} and Mg^{2+} free M2 medium and placed in a 0.5 or 0.2 ml PCR tube. Lysis conditions and reaction conditions were worked out to detect the concerned mutations or DNA sequences in the most efficient and accurate way at the single-cell level. The resulting DNA fragments were further analysed on a polyacrylamide or Metaphor® agarose gel (Liu et al.1994a, 1994b, 1995, Sermon et al. 1997).

5

Diagnosis by the FISH method

The individual blastomeres were first rinsed in medium, then transferred to a 1-2 μl droplet of 0.01N HCl/0.1 % Tween 20 solution on a slide and the FISH procedure as described by Coonen et al. (1994) was used. Double target FISH was performed using directly labelled DNA-probes specific for chromosomes X and Y. The X (Vysis, ?-satellite DNA probe, Spectrum Green) and Y (Vysis, satellite III DNA probe, Spectrum Orange) were used for gender determination. To counterstain the nuclei 4'6-diamidino-2-phenyindole (DAPI) was used. The nuclei were then examined using a Zeiss Axioskop fluorescence microscope with the appropriate filter set (filter 10 for fluorescein isothiocyanate (FITC), filter 02 (DAPI) and Omega filter (FITC/Texas Red) (West et al. 1989, Griffin et al. 1991, Harper et al.1994). All nuclei were observed and FISH results (two green spots in case of the presence of female blastomere or one green and one orange spot in case of a male blastomere) were interpreted by two independent observers.

Embryo transfer, cryopreservation and follow-up

Whenever possible up to 3 unaffected embryos of grade A (no anucleated fragments), B (1 to 20% anucleated fragments) or C (21-50 % anucleated fragments), were transferred per cycle as indicated (female age, rank of trial, embryo quality). Spare unaffected embryos were cryopreserved and transferred in a subsequent cycle. The luteal phase was supplemented by micronised progresterone (600 mg daily) administered intravaginally or HCG (5000 units 5 days after ovum pick-up) administrated intramuscularly and serum HCG was determined from day 10 onwards. Where possible, a close pregnancy follow-up was organised, including regular ultrasound examinations, chorionic villus sampling or amniocentesis to confirm the result of the PID, registration of the pregnancy outcome and clinical evaluation of the child at birth and thereafter (Wisanto et al.1996, Bonduelle et al.1996). If no pregnancy ensued follow-up information on the couples was collected.

Results

So far 61 cycles for preimplantation diagnosis have been performed for 29 patients as reported in table 1. Of these cycles, 36 were performed during the last year. The mean age of the women at their first attempt was 30.4 years, with a range between 24 and 37. The number of attempts per couple ranged from 1 to 5 with an average of 2.1 cycles per couple (see appendix).

The number of cumulus-oocyte complexes recovered per cycle was between 2 and 43, providing a mean of 13.2 (805/61). Fertilisation, i.e., the presence of two pronuclei (2PN) was observed in 456 oocytes which corresponds to a mean of 7.5 per cycle. In 4 cycles there was no further development of the fertilised oocytes and therefore no further analysis. In 333 cleavage-stage embryos between the 4- and the 10-cell stage a biopsy was performed. The mean number of biopsied embryos per cycle was 5.8 (333/57). In 43 (12.9%) of the 333 embryos no diagnosis was possible because of no amplification, inconsistent results or contamination.

One hundred and twenty-nine unaffected embryos, a mean of 2.3 per cycle were available for transfer; except for 1 embryo of grade A, they were all grade B or C. In 12 cycles no embryos could be transferred; in 4 of these because no embryos developed and in the remaining 8 because no unaffected embryos were available. In 16 cycles only 1 embryo was transferred. Unaffected embryos were cryopreserved in 5 cycles and most of these were transferred in three additional cycles but without success.

So far 10 pregnancies have ensued from fresh transfers. One miscarriage has occurred, 4 singleton pregnancies are ongoing and 6 children have been born from the remaining 5 pregnancies. The children are between 3 months and more then 2 years of age. One of them is a boy, the others are girls.

Discussion

The success rate in terms of pregnancies is 10 out of 61 cycles or 16 %. Per transfer the pregnancy rate is 10/48 (21 %) and per couple it is 10/29 (34 %). Numbers are too small to calculate the take-home baby rate but if we subtract the one miscarriage and consider the ongoing pregnancies (n=4) plus the deliveries (n=5), the take-home baby rates are 15% per cycle, 19% per transfer and 31 % per couple. In our regular IVF or IVF/ICSI cycles the pregnancy rate per cycle is currently around 30 % and the take-home baby rate per cycle well over 20 %, and in the world figures for PID the pregnancy rate per cycle was 25 % and per transfer 29 % (Harper, 1996). The lower success rate in this small series cannot be explained by the age of our patients which is quite similar. One of the reasons for a lower pregnancy rate is most probably the higher number of cycles in which none or only 1 unaffected embryo of grade B or C were available for transfer. From our availabe data we therefore decided that cycles for PID with less then 9 cumulus-oocyte-complexes should be cancelled. Another reason for a lower success rate may be a "subfertility" of the myotonic-dystrophy patients due to their disease, since 25 out of the 61 cycles were performed in 11 couples at risk for this disease (Sermon et al. 1997).

None of the 4 couples at risk of CF has become pregnant so far. Two of these had a subfertility problem as well as the genetic risk but, nevertheless one of them has since had two spontaneous pregnancies followed by the birth of non-affected children after CVS. Prior to the pregnancies the couple was intending to have another PID cycle. One couple had 4 cycles so far without success. After CF had been diagnosed in 1 of their 2 children 8 years ago, they waited for the development of PID so as to be able to have at least 1 other healthy child, especially since the wife could not cope with the idea of prenatal diagnosis followed by a possible pregnancy termination. Although this couple was proven to be fertile, the oocytes and embryos produced during the 4 treatment cycles were always low in number and of extremely poor quality.

Pregnancies have ensued in 2 of the 4 couples at risk for CF because the wives of CBAVD-men were carriers. In 1 case the pregnancy occurred during the first treatment cycle after replacement of 3 embryos and a healthy boy now over 2 years of age was born (Liu et al. 1994a). Subsequent cycles were unsuccessful.

For the second couple, 5 cycles were needed to obtain a singleton pregnancy after transfer of 3 embryos.

In 6 out of 10 patients at risk for an X-linked disease, pregnancies have ensued. The mean age of these patients was 28 years. Four of the 10 patients were at risk of DMD. Two of them now have girls. In the first case the pregnancy occurred during the second cycle and the diagnosis was based on a PCR assay detecting the presence or absence of a dystrophin gene deletion. Two embryos were transferred (Liu et al.1995). The girl is now over 2 years of age and healthy. In the second case a triplet pregnancy occurred during the second cycle after transfer of 3 embryos. The triplet was one singleton and one twin (monochorionic, biammniotic) one of which was shown to be an acardiacus between 13 and 14 weeks of pregnancy. Five weeks later selective reduction of the malformed twin was performed extramuros and another 4 weeks later, the children were prematurely born at almost 25 weeks of pregnancy. The morphologically normal twin weighed 450 g and subsequently died. The singleton baby girl weighed 850g and is doing well according to the information we obtained so far. In 2 patients at risk for hemophilia A, 1 healthy girl was born after transfer of 2 embryos and 2 healthy twin girls have recently been born after the replacement of 3 embryos in the second patient respectively. Of the 3 patients at risk of non-fragile-X-linked mental retardation, 1 patient became pregnant after replacement of 3 embryos in the first cycle but a miscarriage occurred. Finally, 1 patient at risk of retinitis pigmentosa is currently pregnant after 1 treatment cycle with transfer of 2 embryos.

Two out of 11 couples at risk of myotonic dystrophy are currently pregnant with singletons, both after a 3rd cycle in which respectively 2 and 4 embryos were transferred (Sermon et al.1997).

The mean age of all the preceding pregnant women was 29.8 years (range 24-37); the mean number of embryos transferred per cycle was 2.5 (range 2 to 3 except in one case where 4 were transferred).

In our population of 29 couples who had requested PID, the indications, apart from the genetic risk, were infertility in the 4 cases with CBAVD, subfertility in 11 cases (most of which belong to the myotonic dystrophy group), a previous history of affected pregnancies which had to be terminated in 8 cases and moral problems with termination of pregnancy in 6 cases. The high pregnancy rate of 60% in the group of patients at risk of sex-linked diseases might be explained by the lack of subfertility problems (only 1 out of 10) and the younger mean age (28 years) of these patients. The one miscarriage occurred in the subfertile couple with a previous history of G4P1A3.

Only the first 4 cycles in couples without CBAVD involved classical IVF. Since then IVF with ICSI has been used for insemination. The aim was to reduce the risk for contamination in PCR reactions from residual sperm-DNA. We still consider this to be the insemination method of choice in PCR- based PID. In FISH-based PID for couples with no known subfertility or infertility, conventional IVF is probably equally valid as an option.

Before starting the treatment, PID patients were asked to agree to a prenatal diagnosis through CVS or amniocentesis to confirm the result of the PID should they become pregnant, since at least in PCR-based assays misdiagnoses have been reported (Harper 1996) and since diagnostic errors may occur as a result of contamination or allele-specific drop-out during the PCR reaction. Of the 10 pregnancies, 1 miscarried before prenatal diagnosis. Two patients pregnant after a FISH-based sex-determination and one patient pregnant after CF-diagnosis declined to have prenatal diagnosis. In 6 cases (1 CVS and 5 amniocenteses) the PID was confirmed or refined (CF carrier boy, non-carrier DMD girl).

The age of the 6 children born so far ranges from 3 months to over 2 years of age. Four of these are girls because female embryos were selected for transfer as a result of a risk of a sex-linked disease. The fifth girl was born to a carrier of Duchenne's muscular dystrophy but the PCR-based PID indicated affected boys (absence of fragment) versus unaffected male embryos and non-carrier as well as carrier female embryos (presence of fragment). This girl and the boy born at term in 1994 were morphologically normal (Liu et al.1994a, 1995). At birth and at 2 years of age their growth and developmental milestones were within the normal range. One of the 4 girls born in 1996 issued from the triplet pregnancy mentioned earlier; she was born at 25 weeks of pregnancy and weighed 850 g. At 4 months of age the girl weighed 3.2 kg and measured 49 cm. According to the parents, who plan to visit us, she was doing fine. The premature birth was probably the result of the selective reduction performed on 1 of the malformed twins at 18 to 19 weeks of pregnancy. The other twin weighed only 450 g at birth and did not survive. The cause of the acardiacus malformation is most probably linked to the twinning process and not to the biopsy procedure. The 3 other girls born in 1996 are doing well according to information obtained from the parents and their physicians. One girl was born at 36 weeks of pregnancy and had a birthweight of 2.4 kg, a length of 47 cm and a head circumference of 32 cm. She is now about 1 year old. The other twin girls were born at 35 weeks of gestation and weighed 2.6 and 2.1 kg respectively; they are now 3 months old. So far, the number of children born is too small to draw any firm conclusions concerning possible problems with morphology, growth or development. As in regular IVF and ICSI, multiple pregnancies should be avoided where possible so as to reduce the risk of complications (Bonduelle et al. 1996, Wisanto et al. 1996, Simpson and Liebaers 1996).

Our PID programme is now well structured and based on a close collaboration between the Centre for Medical Genetics and the Centre for Reproductive Medicine. Before starting, patients are counselled extensively by specialised physicians in both Centres. A nurse-coordinator schedules the cycles and informs the team members who will be involved and especially the laboratories dealing with cycle monitoring, IVF and ICSI, embryo biopsy and FISH or PCR analysis. Patients are asked to come to the clinic for pick-up and on day 3 post-insemination for a possible transfer. The outcome of the embryo diagnosis is discussed with the couple at the clinic. In any case a follow-up visit is scheduled with the geneticist as well as with the fertility specialist so as either to organise a pregnancy follow-up with prenatal diagnosis, ultrasound and finally a baby follow-up or to plan a subsequent cycle. Organising the follow-up of patients from abroad is more complex and the data obtained are less complete.

Possible reasons for the slow development of PID in our centres and elsewhere are probably linked to its experimental character and to the complexity of the procedure at the clinical as well as at the laboratory level. Moreover the take-home baby-rate is low as a result of this complexity and the cost is rather high. Finally, the availability of the procedure in general and of specific procedures for specific diseases is still limited. Nevertheless, the procedure does not appear to be too stressful for many of the patients, since several of them have had repeated PID (see appendix). Further development in diagnostic procedures as well as the evaluation of patient's experience are therefore to be expected. Moreover continuous data collection at the national and international levels will be of great value to correctly appreciate the value of this new procedure (ESHRE Special Interest Group on Reproduction and Genetics, International Working Group on PID).

Table 1. PID in Brussels between February 1993 and February 1997 for monogenic diseases

Disease	Couples	PID indication		Cycles	Transfers	Pregnancies	Miscarriages	Ongoing pregnancies	Births	Children
Cf_a	4	Subfertility	2	9	7	-	–	–	–	–
		History$_e$	1							
		TOP_f	1							
CF_a / $CBAVD_b$	4	Infertile male needing MESA$_g$	4	12	8	2	–	1	1	1
MD_c	11	Subfertility	8	25	22	2	–	2	–	–
		History$_e$	1							
		TOP_f	6							
X-linked$_d$	10	Subfertility	1	15	11	6	1	1	4	5
		History$_e$	6							
		TOP_f	3							
	29			61	48	10	1	4	5	6

$_a$Cystic Fibrosis; $_b$Congenital bilateral absence of vas deferens; $_c$myotonic dystrophy; $_d$X-linked diseases such as Duchenne's muscular dystrophy, Hemophilia A, X-linked mental retardation and retinitis pigmentosa; $_e$previous history of prenatal diagnosis followed by termination of pregnancy; $_f$moral, emotional or religious objection to termination of pregnancy (TOP); $_g$microsurgical epidydymal sperm aspiration.

Addendum

Since the publication of the above article, in total 170 PID cycles have been performed for 84 couples. Twenty-nine pregnancies were established. Five of these were multiple pregnancies.

One pregnancy was terminated because of a misdiagnosis detected at prenatal diagnosis. Seventeen healthy children were born, one acardiacs-twin died. Twelve pregnancies are ongoing.

Genetic indications for preimplantationdiagnosis were for monogenic conditions: several X-linked disorders such as Duchennes Muscular Dystrophy, hemophilia A, Wiskott-Aldrich disease, adrenoleucodystrophy, Charcot Marie Tooth disease, mental retardation, retinitis pigmentosa.

PID was also performed for autosomal recessive and dominant diseases such as myotonic dystrophy, cystic fibrosis with our without (CBAVD), Marfans disease, Charcot Marie Tooth disease, β-thalassemia, 21-β-hydroxylase deficiency, osteogenesis imperfecta and sickle cell anemia.

For chromosomal aberrations, PID has been performed for the velo-cardio-facial syndrome due to a 22q deletion, for a translocation (11;22), for a Yq deletion as well as for Klinefelter patients producing a few spermatozoa in their testes.

The demand for PID has increased over the years. New diagnostic tests are being developed and more centers are offering this new procedure. Evaluation of patients experience with this new procedure is necessary and ongoing.

References

Ao, A., Ray, P., Harper, J., Lesko, J. et al. (1996), 'Clinical experience with preimplantation genetic diagnosis of cystic fibrosis (ΔF508)', *Pren. Diagn.* 16, 137-142.

Bonduelle, M., Wilikens, A., Buysse, A. et al. (1996) 'Prospective follow-up study of 877 children born after intracytoplasmic sperm injection (ICSI) with ejaculated, epididymal and testicular spermatozoa and after replacement of cryopreserved embryos after ICSI', *Hum. Reprod.*, 11(4), 131-159.

Coonen, E., Dumoulin, J.M.C., Ramaekers, F.C.S. et al. (1994), 'Optimal preparation of preimplantation embryos interphases nuclei for analysis by fluorescences in situ hybridisation', *Hum. Reprod.*, 9, 533-537.

Griffin, D.K., Handyside, A.H., Penketh, R.J.A. et al. (1991), 'Fluorescent in-situ hybridization to interphase nuclei of human preimplantation embryos with X and Y chromosome specific probes', *Hum. Reprod.*, 6 (1), 101-105.

Handyside, A.H., Kontiogianni, E.H., Hardy, K. et al. (1990), 'Pregnancies from biopsied human preimplantation embryos sexed by Y specific DNA amplification', *Nature*, 344, 768-770.

Hardy, K., Martin, K.L., Leese, H. et al. (1990), 'Human preimplantation development in vitro is not adversely affected by biopsy at the 8-cell stage', *Hum. Reprod.*, 5, 708-714.

Harper, J.C. (1996) 'Preimplantation diagnosis of inherited disease by embryo biopsy: an update of the world figures', *J. Assist. Reprod. Genet.*, 13(2), 90-95.

Harper, J.C., Coonen, E., Ramaekers, F.C.S. et al. (1994), 'Identification of the sex of human preimplantation embryos is two hours using an improved spreading method and fluorescence in situ hybridisation (FISH) using directly labelled probes', *Hum. Reprod.*, 4, 721-724.

Lissens, W., Sermon, K., Staessen, C. et al. (1996), 'Review: Preimplantation diagnosis of inherited disease', *J. Inher. Metab. Dis.*, 19, 709-723.

Liu, J., Lissens, W., Devroey, P. et al. (1994), 'Amplification of X- and Y-chromosome specific regions from single human blastomeres by polymerase chain reaction for sexing of preimplantation embryos', *Hum. Reprod.*, 9, 716-720.

Liu, J., Lissens, W., Silber, S.J. et al. (1994), 'Birth after preimplantation diagnosis of the cystic fibrosis ΔF508 mutation by polymerase chain reaction in human embryos resulting from intracytoplasmic sperm injection with epididymal sperm', *JAMA*, 272, 1858-1860.

Liu, J., Lissens, W., Van Broeckhoven, C. et al. (1995), 'Normal pregnancy after preimplantation DNA diagnosis of a dystrophin gene deletion', *Prenat. Diagn.*, 15, 351-358.

Sermon, K., Lissens, W., Joris, H. et al (1997,) 'Clinical application of preimplantation diagnosis for Myotonic Dystrophy', *Prenat. Diagn.*, in press.

Silber, S.J., Nagy, Z.P., Liu, J. et al (1994), 'Conventional in vitro fertilization versus intracytoplasmic sperm injection for patients requiring microsurgical sperm aspiration', Hum Reprod ,9, 1705-1709.

Simpson, J.L., Liebaers, I. (1996), 'Assessing congenital anomalies after preimplantation genetic diagnosis', *J. Assist. Reprod. Genet.*, 13(2), 170-176.

Staessen C., Coonen E., Van Assche, E. et al. (1996), 'Preimplantation diagnosis for X and Y normality in embryos from three Klinefelter patients', *Hum. Reprod.*, 11, 1650-1653.

Staessen, C., Janssenswillen, C., Van den Abbeel, E. et al. (1993), 'Evidence of triplet pregnancies by selective transfer of two quality embryos', *Hum. Reprod.*, 8, 1650-1653.

Tournaye, H., Staessen, C., Liebaers, I. et al. (1996), 'Testicular sperm recovery in nine 47, XXY Klinefelter patients', *Hum. Reprod.*, 11, 1644-1649.

Van Steirteghem, A.C., Nagy, Z., Joris, H. et al (1993), 'High fertilization and implantation rates after intracytoplasmic sperm injection', *Hum. Reprod.*, 8, 1061-1066.

Van Steirteghem, A.C., Joris, H., Liu, J. et al. (1995), 'Protocol for intracytoplasmic sperm injection', *Hum. Reprod.*, Update 1, n° 3, CD-ROM.

Verlinsky, Y., Cieslack, J., Ivakhnenko, V. et al. (1996), 'Birth of healthy children after preimplantation diagnosis of common aneuploidies by polar body fluorescent in situ hybridization', *Fertil. Steril.*, 66, 126-129.

West, J.D., Gosden, C.M., Gosden, J.R. et al. (1989), 'Sexing the human fetus and identification of polyploid nuclei by DNA-DNA in situ hybridisation in interphase nuclei', *Mol. Reprod. Develop.* 1, 129-137.

Wisanto, A., Bonduelle, M., Camus, M. et al. (1996), 'Obstetric outcome of 904 pregnancies after intracytoplasmic sperm injection', *Hum. Reprod.*, 11(4), 121-131.

Acknowledgements

Research funds of the university and the F.W.O.-Vlaanderen have made the development of these new procedures possible. Besides the authors and all the other members of the Centres for Medical Genetics and Reproductive Medicine were helpful in taking care of the patients and their embryos. Special acknowledgements go to F. Winter for correcting the grammar and style and J. Heulaerts for typing the manuscript.

2 The various micromanipulative procedures: State of the art, chances, and risks

Dieter Meschede and Jürgen Horst

Micromanipulation has added a new dimension to reproductive medicine. It entails the use of microtools that allow for a precise handling and manipulation of single cells or their subcompartments such as the cytoplasm or nucleus. With various types of micropipettes germ cells or parts of them as well as early embryos can be individually selected, held, drilled, cut, injected, or biopsied. The possible applications of this technology in research, diagnosis and therapy are manifold. Cloning of humans, considered to be on the horizon, would also have to rely on these micromanipulative technologies. But even some currently available techniques such as oocyte cytoplasm donation make conventional in vitro fertilisation (IVF) look like an old-fashioned and almost natural way of inducing pregnancies.

In quantitative terms, intracytoplasmic sperm injection (ICSI) is by far the most important procedure involving micromanipulation (Felberbaum and Dahnke 1997). Its main application is severe male factor infertility, an entity that in the pre-ICSI era had a dismal prognosis for a successful treatment outcome. Centers with ample experience now report clinical pregnancy rates exceeding 30 % per treatment cycle. The fact that this exceeds the natural conception rate in fertile couples illustrates what dramatic progress ICSI represents.

ICSI is supplemented by new techniques for surgical sperm retrieval in azoospermic or severely oligozoospermic men. Patients with obstructions of the seminal ducts may benefit from MESA (microsurgical epididymal sperm aspiration), individuals with non-obstructive azoospermia from TESE

17

(testicular sperm extraction) (Devroey et al. 1994). Both these procedures yield physiologically immature and poorly motile germ cells so that combining them with an ICSI procedure is almost mandatory in order to have a reasonable chance for attaining a pregnancy. Similarly, ICSI facilitates the use of cryopreserved sperm from men with malignant disorders who as a result of radio- or chemotherapy lost their ability to sire children. There is a general trend to go back to increasingly immature developmental germ cell stages for ICSI – in humans normal pregnancies have been induced with spermatids (Fishel et al. 1995), in mice even with secondary spermatocytes which have not undergone the second meiotic division (Kimura and Yanagimachi 1995).

Freezing female gametes or ovarian biopsies has proven difficult, but with technical improvements and the support of micromanipulation such cryopreserved samples may soon become clinically useful. To have a 'cryo-reserve' of eggs or ovarian tissue may in the future enable women to delay childbearing into the postmenopausal age, or have children after fertility-ablating cancer treatment. Cytoplasm donation may be another option for 'reproductively old' women to enhance their fertility potential. Their germ cells can be freshened up with oocyte cytoplasm from a younger donor. This procedure has already resulted in the birth of healthy children (Cohen et al. 1997), but its practical importance remains to be established. The technique does not have any immediate genetic implicatons apart from the remote possibility that mitochondrial disorders could be transmitted. In contrast, ovum nuclear transfer would entail the exchange of the recipient's genome for a donor genome. Possible reasons for the use of this micromanipulative procedure could be advanced reproductive age or an inheritable disorder of the recipient. In genetic terms, ovum nuclear transfer does not differ from the donation of whole oocytes - any offspring resulting from this procedure would not be a genetic child of the recipient. Whether there is any sound clinical rationale for ovum nuclear transfer in humans is unclear.

Finally, cloning humans would entail the use of micromanipulative technology. Cloning is defined as the intentional creation of genetically identical individuals. In that regard, embryo splitting, a procedure employed in veterinary medicine, would qualify as cloning. In less dramatic terms such a procedure could be designated as the artifical induction of a monozygotic twin (or higher multiple) pregnancy. In contrast, cloning in the narrower sense means the creation of a genetically identical copy of an adult individual. As demonstrated in sheep and cattle, mammals can be cloned by inserting a somatic cell nucleus into an enucleated germ cell (Nash 1997). Genetically, cloning means to circumvent the recombination of genes that occurs in meiosis. In natural reproduction this process guarantees that children inherit a non-predictable random sample of their parents' genetic repertoires. The meiotic jumbling of genes is one safeguard for genetic diversity and a driving force of evolution.

Preimplantation diagnosis (PID) can also be counted among the micromanipulative procedures as it entails the sampling of one or a few cells from an early embryonic developmental stage (Lissens and Sermon 1997).

With this cornucopia of micromanipulative procedures already in clinical use or on the horizon, what risks are to be considered? Direct side effects of the hormonal or surgical pretreatment that is required prior to the use of many micromanipulative techniques cannot be discussed here. Concerning the outcome of pregnancies conceived through ICSI, MESA, TESE, injection of spermatids or the use of cryopreserved ova data are still far from sufficient to come to definite conclusions (Bonduelle et al. 1996, Kurinczuk and Bauer 1997). Until now, no convincing evidence has been brought forward that any of these procedures implies health risks for the offspring significantly higher than in natural pregnancies. However, this debate is still ongoing, and patients opting for these treatments need to be fully informed about the incomplete knowledgebase on malformation rates, long-term psychosocial and mental development, and fertility of children conceived with the support of micromanipulative procedures.

Late or even postmenopausal childbearing carries increased obstetric and medical risks. Moreover, having old or very old parents may result in untoward psychosocial and developmental effects on children and adolescents. Obviously, the risk of early loss of one or both parents is increased in such families.

Micromanipulative procedures pave the way for and are one technical cornerstone of PID. So far, it appears unlikely that PID will ever be employed on as broad a basis as conventional prenatal diagnosis. As PID is only applicable in IVF pregnancies, this should preclude its widespread use. It has to be conceded, however, that with improved technology it will become increasingly tempting to subject all IVF or ICSI pregnancies to a genetic 'checkup' through PID. The strongest driving force in that direction is the claim that excluding chromosomal aneuploidies in the in vitro stage enhances the success rate of ICSI (Verlinsky and Kuliev 1996). Behind these more technical considerations looms the basic question of whether it is desirable to diagnose or exclude as many genetic 'flaws' as possible by preimplantation or conventional prenatal testing. The opposing views on this topic are well known, incompatible as ever, and will not be further commented on here.

Since the recent announcements indicating that cloning of mammals is technically feasible, cloning applied to the human species has become the ultimate horror scenario for some, for others the promise of new possibilites which were previously undreamed of. Consensus against cloning humans is still strong, but the flawless frontline already seems to be giving way. It is beyond the scope of this paper to elaborate on the ethical issues arising from endeavors to clone human beings. It may suffice to remark that we do not currently have the slightest idea what medical risks such a procedure would imply for the cloned offspring. The very feasibility of creating a viable mammal from the nucleus of a once fully differentiated somatic cell breaks a basic dogma of developmental biology. It may be envisioned that such clones could suffer prematurely from the ravages of old age, or have an increased rate of cancer, infertility, or other maladies. On the population level, cloning performed on a large scale would reduce genetic diversity by precluding the recombination of genes that under conditions of natural reproduction takes place in every new generation. To what degree this would imperil the long-term genetic health of humankind is a currently unanswerable question.

Table 1. Micromanipulative assisted reproduction: summary of major chances and risks.

chances	risks
• better treatment of infertility	• treatment risks incompletely understood
• parenthood for cancer patients	
• facilitation of delayed childbearing	• facilitation of delayed childbearing
• postmenopausal parenting	• postmenopausal parenting
• starting point for PID	• starting point for PID
• better understanding of gamete and embryo biology	• usage of human embryos for research
• more reproductive autonomy	• new legal dilemmas; assault on human dignity
• avoidance of genetic disease in offspring	• selective embryo transfer; affront to handicapped individuals; loss of genetic diversity
• avenue to germ line therapy	• avenue to germ line therapy
	• avenue to genetic enhancement
	• avenue to genetic engineering at the population level

References

Bonduelle, M., Wilikens, A., Buysse, A., Van Assche, E., Wisanto, A., Devroey, P., van Steirteghem, A. and Liebaers, I. (1996), 'Prospective Follow-up Study of 877 Children Born After Intracytoplasmic Sperm Injection (ICSI), with Ejaculated, Epididymal and Testicular Spermatozoa and After Replacement of Cryopreserved Embryos Obtained After ICSI', *Human Reproduction*, Vol. 11, Suppl. 4, pp. 131-55.

Cohen, J., Scott, R., Schimmel, T., Levron, J. and Willadsen, S. (1997), 'Birth of Infant After Transfer of Anucleate Donor Oocyte Cytoplasm Into Recipient Eggs', *Lancet*, Vol. 350, pp. 186-7.

Devroey, P., Liu, J., Nagy, Z., Tounaye, H., Silber, S.J. and van Steirteghem, A.C. (1994), 'Normal Fertilization of Human Oocytes After Testicular Sperm Extraction and Intracytoplasmic Sperm Injection', *Fertility and Sterility,* Vol. 62, pp. 639-41.

Felberbaum, R. and Dahnke, W. (1997), 'DIR – Deutsches IVF-Register. Ergebnisse der Datenerhebung für das Jahr 1996', *Fertilität*, Vol. 13, pp. 99-112.

Fishel, S., Green, S., Bishop, M., Thornton, S., Hunter, A., Fleming, S. and Al-Hassan, S. (1995), 'Pregnancy After Intracytoplasmic Injection of Spermatid', *Lancet*, Vol. 345, pp. 1641-2.

Kimura, Y. and Yanagimachi, R. (1995), 'Development of Normal Mice From Oocytes Injected With Secondary Spermatocyte Nuclei', *Biology of Reproduction*, Vol. 53, pp. 855-62.

Kurinczuk, J.J. and Bower, C. (1997), 'Birth Defects in Infants Conceived by Intracytoplasmic Sperm Injection: An Alternative Interpretation', *British Medical Journal*, Vol. 315, pp. 1260-6.

Lissens, W. and Sermon, K. (1997), 'Preimplantation Genetic Diagnosis: Current Status and New Developments', *Human Reproduction*, Vol. 12, pp. 1756-61.

Nash, J.M. (1997), 'The Age of Cloning', Time, March 10, 1997, pp. 46-9.

Verlinsky, Y. and Kuliev, A. (1996), 'Preimplantation Diagnosis of Common Aneuploidies in Infertile Couples of Advanced Maternal Age', *Human Reproduction*, Vol. 11, pp. 2076-7.

3 The relation between ICSI and genetic diagnosis from an ethical point of view

Barbara Maier

Introduction

The development of ICSI (Intracytoplasmic sperm injection) has revolutionised the treatment of male infertility by bypassing natural barriers to fertilisation. ICSI and particularly the two sperm retrieval techniques of microsurgical epididymal sperm aspiration (MESA) and testicular sperm extraction (TESE) may cause the transmission of this or other genetic disorders to the next generation. Serious genetic diseases like cystic fibrosis and the heritability of male infertility have become important issues for discussion concerning some subpopulations of ICSI-candidates.

While the mechanical piercing of the oocyte which was initially considered to damage its contents or ultrastructure, does not result in any significant increase in birth defects in ICSI offspring, pregnancies may be obtained with spermatozoa that carry genetic defects (Wisanto et al. 1995, Bonduelle et al. 1996). Thanks to ICSI in the past completely infertile men are able to father their own children. The subsidiary interventions of donor insemination or donor IVF with their special psychosocial implications have been ruled out in a lot of cases by the ICSI method.

But the introduction of ICSI has raised new concerns both for clinicians dealing with male infertility and for ICSI candidates themselves, the couples concerned and their future children. Before the introduction of ICSI, the major question to be asked was whether a man was able to reproduce. Now the question arises whether the same man can have a 'sufficient' healthy child without propagating genetic or epigenetic disorders.

Issues concerning the relation between ICSI and genetic diagnosis

The propagation of genetic defects by the use of ICSI

The disease Cystic fibrosis (CF) may serve as an example for describing the interconnections between ICSI and the manifestation of this serious disease in the offspring of genetically disposed parents.

The subpopulation of infertile men with congenital absence of the vas-deferens and azoospermia may transmit CF to their children provided that also their spouses have the genetic disposition. This is 2 % of men with obstructive azoospermia, a small population indeed, but nevertheless at high risk for CF propagation.

Such men would never have passed on the genetic defect without reproductive assistance in form of epididymal sperm aspiration and the use of ICSI, although a small number had achieved pregnancies by the use of this sperm in conventional IVF.

Genetic screening of this disease is currently available. Couples contemplating a pregnancy are able to know if both are carriers of cystic fibrosis gene-mutation; if so, they face a significant ethical dilemma. Should they proceed with procreation despite the risk of having a child with CF, have preimplantation diagnosis (PID) in order to have unaffected embryos transfered or have prenatal diagnosis (PND) to abort affected fetuses?

Cystic fibrosis is an autosomal recessive metabolic disease described as a triad: chronic obstructive pulmonary disease, exocrine pancreatic insufficiency, and elevation of sodium chloride concentration in sweat. The viscous mucus leads to insufficiency of pancreatic function, maldigestion, cholestatic cirrhosis of the liver and atrecy of vasa deferentia (sterility). People suffer from bronchitis, pneumony and bronchiectasies and may at least die because of cardiopulmonic insufficiency. Cystic fibrosis is the most common children's metabolic disease with an incidence of 1:2500. The incidence of healthy heterocygote carrier is 1:25. Therapy for cystic fibrosis is only symptomatic; it consists of physiotherapy (inhalation, mucolytic substances) diet and antibiotics. The life-expectancy is up to 30 years (Cutting 1996). Living a life suffering from the symptoms of cystic fibrosis means suffering in many respects. This is true for the people concerned as well as for their families.

Parental responsibility plays a role when discussing whether one should consciously risk having a child with cystic fibrosis even if the desire for a child

24

is very strong. Is it part of parental responsibility to undergo screening for carrier-status and if so, have PGD or PND in order to select unaffected embryos or induce abortion of affected fetuses?

The possible propagation of male infertility

ICSI is suspected to facilitate the transmission of male infertility. The pathogenesis of the deletion of the long arm of the Y chromosome is uncertain. There is ample evidence that specific gene-regions on the euchromatic part of the long arm of the Y chromosome have a critical role in spermatogenesis. But further studies are required to determine how frequently the transmission from father to son is performed. However there is a likelihood that a high proportion arise de novo in the affected individual.

According to Tournaye (Tournaye 1997) screening for Y chromosome microdeletions should be mandatory for ICSI candidates with oligozoospermia or azoospermia, since any microdeletion will be inherited by an ICSI-son and may be again associated with reproductive failure.

Although male infertility is not a life-threatening disease or a disabling handicap, couples in whom the infertile male has a deletion of the long arm of the Y chromosome may elect to have PID in order to transfer only female ICSI embryos. But this option does not mean screening of parents but embryo selection, sex-selection for medical reasons.

Another possibility to be offered is common prenatal screening (chorionic villus sampling or amniocentesis) followed by all the implications of induced abortion if testing turns out positive.

But what about the consciously accepted probable transmission of infertility to the next generation? It might be tolerable in the view of prospective parents to have a son with a fertility problem. The father who had himself faced the infertility problem might regard the problem as one which can be solved by his prospective son.

Ethical discussion

Technology assessment from an ethical point of view

The problems arising are not inherent in the technique of ICSI itself but in the treated population.

Micromanipulation is not teratogen probably due to the 'all or none' rule of teratology. Preliminary empirical data provide no evidence for structural abnormalities in live born children after ICSI (2,7 % rate does not deviate from the baseline risk in general population).

But ICSI candidates carry more than the average population chromosomal aberrations and are demanded for karyotype-examination routinely before the beginning of ICSI-therapy (there is a clear inverse relationship between sperm count and the prevalence of karyotypic abnormalities).

Genetic pathology underlies infertility in particular small subpopulations of ICSI candidates. This does not devalue the whole method but demands careful pre-therapeutic clinical examination, consideration of family history and appropriate laboratory studies. Especially karyotyping is seen as a precondition for ICSI by experts and applicants in identifying risk situations for future children.

Counselling and screening as well as follow-up of children born after ICSI are of central ethical concern. The use of counselling and screening must remain voluntary. We have to consider that in a lot of cases not only the infertile man in question but also his spouse is subject to examination, counselling and screening.

For women who have become pregnant after ICSI, invasive prenatal diagnosis by chorionic villus sampling or amniocentesis is available in most centers. For those who do not want invasive prenatal diagnosis, triple testing and high resolution ultrasound are alternatives to be offered.

All this of course does not guarantee the birth of a healthy child.

Access to the ICSI-treatment and physician's responsibilities

Artificial reproductive technologies (ART) should be available to all people with infertility problems without psychosocial discrimination or discrimination on the grounds of genetic risk.

'Any form of discrimination against a person on grounds of his or her genetic heritage is prohibited' according to the Bioethical Convention's article 11 (Convention 1997). Balancing the interests of the child – if it is possible to speak of the interests of future children – with those of people making the decision, it is not so clear how to behave. Risks linked to parental anomalies, including genetic abnormalities, raise the same ethical problems as those of screening in general.

Should in serious risk-cases the performance of ICSI be dependent on screening and judgement of how high the risk of having a child with a severe disease is and how severe the disease for the prospective child would be?

Performing ICSI without prior screening when there is high evidence that both parents could be carriers of CFTR-mutation gene could be judged irresponsible of the medical doctor involved as well as of informed parents.

The physician has a responsibility towards the patients, the infertile couple, but also towards future children. To what extent of severe suffering should prospective children be consciously exposed and by introduction of reproductive assistance? The central ethical concern is the suffering of the future children. It can be avoided by refraining from having just these children by ICSI.

When is birth unfair to the child (Steinbock and McClamrock 1994)? Is it in every aspect better to be than not to be? Is screening then the duty of prospective parents in order to avoid the submission of a child to a miserable life when that could be avoided? Would parents who are not willing to be screened before having children seem to fail to live up to a minimal ideal of parenting?

Is it not up to the responsibility of the physician involved in reproductive assistance to withhold treatment if the birth of a severly disabled child with life long severe suffering is to be expected? A child affected by cystic fibrosis is exposed to suffering in many aspects and causal therapy is not available. The disease leads to early death under very bad circumstances.

Autonomy of clients seems to be restricted for the sake of responsibility for the offspring. Balancing of rights and duties in reproduction means taking into consideration what the life of future children would be like. Duties of prospective parents coincide with the duties of physicians involved. If there are different views, parents as well as physicians are to decide responsibly according to their convictions. In spite of non-discrimination-principles, physicians are under no obligation to act in favour of full autonomous choice of infertile people against their own conscience.

Generally parents and physicians agree with regard to prospective children, but if there are essential differences no physician should be obliged to perform ICSI against his or her convictions.

Genetic counselling in reproductive medicine

Genetic counselling in reproductive medicine faces common counselling difficulties as well as specific ones.

Nondirectiveness seems to be the supreme goal of the counselor in providing clients with information and responding to their questions and concerns. Nondirective counselling should assure autonomous decision making but is not without problematic implications itself (Terrell White 1998). The meaning of autonomy in genetic counselling is not defined in the literature. Nondirectiveness guides counselors to focus on 'objective' medical facts rather than on psychosocial issues because the latter are more influenced by values and value-expressions. This has been shown by several empirical studies (Frets, Niermeijer 1990). People facing genetical problems and needing decision making on that are more interested in psychosocial issues than in information only about medical facts.

The perception of risk has been found to be associated with clients' prior knowledge of, or experience with, the disorder in question. Other factors known to contribute to reproductive decisions include clients' desires for children: perceptions of burdens – emotional, physical, financial, and social; reproductive history; confidence in parenting ability; clients' age; timing of testing; and the anticipated responses of other children and relatives to decisions (Terrell White 1998, pp. 9-10).

Genetic screening in infertile men and their spouses

Screening is proposed by providers as well as applicants for several subpopulations of ICSI-candidates. But should we go so far as to say that screening should be a precondition for ICSI in certain cases? What about the criteria and guidelines for preconditioning?

According to publications of the scientific community and opinions of practitioners screening is the safer method to avoid transmission of genetic disorders to a certain degree and may be carried out on different levels:

- on the level of the prospective parents, who are able to decide consciously for themselves and inevitably involve their prospective children. They give informed consent willing to know about their genetic constitution and the implications.
- on the level of PID. Embryos are examined and chosen for transfer if not affected.
- on the level of prenatal diagnosis (chorionic villus sampling/amniocentesis) as the ethically most questionable because of the abortion consequences.

Decisions and possible implications

a) What about reproductive autonomy? What about reproductive responsibility of prospective parents and their duty of beneficience towards prospective children?

'Give me children or I shall die' (Cohen 1996) is the title of a paper dealing with new reproductive technologies and harm to children. The paper concentrates on reproductive technologies inducing serious illness and disorders in a small but significant proportion of children who are born when using them. Analysing the application of reproductive technologies the author concludes: 'If these technologies were found to do so, it would be wrong to forge ahead with their use' (Cohen 1996, p. 19).

The 'harm to children' argument should be introduced into the discussion when contemplating a pregnancy by ICSI through a father/mother at risk of transmitting disorders or diseases. Pro-reproductive-arguments are based on the 'interest-in-existing' argument, which assume that children with an interest in existing are waiting in a spectral world of non-existence where their

28

situation is less desirable than it would be were they released into this world (Cohen 1996, p. 20).

Parental responsibility attempts to refrain from having children unless certain minimal conditions are satisfied. Before embarking on so serious an enterprise as parenthood people should think about the consequences for their offspring (Steinbock and McClamrock 1994). It might amount to a failure to engage fully in the (not just financial) planning that is part of a parent's commitment to his or her children. Whether one has a moral responsibility to know one's genetic condition, and the strength of that responsibility, will depend upon the particulars of the situation. In all likelihood, however, a person's responsibility to know will not depend upon the strength of his or her desire to know or not to know.

If we are to make responsible decisions about accepting or refusing medical information, we must begin by acknowledging that these decisions affect others as well as ourselves. But judgements about the consequences are inescapably subjective. They are subject to the prospective parents' decision-making and it is up to them what risks they judge worth taking for their children. It is up to the doctors involved to balance the risks for future children, to accept patients for ICSI treatment or to refuse them.

In this context it is of great importance to underline that it is not necessarily a reproach to disabled children who are already born if decisions are made against knowingly conceiving children who would have the same disabilities (Cohen 1996, p. 25).

Counselling about ICSI procedures as well as the chances and limitations of screening have an important ethical impact on the assessment of the whole technology. For a subpopulation of ICSI-candidates the link between reproductive medicine and genetics has become intensive. The question for them is not only whether to have a child or not but whether to have a 'sufficient' healthy one or none. What sort of handicap will be too bad? Will infertility be too bad a handicap or one to be compensated? CF will lead to a life of severe suffering without hope for essential therapy or final release from severe symptoms and probable death in the late twenties. Is that 'fate' to be imposed on people if we know it will be theirs when coming into existence?

b) Follow-up of children born after ICSI has to be an integral factor of ICSI treatment. ICSI couples usually agree to a prospective follow-up of pregnancies and children; almost all have undergone prenatal diagnosis by chorionic villus sampling or amniocentesis (Bonduelle 1996). Once children are born and have grown older, follow-up might cause several difficulties: depending on the extent to which children have learned about their origin from their parents. Parents cannot be obliged to inform their children even when they probably carry (epi)genetic disorders.

Follow-up should be performed without discrimination. By what means could this be carried out? Is it in the child's interest to be informed or not? When would information be best provided? Until now, ICSI children have not reached adolescence age, the most vulnerable age in this respect.

Children should be asked for informed consent to be followed up when they have reached a mental stage in which they are able to consent. They can refuse or participate like any other adult. Privacy and confidentiality of families concerned have to be respected anyway. These issues have to be integrated into counselling of ICSI candidates and their wives and consciously be reflected in decision making.

Conclusion

Although in principle access to ART should be open to all infertile clients without any discrimination parents as well as physicians should focus on the 'fate' of prospective children. Beneficience and responsibility are task of medical doctors as well as parents to be.

In awareness of the contradiction of not discriminating against people with genetic risk and nevertheless withholding ICSI-treatment under certain conditions (e.g. severe suffering of the prospective child), we have to provide strong arguments against providing treatment – the strongest in practice would be the severe suffering argument.

References

Bonduelle, M. et al. (1996), 'Prospective Follow Up Study of 423 Children Born After Intracytoplasmic Sperm Injection', *Human Reproduction*, Vol. 11, No. 7, pp. 1558-64.

Cohen, C.B. (1996), '«Give Me Children or I Shall Die!» New Reproductive Technologies and Harm to Children', *Hastings Center Report*, March-April 1996, pp. 19-27.

'Convention For the Protection of Human Rights and Dignity of the Human Being with Regard to the Application of Biology and Medicine: Convention on Human Rights and Biomedicine' (Adopted by the Committee of Ministers on 19. Nov. 1996), *Human Reproduction*, Vol. 12, No 9, pp. 2076-80, 1997.

Cutting, G.R. (1996), 'Cystic Fibrosis', in: Rimoin, D.L., Connor, J.M. and Pyaritz-Reed, E. (eds), *Principles and Practice of Medical Genetics*, pp. 2686-705.

Frets, P.G., Niermeijer, M.F. (1990), 'Reproductive Planning After Genetic Counselling: A Perspective from the Last Decade', *Clinical Genetics,* Vol. 38, pp. 295-306.

Steinbock, B. and McClamrock, R. (1994), 'When is Birth Unfair to the Child?' in: *Hastings Center Report*, Vol. 24, No 6, pp 15-21.

Terrell White, M. (1998), 'Decision-Making Through Dialogue: Reconfiguring Autonomy in Genetic Counseling', in: *Theoretical Medicine and Bioethics*, Vol. 19, No 1, pp. 5-19.

Tournaye, H. et al. (1997), 'Heritability of Sterility: Clinical Implications', in Barratt, C. et al.(eds), *Genetics of Human Male Fertility*, pp. 123-44.

Wisanto, A. et al. (1995), 'Obstetric Outcome of 424 Pregnancies After Intracytoplasmic Sperm Injection', *Human Reproduction*, Vol. 10, No. 10, pp. 2713-8.

4 Modification of IVF application and access to IVF services by PID?

Brian A. Lieberman

Introduction

In vitro fertilisation (IVF) and intracytoplasmic sperm injection (ICSI) services were established to provide treatment to infertile couples. The technology used to provide these therapeutic services may be adapted to a screening and preimplantation diagnostic programme for genetic disorders. Prior to the introduction of these services detailed consideration needs to be given to the ethical implications of the proposed developments. The services require additional resources, suitably trained personnel and a central laboratory to undertake the appropriate genetic testing on a single blastomere.

It is necessary to consider the groups of people who may benefit from genetic screening.

Pre-treatment screening

Pre-treatment screening is highly desirable as it provides important information to the prospective parents. These individuals are then able to exercise choice, to avoid the birth of such offspring by using donated gametes or to proceed with treatment in the knowledge that their children may inherit the disorder.

Pre-treatment screening is indicated in individuals with possible genetic abnormalities which would not have been transmitted to their offspring without IVF/ICSI services. Examples include gene deletions on the Y chromosome in males with severe oligo- and azoospermia and screening for cystic fibrosis in males with congenital bilateral absence of the vas deferens.

Preimplantation diagnosis (PID) for known single gene disorders

In this group of people the existence of the single gene defect is usually known after the birth of an affected individual. The prevention of the birth of another affected individual is possible given the availability of suitable laboratory techniques.

PID for fertility treatment

It is highly desirable both in terms of resources and efficiency to improve the outcome of IVF treatment. The low rate of successful implantation with IVF is thought to be due to a number of factors. These include 'poor quality' embryos, embryos with abnormal karyotypes and abnormalities of the endometrium.

Routine karyotyping of embryos is not current practice. This would require a major reorganisation of IVF techniques moving towards the routine replacement of a single blastocyst. The replacement of a single, chromosomal normal blastocyst would represent a major advance both in terms of increasing the rate of implantation and reducing the risk of a multiple birth.

Ethical implications of screening programmes:

1   Prior to the introduction of a screening and diagnostic programme clinics should give detailed consideration to the ethics and problems associated with the screening for inherited genetic disorders.

•   Medical investigations generally involve an individual, the patient. Human genetic tests differ from most others undertaken in clinical medicine, as they may reveal important information about relatives and thus have a great impact on families.

•   Will the service restrict screening to inherited recessive disorders which do not have any significant direct health implications for the patients or gamete donors but which may have important implications for their offspring e.g. cystic fibrosis?

•   Will the clinic offer to screen more extensively and to include those disorders which may manifest in the individual being tested in later life? These include inherited dominant and X linked disorders, chromosomal disorders, adult onset genetic disorders regardless of inheritance, or the genetic components of multifactorial diseases including somatic mutations.

2   Clinics should notify patients and gamete donors of the availability of genetic screening. It is important for these persons to know what tests are available and that testing may reveal previously unsuspected defects.

• Persons undergoing IVF/ICSI are often mistaken in their beliefs about the ability of the embryologists to detect abnormal embryos and to exclude those carrying a genetic disorder. Counselling prior to IVF should inform the couples about genetic screening tests available generally and in addition those tests which may be important in their particular circumstances e.g. Tay Sachs disease, beta thalassaemia.

3   Clinics that provide genetic testing should ensure that suitably trained persons are available to counsel those requesting genetic screening.

• These individuals should understand the nature of the tests to be used, their *scope* and limitations, and the accuracy, implications and use of the result. The counsellors should possess the interpersonal skills necessary to impart this information to the individuals being screened.

4   Patients and gamete donors must be informed of the result of the screening test and there must be arrangements in place for them to receive post test counselling.

• The test result may have implications for the family as well as the individual being tested. The result may cause anxiety in otherwise healthy individuals. Confidentiality must be protected but the person being tested must understand the probable implications for other family members. In particular for IVF services screening for the BRCA1/2 gene and Huntington disease need to be considered.

• Written information and fact sheets for the more common disorders should readily be available ideally before and at the time of the initial consultation.

• Modification and access to IVF /ICSI services.

Resource implications

Preimplantation diagnostic services: In principle prevention of the conception of a fetus with a profound disorder is preferable to abortion or the long term care of a severely disabled individual. It could thus be argued that the prevention of the birth of a child with a severe disability and shortened life expectancy is an appropriate use of public funds. The funding of genetic screening and PID programmes may thus be seen as different to the treatment of the infertile although both require the use of IVF technology.

Routine IVF services: Theoretically the routine culture and transfer of human blastocysts would increase the implantation rate and reduce the need for the transfer of multiple embryos. This raises the possibility of routine embryo biopsy at the 4-8 cell stage to determine the karyotype. Only blastocysts with normal karyotypes would be replaced. Should this become common practice it would have major implications for preimplantation genetic diagnostic services.

Funding remains an issue certainly within the UK, although the situation may differ within Europe. It is unlikely that comprehensive PID services will be established within the private sector, as the laboratory genetic facilities are all state or university funded. The private sector provides the majority of IVF services. The development of 'satellite and transport' services is the only realistic option. This would entail the counselling, IVF and embryo biopsy at the clinic. The blastomere is then transported to the genetic centre for testing. Another possible but more complicated scenario is the freezing of the embryos, their transport to the genetic centre for thawing, biopsy and testing. The replacement may be undertaken at the clinic or genetic centre.

5 Examples for possible PID indications – scientific background and reflections on effects

Ulrike A. Mau

As yet, PID is an experimental – costly and technically demanding – procedure at an early stage of development. Less than 100 children are born world-wide after PID. The German 'Embryonenschutzgesetz' prohibits physicians from doing PID on totipotent cells.

The procedure as such has advantages: A result is available even before the pregnancy is in utero; problems like conventional prenatal diagnosis, its abortion risk and an eventual late termination of the pregnancy do not arise. This means for the couple and the medical professional: no pregnancy on probation! Only a genetically normal embryo (with respect to the particular disease under consideration) is implanted. The overall general risk of 3-5 % for inborn mental and/or physical disabilities of course remains! So the aim cannot be to implantate an absolutely normal embryo, but a normal embryo concerning the particular disease.

But we must not neglect the problems of PID: It requires a complex and distressing procedure of medically assisted reproduction. Results may not be totally reliable. Lissens and Sermon (1997) discussed among others the problem of allelic drop-out, i.e. the non-amplification (PCR) of one or both alleles in a heterozygous single cell. Another problem is that a postimplantation genetic change such as mosaicism would remain a possibility after performing PID.

In spite of these problems and of course the ethical problems which in my opinion arise, we should not reject the PID-technique in general.

I will present some real-life cases from our Division of Clinical Genetics, where I would like to show different aspects of doing or not doing PID. Deliberately I will confront you in detail with symptoms, development and prognosis. It is quite easy to discuss ethical questions on a theoretical basis – ignoring reality with its pain, grief, sorrow and sometimes hopelessness as we see it as medical professionals.

Case 1: Cerebro-hepato-renal syndrome (Zellweger syndrome)

Clinical findings

Jonathan (name changed) was the first child of healthy non-consanguineous parents. The mother was 27 years, the father 29 years old. Pregnancy and delivery were uneventful.

At birth Jonathan was a little bit smaller than other newborns. A profound muscular hypotonia was striking: Jonathan did not move actively and he was not able to react properly to different stimulations as normal babies do (non-responsiveness). He was cerebrally depressed and sucking and swallowing reflexes were absent. Therefore normal feeding was impossible and feeding by gastrostomy was necessary throughout life. Jonathan displayed different craniofacial dysmorphic features: a high bulging forehead, wide open fontanels and sutures, puffy eyelids, mongoloid slants, ocular hypertelorism, epicanthic folds, glaucoma, cataracts, optic nerve dysplasia, low set dysplastic ears, a high arched palate with cleft of the soft palate. Other features included a cryptorchidism, thymus hypoplasia, and camptodactyly. Soon after birth hepatomegaly (increase of liver-size) developed with jaundice and melena (blood in faeces). There was an extreme failure to thrive. Jonathan showed no psychomotor development at all. The parents were not able to identify any sign of motion in his motionless little face. They learned how to feed him through the gastrostomy but his convulsions, which started soon after birth, were terrifying for them – especially because they were drug-resistant. Additionally Jonathan had some attacks of respiratory arrest. Repeated infections of the respiratory tract occurred (the thymus hypoplasia can lead to immunodeficiency) and finally Jonathan died at the age of 8 months.

Genetic background

Zellweger syndrome is a disorder of the peroxisomes. Peroxisomes are small intracellular organelles which perform a multitude of metabolic functions. Abscence or marked diminution of peroxisomes has, therefore, a profound and complex impact on the metabolism which is barely compatible with a longer postnatal survival. There is no treatment, except symtomatic. Life expectancy is severely curtailed: 70 % of the children die within the first 3 months and most within the first year.

Occurrence of Zellweger syndrome is about 1 : 25000-50000 live births. Males and females are equally affected. The disease is determined by a single gene inherited in an autosomal recessive manner. This means that both healthy parents carry a chromosome with a hidden gene defect and one with the normal gene (see figure 1). Only one chromosome of each parent is transmitted to a child. So there are only 4 possibilities to pass the chromosomes to offspring. A child will be healthy (homozygous or heterozygous) in 75 %, a child will have Zellweger syndrome in 25 %.

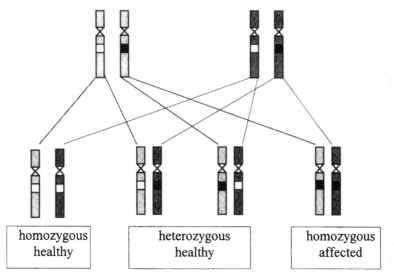

Figure 1: Autosomal recessive inheritance (□ normal gene, ■ defective gene)

Prenatal diagnosis

After the birth of an affected child prenatal diagnosis is possible, e.g. amniocentesis with a special test (proof of elevated long-chain fatty acids). If the fetus should be affected the pregnancy might be in the 18th week of gestation (or even later). The pregnancy is evident for others, the mother already starts to feel foetal movements. If the fetus is affected very few couples opt for having the child. According to our experiences (and experiences of others) most couples choose termination of the pregnancy in similar situations. Termination of pregnancy means to start labour by drugs. At this stage of pregnancy it is usually not easy to produce labour (it takes 2-5 days). The woman experiences a 'normal' birth of a child that is too small and immature to survive. It usually dies during the procedure.

But let us return to Jonathan and his parents. If this German couple wishes to obtain a healthy child there is only the possibility 'to try again and hope'. What are the typical decisions of couples in a similar situation? If doing research work on literature about psychological aspects of reproductive decision making of couples with a genetic risk one can find some interesting facts: A variety of factors influence the reproductive decision and the frequently contradictory conclusions. Couples tend to make decisions that seem to be irrational for an outsider. Some authors found that even couples with a high genetic risk who had no children during counselling were more likely to plan a pregnancy than those who already had children (Bocsknov 1979, Frets et al. 1990a). The desire to have children and the absence of personal experience with the disorder (no close relative being affected) are important single factors for the decision to opt for having children after genetic counselling. Data from Frets et al. (1990b) showed that the magnitude of the genetic risk is of only relative importance in reproductive planning. In fact their results demonstrated that the desire to have children is more important than the magnitude of the genetic risk. Decision for artificial insemination, adoption or not to have any (more) children was the exception. Counselees tend to take high risks even when prenatal diagnosis is not available. The authors stated: "An explanation for this apparent disregard for the consequences might reflect an unconscious reaction to the 'unbearable' feeling of lowered self-esteem, due to the hereditary nature of the disorder". This shows that taking an informed decision in such a high risk situation is a very complicated process. It involves much more than the 'rational' assumption that one should avoid further reproduction in the face of a high risk. Another interesting observation of Frets et al. (1990b) is that couples at risk for a defect resulting in early death mainly opted for having children whereas couples at risk for a prolonged illness were more afraid to take the risk.

Working as a genetic counsellor or gynecologist you know that these decisions are 'normal' and this fact makes it sometimes very difficult to understand why the PID-technique is rejected in Germany. A lot of pain could be prevented. And now my question: if PID were be possible and reliable in the above case with Zellweger syndrome, would it be ethical and human to refuse PID to this couple?

The intention of PID in the first case is to prevent one special risk of an individual couple. The intention of PID in the second situation is somehow different.

Case 2: PID in infertile couples prior in-vitro fertilisation (IVF) with intracytoplasmic sperm injection (ICSI)?

First let me give you some details, numbers and statistics:

10-15 % of all couples are sterile, so this is a huge number of 'patients'.

Male infertility (low sperm count, bad mobility and/or morphology) is primary indication for IVF plus ICSI.

Chromosome analyses of such males and their spouse show a higher rate of chromosomal abnormalities (about 6-15 % in males, 3-5 % in females, see Mau et al. 1997).

These sterile couples belong to a more or less high-risk group per se. Besides the general risk[1] of 3-5 % for an inborn mental/physical disability in a child, those couples with a chromosomal anomaly have an additional risk for unbalanced offspring. Till now it is unknown, if there is an increased risk because of the ICSI procedure compared to pregnancies in fertile couples with the same anomaly (natural selection from injection onwards might work as good as in fertile couples).

Plachot et al. (1988a) carried out a multicentric study in which they analysed the chromosomal status of unfertilised and fertilised oocytes. The average rate of anomalies in unfertilised oocytes was 26 % and 29 % of the embryos had chromosome anomalies. Interestingly, maternal age increased the rate of aneuploidy significantly: 38 % in patients over 35 years versus 24 % in younger patients. Provided that natural selection against unbalanced embryos works as sufficient as in fertile couples, one should expect a lower implantation rate or a higher abortion rate respectively. This seems to be true. The high rate of chromosome disorders in early life after IVF let Plachot et al. (1988b) raise the ethical question of the opportunity of carrying out a genetic control of normality in human embryos at the preimplantation stage.

In fact Gianaroli and coworkers (1997) carried out PID of aneuploidy for chromosomes X, Y, 13, 18 and 21 on 196 embryos from 36 infertile patients classified with poor prognosis (due to maternal age, repeated IVF failures or mosaic karyotype). The percentage of abnormal embryos was comparable in the three groups (63 %, 57 %, and 62 % respectively). Following PID, 28 patients had at least one embryo transferred that appeared normal by fluorescent in-situ hybridisation (FISH). Four clinical pregnancies resulted, with an implantation rate of 10 % per normal embryo. Gianaroli et al. concluded that the high rate of chromosomally abnormal embryos may have been the cause of implantation failure in previous IVF cycles of the group of poor prognosis patients. They discuss that transferring embryos with a normal FISH complement could improve the chance of pregnancy in this category of patients. Figure 2 tries to show the scenario.

41

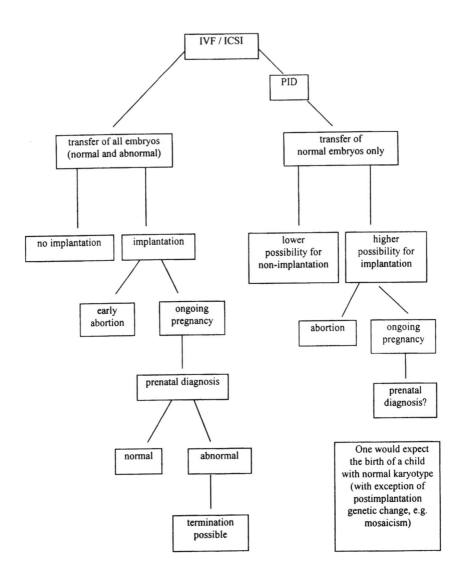

Figure 2: **Flowchart of the different options in IVF/ICSI with or without PID**

So, should we do PID routinely in IVF and/or ICSI? I think only couples with a high genetic risk (and for whom termination would not otherwise be acceptable) might be suitable for PID.

But where are the limits? Who is drawing the line? Which couple/s is/are 'privileged' to get PID and which not and why? Which disease is harmful enough to justify such an invasive and cost-intensive method? Do we need a catalogue of diseases pro/contra PID? Is there a difference between fertile couples and infertile couples with IVF/ICSI indication? The latter get IVF anyhow (so there would not be an extra risk, as in fertile couples). How about PID on embryos at risk for late-onset disorders like Chorea Huntington? How about minor disabilities e.g. microdeletions of the Y-chromosome (which means, that a male is most probably infertile)?

In offering PID can we avoid 'social duty'? Do couples really have the choice – maybe on the basis of an informed consent? Who decides which couple/s gets PID? Should it be a team of specialists as for organ-transplantation? Or should it be just the physician who performs IVF?

There are definitely a lot of aspects that have to be discussed very carefully in the future. But if the PID technology improves, it might in due course prove useful for couples at high risk for unbalanced conceptions or an embryo with a serious monogenetic disease, but scarcely for fertile couples at relatively low genetic risk.

Note

1 The general risks for any healthy couple (presumably world-wide) of having a child with a congenital mental/physical disability (3-5 of 100 newborns). Usually these disorders are not foreseeable or preventable. Reasons may be
    a. acquired during pregnancy (i.e. infections, alcohol, oxygen starvation during delivery)
    b. a chromosomal aberration (i.e. Down's syndrome) (only 1/10 of the general risk attribute to chromosomal aberrations)
    c. single gene defects (i.e. Zellweger syndrome, hemophilia, cystic fibrosis etc.) (about 1/5 of the general risk attribute to gene defects; every healthy person carries 5-10 hidden gene defects!)
    d. multifactorial inheritance: concurrence of hereditary disposition and environmental factors (i.e. hay-fever, congenital isolated heart defect, neural tube defect etc.)
    e. disabilities and/or mental retardation of unknown origin
    The frequency of chromosome abnormalities at gametogenesis and during pregnancy is shown in figure 3.

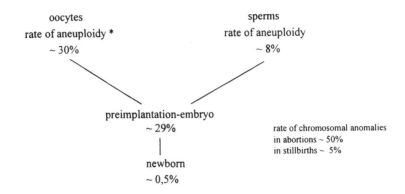

oocytes
rate of aneuploidy *
~ 30%

sperms
rate of aneuploidy
~ 8%

preimplantation-embryo
~ 29%

rate of chromosomal anomalies
in abortions ~ 50%
in stillbirths ~ 5%

newborn
~ 0,5%

Figure 3: **The frequency of chromosome abnormalities at gametogenesis and during pregnancy, demonstrating the effectivness of natural selection.**

* This number is subject to some doubt; the women sampled in most studies are of older age, the process of stimulating ovulation might itself cause nondisjunction, and the oocytes analysed are those which failed to fertilise. Hassold et al. (1993) note that in four studies of unstimulated oocytes (which may better reflect nature) aneuploidy rates were 1.5%, 0%, 3%, and 20% respectively.

References

Bocsknov, N.P. (1979), 'Genetic Counselling in the U.S.S.R.', *Prog Clin Biol Res,* Vol. 34, pp. 31-40.

Frets, P.G. (1990a), *The Reproductive Decision After Genetic Counselling,* Koninklijke Blibliotheek, Den Haag.

Frets, P.G., Duivenvoorden, H.J., Niermeijer, M.F., van de Berge, S.M.M. and Galjaard, H. (1990b), 'Factors Influencing the Reproductive Decision After Genetic Counselling', *Am J Med Genet,* Vol. 35, pp. 496-502.

Gianaroli, L., Magli, M.C., Munne, S., Fiorentino, A., Montanaro, N., Ferraretti, A.P. (1997), 'Will Preimplantation Genetic Diagnosis Assist Patients with a Poor Prognosis to Achieve Pregnancy?' *Hum Reprod,* Vol. 12, No. 8, pp. 1762-7.

Hassold, T., Hunt, P.A., Sherman, S. (1993), 'Trisomy in Humans: Incidence, Origin and Etiology', *Curr Opin Genet Devel,* Vol. 3, pp. 398-403.

Lissens, W., Sermon, K. (1997), 'Preimplantation Genetic Diagnosis: Current Status and New Developments', *Hum Reprod,* Vol. 12, No. 8, pp. 1756-61.

Mau, U.A., Bäckert, I.-T., Kaiser, P., Kiesel, L. (1997), 'Chromosomal Findings in 150 Couples Referred for Genetic Counselling Prior to Intracytoplasmic Sperm Injection', *Hum Reprod,* Vol. 12, No. 5, pp. 930-7.

Plachot, M., Veiga, A., Montagut, J., de Grouchy, J., Calderon, G., Lepretre, S., Junca, A.M., Santalo, J., Carles, E., Mandelbaum, J. et al. (1988a), 'Are

Clinical and Biological IVF Parameters Correlated with Chromosomal Disorders in Early Life: A Multicentric Study', *Hum Reprod,* Vol. 3, No. 5, pp. 627-35.

Plachot, M., de Grouchy, J., Junca, A.M., Mandelbaum, J., Salat-Baroux, J., Cohen, J. (1988b), 'Chromosome Analysis of Human Oocytes and Embryos: Does Delayed Fertilisation Increase Chromosome Imbalance?' *Hum Reprod,* Vol. 3, No. 1, pp. 125-7.

6   Should there be a uniform list of genetic diseases allowing access to PID?

Hansjakob Müller

Introduction

The last few years have seen a remarkable growth in the understanding of genetics as applied in medicine and rapid advances in the technology for the detection of mutations leading to genetic diseases. This development must also be considered with regard to the regulation of the use of new methods in medically assisted reproduction, particularly when intracytoplasmic sperm injection (ICSI) is employed. This latter technique has also engendered an ethical debate of its own. Genetic defects leading to disease or a predisposition thereto are already present in gametes before conception. They can therefore be detected from that point on, or in the first embryonic stages after conception (for summary see Müller 1998).

Prenatal diagnosis (PND) and preimplantation diagnosis (PID) – also called preimplantation genetic diagnosis (PGD) – face future parents with the problem of selecting their offspring according to health quality criteria. This is generally seen as morally ambivalent. It is therefore hardly surprising that there are repeated demands for a definition of the genetic diseases allowing access to PND and PID and the compilation of these diseases into a restrictive list. Such a list has been discussed among others in the drafting of the Council of Europe guidelines on medical genetic testing and also within national committees of experts, as in the Netherlands (1989) or recently in the Swiss committee of experts that was charged with drawing up a preliminary draft for a federal law on genetic testing in humans.

ICSI allows a genetically induced inability of sperms to effect natural fertilisation to be passed on to the next generation. However, the question of whether one should establish a list of genetic defects occurring in the infertile couple, in the case of which ICSI is not authorised, has hardly been considered.

Considerations relating to the creation of a list

The ultimate goals of genetic testing are the treatment, cure and prevention of genetic diseases. Unfortunately, however, effective medical support lags behind the ability to detect genomic mutations leading to genetic disease or an increased susceptibility to disease. Early genetic diagnosis and the prevention of the birth of severely handicapped offspring offer prospective parents the opportunity to avoid being burdened by genetic disorders and to plan their family with greater reproductive confidence (Pembrey 1998).

There is general agreement that PND including PID should only be considered for the diagnosis of severe, untreatable genetic disorders and birth defects in the newborn or infant. However, it is already proving difficult to produce a generally acceptable definition of the term 'severe'. In the evaluation of individual symptoms, the boundary between 'normal' and 'pathological' is a fluid one. Even in clinically quite well defined syndromes such as trisomy 21 (Down's syndrome), most of the symptoms overlap with ones more or less frequently seen in the average population. The view taken of a disease depends not only upon biological and medical but also upon social and personal factors whose influence can change within a short period of time. Values relating to genetic disorders also vary in different families, societies or ethnic groups. Self-help organisations have a growing influence on the acceptance of a given syndrome, not only among those affected and their relatives but also in society at large (Zerres and Rübel 1993).

The evaluation of health and disease is also influenced by technical progress in medicine. Advances in genetic testing methologies are making the detection of genetic defects that will lead to mild disorders in the child, such as X-gonosomal recessive inherited ichthyosis or disorders with a late onset such as Huntington's disease or familial colorectal and breast cancer, increasingly possible (Müller 1993). In addition, we are living in a time when parents are having fewer children and having them later in life. This could lead to an increased emphasis on having offspring who are not only healthy but also have certain desired characteristics. Pressure could therefore be exerted to use PID for other reasons than for the avoidance of serious genetic disease. This tendency is illustrated by the use of ominously fashionable terms like 'designer children', 'designer genes' or 'genetic perfectibility'. In order to counteract this trend, it is neccessary to seek measures other than a list of this kind.

The problems of establishing such a list are illustrated in the next section primarily on biological and medical grounds. When drawing up laws or guidelines, scientists and biologists must continually point out that many aspects of human beings simply do not fit into a rigid pattern. Furthermore, reference is also made to the list's effects on reproductive genetic counselling.

The nature of genetic disorders

With regard to some diseases resulting from a genetic defect, a broad consensus in favour of their inclusion in such a list could undoubtedly be obtained because PND or PID can reliably predict the relevant disease or handicap and its degree of severity. This will be illustrated below, taking as an example a representative of each of the main classes of genetic disease.

Triploidy, the occurrence of three haploid chromosome sets, is occasionally observed during IVF procedures, mostly as a result of fertilisation with two sperms. Early spontaneous abortion is usual. However, a triploid conceptus is occasionally live born. Affected neonates have a markedly low birthweight, a disproportionately small trunk as compared with head size, syndactyly and multiple congenital malformations. Triploidy is generally not compatible with survival past the neonatal period.

Trisomy for most autosomal chromosomes is lethal at an early embryonic stage. However, trisomy 21, 18 and 13 and a few other types have been described in full-term births. The clinical picture of trisomy 13 includes multiple dysmorphic features and malformations including congenital heart disease. About one half die within a month. Only 10 % survive beyond the first year, and these show profound developmental retardation.

Some single-gene disorders are also incompatible with prolonged life. Type I spinal muscular atrophy is inherited as an autosomal recessive trait. It is caused by a variety of mutations in the SAMN gene. The disease is characterised by progressive weakness due to anterior horn cell loss, reduced or absent tendon reflexes and fasciculation. Death usually occurs by the age of 3 years. Another autosomal recessive trait which leads to early death is Tay-Sachs disease, frequently occurring in Ashkenazi Jews. Mutations in the gene for serum beta-N-acetylhexosaminidase A (HEXAA) lead to progressive neurological abnormalities and the characteristic cherry-red spot in the macula.

Anencephaly belongs to the entity of multifactorially caused neural tube defects. The skin and cranial vault are missing; the exposed nervous tissue degenerates. Stillbirth or neonatal death invariably occurs.

For genetic and medical reasons, the continued compilation of such a list soon becomes difficult. In many genetic disorders the clinical consequences even of defined mutations in the genome and their effects on the expectation and quality of life cannot be accurately predicted. For a long time our

49

understanding of monogenic hereditary diseases was determined by those whose gene product is at the end of a metabolic process. If this is missing or altered, a specific function will be lacking, resulting in defined clinical consequences. We are progressively gaining a knowledge of genes which, in a figurative sense, act as a single instrument in a complex biological orchestra or which perform the role of a conductor (e.g. transcription factors) that controls the activity of other genes. A mutation of these genes may prove harmful only in specific periods of life, i.e. parts of the concert. Their manifestation is often influenced by other genetic or environmental factors. In the language of genetics, these situations are described with such terms as penetrance, expressivity or modifiers.

Autosomal dominantly inherited disorders can exhibit reduced penetrance and 'skip' generations, i.e. the disorder is not expressed at all in some individuals who carry the mutated gene. Expressivity refers to the variation of the severity of a given genetic trait. Neurofibromatosis type I (NF1 = Recklinghausen's disease) displays multiple café au lait patches, skin neurofibromata, but also more severe symptoms such as seizures and optic pathway gliomas or spinal cord or root compression. NF1 is inherited as an autosomal-dominant trait with almost full penetrance but very variable expression. Modifiers are defined genetic and environmental factors that influence the manifestation of a genetic trait. They are considered responsible for the fact that not all members of a family with the same mutated gene predisposing to cancer develop the same tumour in the same period of life.

In addition, a number of genes at different loci can result in similar disease pictures. A single gene can be mutated at a different locus from the one initially suspected and tested. The so-called genetic heterogeneity presents a major challenge to genetic diagnostics.

Disease and the feeling of being ill are not one and the same thing. It has already been pointed out that there are large differences in the subjective perception of disease symptoms by patients and their relatives who are clinically affected to the same or a very similar degree, and also in the ability to cope with a given genetic fate. The latter can also change rapidly during short periods of life, as for instance as a result of the early death of an affected relative.

Finally, such a list would be constantly outdated due to the rapid advances in research into the human genome. Its composition would have to make regular allowance for advances in therapy which influence the seriousness of the relevant diseases. It also could, therefore, adversely affect the objectives of therapeutic research by diverting attention away from efforts relating to the listed diseases. Patients would be directly affected by such developments.

Technical prerequisites

In clinical medicine it is essential to obtain an accurate diagnosis. This particularly applies to medical genetics. Although it seems impossible to establish a list of disorders warranting access to PID, one can define the technical conditions whose fulfillment is a prerequisite for the carrying out of PID.

The safety and effectiveness of genetic tests should be established before they are used routinely. PID is still in its infancy (Nagy et al. 1998). Misdiagnosis is a recurrent problem of PID due to the limitations of fluorescence in situ hybridisation (FISH) or polymerase chain reaction (PCR) when only single cells can be used (Gibbons et al. 1995). Pilot studies are required of any new test before its wide-scale application. It is important that the centres offering this testing should cooperate to allow a rapid gathering of the data by which accuracy and innocuity can be assessed (Harper 1996).

Reproductive genetic counselling

All bodies that have concerned themselves with the application of genetic testing for medical purposes have come to the conclusion that such testing must be accompanied by genetic counselling. Genetic counselling is the support given by the medical profession to help individuals, couples and entire families to get to know and understand relevant aspects of their personal medical genetic problems. Its goal is to enable people to make informed and independent personal and familial health decisions.

In our European societies autonomy outweighs most public health considerations. With regard to PND and PID, a choice between the various morally accepted courses of reproductive medicine should be permitted. Voluntariness should also be the cornerstone of related genetic testing. A list of the diseases giving access to PID would not take due consideration of the individual concerns and needs of persons seeking counsel and would clearly prevent the observance of the principles of autonomy and voluntariness. The principle of non-directive counselling, which has a strong and continuing tradition and is considered to be of special importance for reproductive decisions, could no longer be upheld in connection with PID. In the context of PID a 'case by case' approach would also have the advantage of minimising explicit reference, with resultant stigmatisation, to a model of severe handicap versus normality (European Commission 1996).

Conclusion

PID is inevitably linked with the concept of selection. The creation of a list of disorders for which PID is permitted would generally assign a higher value to some lives than to others. It would exert social and economic pressure to avoid producing children with the listed genetic disorders. The autonomy of the affected subjects would be drastically impaired and the danger of eugenic abuse increased. Above all, such a list should not allow any form of prenatal genetic testing or any reproductive choice to be simply regarded as 'correct' or 'false'. Parental options have to be respected and protected insofar as they fulfil the moral demands of the society. Our high regard for human diversity as well as the tolerance for people with disabilities must not be jeopardised.

Even if this contribution shows that – from the medical genetic point of view – it is not possible to establish an acceptable comprehensive list of diseases warranting access to PID or PND, this certainly does not mean we should not try to formulate ethical principles to guide persons seeking counsel and the medical profession in the application of PID. The way to a responsible application of ICSI and PID is not through a rigid scheme of authorisations and prohibitions, but through a process of guidance by measures aimed at fostering a sense of responsibility in all concerned.

References

Committee of the Health Council of the Netherlands (1989), *Heredity: Science and Society. On the Possibility and Limits of Genetic Testing and Gene Therapy. Report*, The Hague, December 29, pp. 79-80.

Counseil de l'Europe (1992), *Recommandation du Comité des Ministres aux Etats membres sur les tests et le dépistage génétiques à des fins médicales.*

European Commission (1996), *The Ethical Aspects of Prenatal Diagnosis. Opinion of the Group of Advisers on the Ethical Implications of Biotechnology*, Brussels.

Gibbond, W.E., Girlin, S.A. and Lanzendorf, S.E. (1995), *Strategies to Respond to Polymerase Chain Reaction Deoxyribonucleic Acid Amplification Failure in a Preimplantation Genetic Diagnosis Program, Am J Obstet Gynecol*, Vol. 172, pp. 1088-96.

Harper, J. (1996), *Preimplantation Diagnosis of Inherited Disease by Embryo Biopsy. An Update on the World Figures, J Assist Repro Genet*, Vol. 13, pp. 90-5.

Müller, Hj. (1993), *Predictive Genetic Testing: Possibilities, Implications, Limits* in Haker, H., Hearn, R. and Steigleder, K. (eds), *Ethics of Human Genome Analysis, European Perspectives.* Attempto: Tübingen, pp. 136-46.

Müller, Hj. (1998), *Connecting Lines From a Medical Point of View*, in Hildt, E. and Mieth, D. (eds) *In Vitro Fertilisation in the 1990s,* Ashgate: Aldershot, pp. 281-92.

Nagy, A.-M., De Man, X. et al. (1998), *Scientific and Ethical Issues of Preimplantation Diagnosis, Ann Med,* Vol. 30, pp. 1-6.

Pembrey, M.E. (1998), *Ethical Issues in Preimplantation Diagnosis? Europ J Hum Genet*, Vol. 6, pp. 4-11.

Zerres, K. and Rüdel, R. (eds) (1993), *Selbsthilfegruppen und Humangenetiker im Dialog. Erwartungen und Befürchtungen,* Enke: Stuttgart.

7 Nuclear transplantation – medical and ethical aspects

Gerd Richter and Matthew D. Bacchetta

As the result of dramatic advances in molecular biology and reproductive medicine, gene therapy, although in its infancy, is becoming a viable option in the medical armamentarium. In this paper, we review and consider aspects of the medical and ethical issues concerning advances in artificial reproduction, frameworks for ethical analysis, and problems with oocyte donation. One area of special interest involves mitochondrial DNA (mtDNA) and recent proposals to treat mitochondrial diseases. In the current debate regarding the different possibilities for gene therapy, it is presupposed that genetic manipulations are limited to the nuclear genome (nDNA). Given recent advances in genetics however, the mitochondria genome of eukaryotic cells must be considered as well.

In an effort to explain and suggest mtDNA manipulations, Rubenstein *et al.* proposed a protocol for treatment of a mitochondrial genetic disease. It is a nine step protocol at the germline level, and is called *in vitro* ovum nuclear transplantation (IVONT). This proposal is the first protocol ever to use germline intervention for human disease and provides the first method to apply germline manipulation to future persons as a preventive intervention. As a review of their approach, we start with a brief overview of the mitochondrial genome, explain the IVONT-protocol in detail, present a new classification schema for genetic interventions in the human genome, and raise some questions about medical and ethical problems in regard to this particular IVONT-protocol and to the subject of therapeutic nuclear transplantation in general, especially that which requires oocyte donation. IVONT is a paradigmatic case for genetic interventions.

During the early conceptualisation of gene therapy, LeRoy Walters developed a two-dimensional framework that provided the paradigmatic outline of the ethical debate about gene therapy (Walters 1986, 1991). His framework, which contains four major classifications or types, elucidates and facilitates the discernment of important ethical issues and differences in genetic interventions. Conceptually, these classifications are split along two dimensions: the type of cell intervened in or altered, and the intended outcome of the intervention, (see Figure 1). The first focuses on whether somatic or germline cells are manipulated. The second part considers whether the intention of the genetic alteration is therapeutic/preventive or an enhancement of capabilities, i.e. eugenically positive.

Dimensions of gene therapy

	somatic	germline
Therapy/Prevention	1	2
Enhancement	3	4

Figure 1.: LeRoy Walters' ethical framework of gene therapy

Type 1 represents genetic interventions in somatic cells where the intention of the transformation is therapeutic or preventive. The goal of type 2 genetic manipulations seeks not only to prevent a disease from occurring in a particular individual as in type 1 but also to enable that person to pass her transformed DNA onto her progeny. Therefore, the cell type or tissue of interest are the reproductive cells, such as spermatozoa, its precursors, and eggs. Totipotent embryonic cells at the 8- or 16-cell cleavage stage are also potential target cells for type 2 genetic interventions because of their ability to effect inheritable change in an organism's DNA. This type of manipulation would most logically follow after preimplantation diagnosis utilising one of the totipotent cells. This alteration changes the DNA of a pedigree or family line permanently. In the international literature, type 2 interventions, i.e. germline manipulation on the genetic level in order to prevent genetic diseases in future persons, are called germline gene therapy.

This is misleading because 'therapy' by definition implies treatment of an individual for an identifiable disease. Genetic manipulation in germline cells ought never be called therapeutic, because an individual who is supposedly affected by the disease does not exist (Richter and Schmid 1995). Genetic interventions in germline cells are preventive strategies for potential diseases of potential persons. A more appropriate term, germline gene manipulation, would limit space for disingenuous suggestions in public discourse about gene transfers in humans (Torres 1995). Both type 3 and 4 manipulations attempt not only to correct deleterious genes but also to enhance 'normal' genes. Type 3 manipulations enhance the genotype at the somatic level so that any improvements incorporated into an individual cannot be passed to his or her progeny. The type 4 genetic intervention, or germline transmutation, would take this a step further and pass the change on to future generations.

Mitochondrial genome

Although Walters' typology of genetic interventions proved useful, advances in medical science and technology have led to its obsolescence. Our growing knowledge about the mitochondrial genome has strained the limits of his framework's adequacy and usefulness. Thinking about the possibilities of gene transfers, we have not only to consider the difference of somatic vs. germline cells, but also the existence of the two human genomes, the nuclear and the mitochondrial genome.

Mitochondria contain their own genomes, which encode a small percentage of the macromolecules found within the cell's organelle. Human mitochondrial DNA has been completely sequenced, it is circular and contains 16,569 bp for 37 genes. Most mitochondria have 5 to 10 copies of mtDNA, an important distinction compared to the nuclear genome, which exists as a single copy in each cell. Furthermore, there are hundreds to thousands of mitochondria within each eukaryotic cell. The mammalian mitochondrial genome is also noteworthy for its density of information coupled with a lack of redundancy; i.e. there are no introns and in several instances the first nucleotide of one gene is also the last nucleotide of the preceding gene. The genes encoded by human mtDNA are 13 polypeptides, two ribosomal RNAs and 22 tRNAs that create and form parts of the respiratory chain. Additional respiratory chain polypeptides are encoded by the nuclear genes as are all the other polypeptides that contribute to mitochondrial structure and function. Thus, mitochondria are the products of both nuclear and organelle genomes.

Another important characteristic of the mitochondrial genome is that mtDNA has a very high sequence evolution rate that is 10-20 times higher than that of the nuclear genome, so the mtDNA tends to mutate about 10 times faster than nDNA. It is presumed that the difference is caused by a lower fidelity of DNA replication and a less accurate DNA repair mechanism in mitochondria. See Figure 2 for a summary of mitochondria.

Given the high density of information, the mutation rate and low redundancy, the mitochondrial genome provides a rich breeding ground for diseases caused by mitochondrial gene defects. Regarding mitochondrial diseases with mtDNA etiology, there are four different groups: *missense mutations* in polypeptide genes (i.e. LHON Leber's hereditary optic neuropathy); *protein synthesis mutations* in tRNA (i.e. MELAS mitochondrial encephalomyopathy, lactic acidosis, and stroke-like episodes) and in rRNA genes (aminoglycoside-induced and nonsyndromic cochlear deafness); *insertion-deletion* mutations; and *copy number mutations* (mtDNA depletion syndrome) (See Figure 2).

The mitochondrial Genome

Geneproducts of mtDNA:	Sites of mutation in inherited mitochondrial diseaeses
- 13 Polypeptides	- missens-mutations (polypeptide-gene
- small (12S) and	- pointmutation within tRNA-genes
- large (16S) rRNA	- pointmutation within rRNA-genes
- 22 tRNAs	- mtDNA-Insertions
	- mtDNA-Depletions

Figure 2.: Characteristics of the mitochondrial genome

Potential interventions in the mitochondrial genome

The recent proposals of mitochondrial transfection (Seibel et al. 1995) and the IVONT protocol for mitochondrial disease (Rubenstein et al. 1995) provide further evidence that Walter's framework is obsolete. Seibel et al elucidate and enumerate a number of possibilities within the realm of genetic therapy targeted at mtDNA. By coupling DNA fragments to short mitochondrial leader peptides, they demonstrated a means for delivering genes, antisense-RNA, or antisense-DNA into mitochondria via a mitochondrial peptide pathway.

Rubenstein et al.'s proposal of IVONT is a nine step protocol at the germline level for the preventive procedure of mitochondrial genetic diseases, such as mitochondrial encephalomyopathy, lactic acidosis, and stroke-like episodes (MELAS). Essentially, the IVONT procedure would transfer the nucleus of a cell with defective mitochondrial DNA into the cytoplasm of an enucleated ovum with normally functioning mitochondria. Thus, the newly created cell has the potential to develop without the mitochondrial DNA disease, yet retains the nuclear DNA potential.

In their paper, Rubenstein and colleagues endeavored to create a method through which mitochondrial genetic intervention can be properly evaluated. They suggest a means of improving upon Walters' two dimensional framework by offering a protocol to evaluate the ethical issues of human mtDNA interventions that complements and works within his framework without fundamentally challenging its appropriateness (Rubenstein et al. 1995).

Central to this modification is their concept of 'cellular penetration' as the metric upon which to compare the efficacy and ethics of 'future strategies' of genetic interventions. Although they focus their attention on type 2 genetic interventions, their supplement to Walters' work could be applied to each of his types. Their conception of cellular penetration as a graded metric is based upon 'the depth of cellular penetration to accomplish DNA manipulation'. They subclassify cellular penetration into three gradation levels. Level 1 represents 'the outermost level' where DNA could be accessed by penetrating the cell membrane. Level 2 therapy penetrates both the cell membrane and nuclear membrane to effect its therapeutic intervention. Level 3 therapy embodies 'the direct manipulation of specific DNA sequence on one chromosome'. As genetic intervention progresses from level 1 to level 3, it must pass more stringent ethical muster. Rubenstein et al. argue that the increasing ethical scrutiny is a function of 'the higher risk, effort, and cost to generate a successful protocol', which correlates with the progression from level 1 to 3.

Several problems arise with this modified framework of Walters. To effect a cure of a mitochondrial disease such as MELAS syndrome would require either a mitochondrial transfection vector protocol or something like the IVONT protocol to effect a complete exchange of all extranuclear DNA. This is feasible only if all other cytoplasmatic structures, including all membrane components, could be exchanged. More specifically, the transfection vector protocol involves transporting the wild-type DNA through the cell's membrane, transporting it through the mitochondria's membranes, and incorporating it into mtDNA. Effecting a cure of a nuclear genetic disease such as cystic fibrosis in a fashion similar to the mitochondrial example would require transporting the wild-type DNA through the cell's membrane, transporting it through the nuclear membrane, and incorporating it into the nDNA. Using Rubenstein et al.'s classification scheme, it is unclear how to differentiate adequately between these two, certainly in regard to risk, effort, cost, and benefit. Although they recognise these differences, their protocol fails to provide a means to differentiate accurately, consistently, and coherently between two obviously different interventions. Thus, the fundamental ethical concerns of these two examples do not turn on the idea of cellular penetration.

Indeed, the subclassifications of cellular penetration fail not only to provide an appropiate framework through which to evaluate and analyse these issues, but also misdirect our attention away from the fundamental issues and risks of genetic interventions. The fundamental ethical questions that we must confront have less to do with penetrating cellular membranes, nuclear membranes, and mitochondrial membranes than with the risks, effects, and intended uses of genomic manipulation of nDNA and mtDNA and whether these effects are bounded, e.g. somatic, or unbounded in duration, e.g. germline. As for accounting for the scientific challenges, we doubt cellular penetration works as an adequate direct or surrogate metric of the ethics of the technology employed to accomplish specific interventions. With these doubts in mind, Rubenstein et al.'s subclassification remains dubious and the obsolesence and limitations of Walters' original framework is apparent.

A new classification schema

To solve the contemporary ethical challenges of advances in genetics requires a more drastic modification of Walters' four types of potential genetic interventions. As opposed to the two-dimensional approach offered by Walters, we add a third dimension that demarcates between nDNA and mtDNA interventions (Bacchetta and Richter 1996) as well as an additional subclassification along the intervention axis (see Figure 3). The third dimension is necessary to accommodate the application of various technologies that effect changes with respect to either the mitochondrial or nuclear DNA, which both Walters and Rubenstein et al. fail to consider. The addition of a separate subclassification, i.e. a demarcation between therapy and prevention, represents a modification of our earlier framework in deference to points made by Parens (Parens 1998), and it also better accounts for Richter's and Schmid's position that germline interventions are limited to prevention (Richter and Schmid 1995). Parens parses well the language of genetic intervention while acknowledging the ambiguity which is inherent to the discourse of any controversial topic. We agree that the fact that distinctions are 'wrenched from the context in which we articulated them' is as old as language itself. Yet, taking a pragmatic approach to the affairs within and outside the clinic (Fins et al. 1997), we attempt to make our classification scheme clear while accepting that a continual discourse within our political and democratic institutions is essential to resolve our differences and hone our ideas and values.

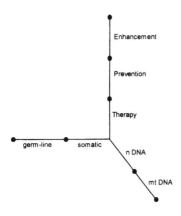

Figure 3.: Dimensions and classifications of interventions into the genome

We suggest that separating therapy and prevention has value because it maintains a distinction between disease and predisposition to disease, which facilitates a more thorough examination of the ramifications of interventions aimed at each. More specifically, therapy aims to treat and restore normal function as well as possible in the case of an existing disease with its diagnostic signs and symptoms. Prevention, on the other hand, is aimed at a disease not yet manifest, regardless of predisposition or potential for its development. This demarcation permits the incorporation of more subtle genetic issues in the discourse such as the level of penetrance of various genetic disorders. Enhancing interventions intend to improve capacity beyond normal, i.e. average capabilities. Admittedly, any definition of normal human physiology and capacity is less than unequivocal, but yielding to pragmatic constraints it works as a starting point for further discussion. We remain optimistic that we can reach an approximate consensus about most aspects of normal human physiology even though we may never agree on psychological factors of health.

In Figure 4, all theoretically possible genetic interventions can be imagined as cubes within a three-dimensional matrix defined by the dimensions of cell type, intention, and targeted genome. This format results in 12 cubes defined as follows: 1) somatic therapy with nDNA, 2) somatic therapy with mtDNA, 3) somatic prevention with nDNA, 4) somatic prevention with mtDNA, 5) somatic enhancement with nDNA, 6) somatic enhancement with mtDNA, 7) germline therapy with nDNA, 8) germline therapy with mtDNA, 9) germline prevention with nDNA, 10) germline prevention with mtDNA, 11) germline enhancement with nDNA, and 12) germline enhancement of mtDNA. There are, however, limitations to the possible types of interventions.

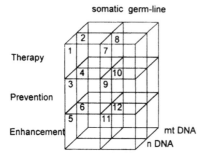

somatic germ-line

Figure 4.: Theoretically possible genetic interventions into the human genome:
cube 1: somatic gene therapy with nDNA
cube 2: somatic gene therapy with mtDNA
cube 3: genetic prevention with nDNA of somatic cells
cube 4: genetic prevention with mtDNA of somatic cells
cube 5: genetic enhancement with nDNA of somatic cells
cube 6: genetic enhancement with mtDNA of somatic cells
cube 7: germline therapy with nDNA
cube 8: germline therapy with mtDNA
cube 9: genetic prevention with nDNA of germline cells
cube 10: genetic prevention with mtDNA of germline cells
cube 11: genetic enhancement with nDNA of germline cells
cube 12: genetic enhancement with mtDNA of germline cells

Utilising our previously stated definitions, we conclude that therapeutic interventions are limited to organisms with diseases, and thus, there are no therapeutic interventions on germline cells, only preventive (Richter and Schmid 1995). Furthermore, we reject claims that mtDNA can be enhanced beyond normal physiologic capacity. Thus, the actual types of genetic interventions are limited to those shown in Figure 5, which represents a change to our earlier framework (Bacchetta and Richter 1996) (Richter and Bacchetta 1998). It also differs greatly from Walters' original matrix, yet it recognises and accommodates the potential feasibility of mtDNA manipulation by new techniques that can gain access to mtDNA as well as parsing of therapy and prevention.

Conspicuously absent are cubes 6 and 12, which would be categories for mtDNA enhancement at somatic and germline levels. This is appropriate given the limited and highly compressed nature of mtDNA and the demonstrated unique characteristics of the mitochondrial genome that make it an unlikely candidate for enhancement. Cubes 7 and 8 are expunged from our previous framework because it is impossible to give therapy to a germline cell. Interventions in germline cells are limited to prevention and enhancement. This distinction is important because it permits a more precise discussion about the allocation of scarce resources between persons with a diagnosed disease and future persons with a predisposition for a disease. In the often fierce battles surrounding the distribution of money for research and treatment, this distinction matters and will become increasingly significant as advances are made in genetic engineering. To whom we ought to dedicate scarce resources, persons or future persons, is a challenging social, political, and ethical issue, and we are in the forefront of the debate attempting to grapple with it.

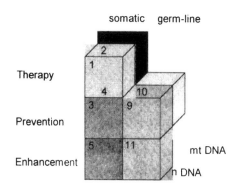

Figure 5.: Actual feasable types of genetic interventions into the human genome:
cube 1: somatic gene therapy within nDNA
cube 2: somatic gene therapx within mtDNA
cube 3: genetic prevention within nDNA of somatic cells
cube 4: genetic prevention within mtDNA of somatic cells
cube 5: genetic enhancement within nDNA of somatic cells
cube 9: genetic prevention within nDNA of germline cells
cube 10: genetic prevention within mtDNA of germline cells
cube 11: genetic enhancement within nDNA of germline cells

Ethical evaluation with the new framework

To proceed with an ethical analysis using this classification schema (Figure 6), there are currently six basic categories of genetic interventions that progress as follows: 1) therapeutic somatic gene intervention involving nDNA and mtDNA aimed at treating a diagnosed disease; 2) preventive somatic gene intervention intended to prevent a disease in a person with a predisposition for developing one; 3) preventive germline manipulation of mtDNA; 4) enhancement of nDNA in somatic cells; 5) preventive intervention in nDNA in germline cells; 6) enhancement of nDNA in germline cells. Each step or progressive category of genetic intervention requires a distinct ethical justification with increasing demands from the first through the sixth. And it is certainly imaginable that there may be situations where no ethical justification for one of these genetic interventions can be provided.

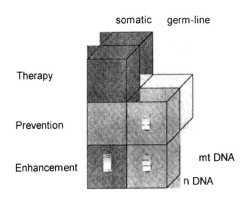

Figure 6.:Ethical justification (increasing demands of ethical justification from 1 through 6):

    1: therapeutic somatic gene intervention involving nDNA and mtDNA
    2: preventive somatic gene intervention involving nDNA and mtDNA
    3: mitochondrial germline gene manipulation
    4: enhancement of nDNA in somatic cells
    5: preventive intervention within nDNA of germline cells
    6: enhancement of nDNA in germline cells.

Undeniably, this new framework is significantly more complex than Walters' original, yet the science of genetics has become more complicated and so has the ethical analysis. The order of the progression is not intuitively obvious either. Why are we more willing to permit germline *mtDNA* interventions than somatic enhancement, especially after noting the risks associated with germline manipulation? And why suggest that somatic enhancement requires less stringent ethical justification than germline prevention within nDNA? We take this position because enhancement of any variety is morally unsavory though not necessarily proscribed, and frought with more profound social, cultural, and economic ramifications than preventive strategies for mitochondrially-based disease. Yet at the same time, we find somatic enhancement of nDNA less problematic than preventive interventions with germline nDNA because somatic interventions lack inheritability. Germline manipulations of nDNA are significantly more complex, with a potential impact and duration far beyond our current understanding or technological capability.

So how do we arrive at such a seemingly tangled progression? Our essential ethical concerns, as illustrated in Figure 4, are: 1) *inheritability*, i.e. risks to future persons and the moral repugnance of the steps to correct mistakes which require negative eugenics; 2) *enhancement* which risks exacerbation of existing social, cultural, political, and economic inequities; 3) *type of DNA* because, in general, there is greater risk in working with nDNA given that it carries nearly all of the genetic information and its operation is vastly more complex than mtDNA; and, 4) *technological complexity* of the intended intervention because different methods carry different risks. This factor prevades each of the previous concerns and is relevant to each type of intervention. It is a long-standing problem that ethical discourse gives parsimonious treatment to differences in various technologies, their capacities and limitations. This discourse not infrequently lacks the scientific rigor commensurate with discussing a topic intelligently, and not understanding the science limits one's ability to speak intelligently on the ethical issues (Bacchetta and Richter, in press).

A paradigmatic case: the IVONT protocol

Within the IVONT protocol, a number of medical and ethical problems arise. 'Medical' problems, include animal modeling, technical challenges, development of autoantibodies, preservation, and embryo development. A protocol such as IVONT should be performed initially in an animal model of mitochondrial disease prior to its use in humans. Somatic gene therapy had extensive animal model testing before the first clinical trial. Unfortunately, a good animal model does not currently exist for any mitochondrial disorder. A mtDNA deletion similar to those found in the Kearns-Sayre and Pearson syndromes was found in wild mice, so it is known that such deletions can be propagated in a mouse model. Unfortunately this particular line of mice no longer exists, and no other mtDNA mutations have been observed since, in mice or any other mammals.

Currently, it is difficult to ensure mitochondrial purity in nuclear (nDNA)-cytoplasmic exchange. Development of nondestructive techniques to isolate clean, mitochondria-free nuclei seems to be lacking. Another concern of IVONT might be the development of autoantibodies. Although anti-mitochondrial antibodies are known to exist and can cause significant diseases such as primary biliary liver cirrhosis, it is unknown whether this form of germline intervention would elicit an autoimmune reaction, potentially leading to future cases of liver disease.

Prior to IVF the patient and the woman donating the oocytes will need to have synchronous menstrual cycles, because the ability to freeze and then successfully thaw ova has not yet been developed. The technical challenge of cryopreservation follows from the larger size of oocyte and the extensive amount of fluid in it. At this point medical and ethical problems will have an overlapping area of concern. Once the ability of freezing and thawing is developed, egg banking will occur and the same issues that currently surround cryopreservation of sperm and embryos will arise. Commercial ova banks, which may or may not be associated with sperm and embryo banks, will need to be established. Undoubtedly, such banks will both buy or procure eggs from women and then resell them to doctors and couples in need of an egg donation. The main issues will then concern the precise nature of the arrangement between the donor and the bank regarding subsequent use, and whether the bank will be responsible for genetic and infectious disease screening, any rearing costs of offspring, or other possible liability factors.

Because normal development of an embryo to term is critically dependent upon the initiating events at the time of fertilisation, close attention must be given to the effect of IVONT on embryonic and postnatal development. Therefore, long-term follow up studies are not only necessary but mandatory. The impact of developmental problems may not manifest for many years in children created and conceived through such techniques. With that said, an important result concerning embryonic development appeared in a recent case report of the birth of a child following oocyte cytoplasmic donation at the time of fertilisation (Cohen et al. 1997). The purpose of this intervention was to treat the maternal gamete's presumably defective cytoplasm/mitochondria with donor cytoplasm.

Donor oocyte program

In Figure 7, there is a summary of the requirements of the oocyte donation programs at four American fertility centers: the University of Washington Medical Center in Seattle, the private university affiliated Montefiore Hospital/Albert Einstein Medical Center in the Bronx, New York, IVF America in Boston, and the Huntington Reproductive Center in Pasadena, California (Cohen 1996). Donors have to be healthy women between the ages 21 and 35, be interviewed and answer questions about their motivation for donating, their sexual and medical history, and undergo a physical examination with blood tests. The blood tests include a complete blood count, ABO-Rh and antibody screening tests, and blood chemistry. The donor is also screened for socially and sexually transmitted diseases such as Mycoplasma hominis, Ureaplasma urealyticum, gonorrhea, syphilis, toxoplasmosis, CMV, herpes, hepatitis, rubella, and HIV. Psychological counseling and formal testing are performed, and sexual abstinence and monogamy during the stimulation and retrieval process are required.

Donor Oocyte Program

- donors: healthy women aged 21-35
- interviews and questionnaires: motivation of donation, life style of donors and their partners, sexual life style etc.
- medical history, physical exam, baseline blood count, chemistry, ABO-Rh and antibody screening tests
- genetic counseling, genetic screening
- socially and sexually transmitted diseases: Mycoplasma hominis, Ureaplasma urealyticum, Neisseria gonorhoe, syphilis, toxoplasmosis, CMV, herpes, Heatitis A,B,C, and possible D and E, rubella, immune deficiency virus disorder
- Psychological counseling and formal testing
- monogamy and sexual abstinence at times during the donation treatment cycle.

Figure 7.: Donor oocyte program

Potential medical risks to oocyte donors

There are major differences between oocyte donation and sperm donation with respect to recruitment, motivation, number of collections, method of obtaining gametes, potential medical risks to the donor from the collection procedures, and psychological screening. The method of retrieving sperm gametes is very easy compared to oocyte retrieval via an ultrasound-guided transvaginal ovarian puncture and needle aspiration of follicles under local analgesia or anesthesia. With the use of prophylactic antibiotic therapy, an associated ascending infection process in the oocyte donor, although rare, can occur. A pelvic infection following an egg retrieval could culminate in infertility and sterility. Bleeding from the retrival process is another potential complication.

A long term, and poorly understood, concern involves the potentially increased risk of ovarian cancer in patients exposed to several cycles of ovulation induction. At present, the scientific evidence for this appears clouded because of methodological flaws in the original study. Nevertheless, infertility specialists should use caution and limit the maximum number of hormonal stimulations of oocyte donors. Also, oocyte donors should be advised about the risk of ovarian hyperstimulation, a syndrome induced by the ovulatory drugs that could represent a life-threatening situation for them. Furthermore, if an oocyte donor experiences an unprotected sexual encounter around the time of egg retrieval and the infertility specialist fails to retrieve all eggs, the donor may face the possibility of pregnancy. Therefore, caution should be exercised to avoid overstimulating the donor, and barrier contraception should be advised if the donor engages in any sexual activity around the time of egg retrieval (see Figure 8).

Potential Medical Hazards to Oocyte Donors

- associated ascending infection process (transvaginal ovarian puncture and needle aspiration of follicles under drug analgesia and/or anesthesia)
- pelvic infection
- infertility and sterility
- risk of ovarion cancer in women exposed to several cycles of ovulation induction
- syndrome of ovarian hyperstimulation
- possibility of pregnancy by unprotected sexual encounter around the time of egg retrieval.

Figure 8.: Potential medical hazards to oocyte donors

Ethical problems concerning egg donation

One of the major ethical concerns regarding egg donation is commodification. Here there is much ethical confusion (Cohen 1996), and significant practice and legal differences among various countries only serve to highlight further the moral ambiguity surrounding this practice. For instance, clinics in the U.S. pay their egg donors whereas Germany prohibits any form of egg donation. Naturally, there is a concern that the current practice in the U.S. threatens to commodify egg donation and risks exploitation of women. The most common position defending this practice is that clinics reimburse women for their time lost in the labor market and the inconvenience of the donation procedure, but do not pay them for the product, i.e. their eggs.

This position has become increasingly difficult to defend as the fee paid to donors has steadily risen. It is arguable that by paying donors $2,500 per donation with recent payments reaching as much as $5,000 (Kolata 1998), America has begun a de facto experiment with the ethical acceptability of commodification, and it is disingenous to suggest otherwise. Thus, a real concern arises about whether the U.S. has given adequate consideration to this issue.

The social, legal, and ethical issues of egg donation and commodification are well covered in Cohen's book on egg donation (Cohen 1996). Some of the more distressing risks noted include the following: the potential for exploitation of women; increased rates of infection and inheritable disease from donors who have chosen to lie about their past social, family, and medical histories to avoid exclusion from donation; and exacerbation of social inequalities. Taking a pragmatic approach (Fins et al. 1997, Miller et al. 1996) to this problem and formulating the U.S. position on commodification as a moral hypothesis, it would behove those involved with artificial reproduction to study and investigate this issue more intelligently to gain insight into its ethical acceptability, regardless of whether one currently agrees with this practice.

Several hypotheses are worth examining to understand better the social and ethical impact of commodification. For example, under what conditions and for what reasons do women donate their eggs – money, beneficence? Is it true that poor women are the usual donors and wealthy women the recipients? If this is the case, does it matter? Do donors feel exploited? Is the screeening process for donors a subterfuge for eugenic practices? Does commodification encourage donors to lie about their family and medical history, and thus increase the risk to recipients by enticing 'undesirable' women to donate? In regard to the last question, one could argue the increased risk simply reflects the market's risk-reward relationship at work, and recipients ought to share in more of the risk associated with the increased demand.

Clearly, these questions and others like them are much easier to ask than to answer. At this point, the hard work of ethics lies not in the contemplative tower, but in the trenches digging for the answers to these questions. Our society needs to understand better what the enterprise of artificial reproduction is about, simply making babies for couples who cannot, for whatever reason, conceive naturally, or who fear the consequences of the natural lottery, i.e. having a child with a technologically avoidable genetic disease like cystic fibrosis. Or is it much more than this single and simple aim?

Conclusion

We offer a new framework within which to analyse the ethics of genetic engineering in humans. It differs significantly from Walters' original schema as well as from Rubenstein et al.'s. It also represents a modification of our previous framework although the salient features are the same. It accounts for the three dimensions of genetic interventions: type of DNA, aim/intention of the intervention, and cell type. In essence, there are two DNAs to consider, nDNA and mtDNA; two cell types, somatic and germline; and, three types of goals for genetic manipulation, therapy, prevention, and enhancement. Futhermore, each of type of intervention has concommitant risks associated with the requisite technology, which must be part of the ethical evaluation.

The increased sophistication of this ethical framework is made necessary because of advances in genetic engineering and the inchoate debate regarding the allocation of resources to existing persons and future persons. In their paper, Rubenstein et al. suggest a form of genetic intervention targeted at mitochondrial disease, and attempt to create an ethical framework based on the concept of cellular penetration. Their framework is inadequate for a number of reasons, primarily because it does not accurately account for the technologic challenges of genetic engineering, and does not provide a useful means with which to distinguish important ethical differences between various types of genetic interventions.

Finally, we briefly review the role of egg donation in the enterprise of artificial reproduction and the de facto commodification of egg donation in the U.S. We suggest that it is time to give pragmatic consideration to the ethical acceptability of this practice, primarily in regard to its risk to women, in general, and donors, recipients, and potential offspring, specifically.

References

Bacchetta, M.D. and Richter, G. (in press), 'Contemporary Ethical Analysis: A Shortfall in Scientific Knowledge', *Politics and the Life Sciences.*

Bacchetta, M.D. and Richter, G. (1996), 'Dimensions and Classifications of Interventions into the Human Genome', *Cambridge Quarterly of Healthcare Ethics*, Vol. 5, pp. 450-7.

Cohen, C.B. (ed.), *New Ways of Making Babies: The Case of Egg Donation*, Indiana: University Press.

Fins, J.J., Bacchetta, M.D., Miller, F.G. (1997), 'Clinical Pragmatism: A Method of Moral Problem Solving', *Kennedy Institute of Ethics Journal*, Vol. 7, pp. 129-45.

Kolata, G. (1998), 'Price of Donor Eggs Soars, Setting Off A Debate on Ethics', *The New York Times*, Feb 2.

McKinley, J. (1998), 'The Egg Woman', *The New York Times*, May 17.

Miller, F.G., Fins, J.J. and Bacchetta, M.D. (1996), 'Clinical Pragmatism: John Dewey and Clinical Ethics', *The Journal of Law and Health Policy*, Vol. 13, pp. 27-51.

Parens, E. (1998), 'Is Better Always Good? The Enhancement Project', *Hastings Center Report*, Supplement to Jan-Feb. 1998 issue.

Richter, G. and Bacchetta, M.D. (1998), 'Interventions in the Human Genome: Some Moral and Ethical Considerations', *Journal of Medicine and Philosophy*, Vol. 23, pp. 303-17.

Richter, G. and Schmid, R. (1995), 'Gentherapie – eine medizinische und ethische Standortbestimmung', *Deutsche Medizinische Wochenschrift*, Vol. 120, 1212-8.

Rubenstein, D.S., Thomasma, D.C., Schon, E.A. and Zinaman, M.J. (1995), 'Germline Therapy to Cure Mitochondrial Disease: Protocol and Ethics of in Vivo Nuclear Transplation', *Cambridge Quarterly of Healthcare Ethics*, Vol. 4, pp. 316-39.

Part Two
PERSONAL INTERESTS AND MORAL IMPLICATIONS

1 Ethics of preimplantation genetic diagnosis

Guido de Wert

Introduction

Assisted reproductive technologies (ART) can help prospective parents to reach their parental goals. Techniques are constantly being developed or improved which can circumvent sub-/infertility. Furthermore, developments in (prenatal) diagnostic techniques make it increasingly possible to avoid the birth of a severely handicapped child. While it is widely acknowledged that ART can contribute to human well-being, it is at the same time recognised that the 'reproductive revolution' raises a wave of moral questions concerning the responsibilities of prospective parents, the scientists involved, and society as a whole.

This chapter concentrates on ethical aspects of preimplantation genetic diagnosis (PID), which illustrates perfectly the confluence of ART with molecular biology.

Ethical analysis

PID as well as other developments in reproductive genetic technology can be analysed from different ethical perspectives and at different levels. A clinical ethics perspective concentrates on (micro-)ethical issues which need to be discussed in order to promote 'good clinical practice'. A socio-ethical perspective, on the other hand, is concerned with the relationship of reproductive genetic technology to society, and may question the very introduction of these technologies in view of adverse social changes that they might bring about. Although my analysis relates primarily to the first perspective, I want to briefly mention two concerns which are of paramount importance at the socio-ethical level of analysis.

First, there is a concern that the introduction and increasing use of reproductive genetic technologies will endanger respect for reproductive autonomy, that it will result in a (more or less subtle) societal pressure on prospective parents to make use of the available 'preventive' options. This concern is difficult to evaluate. In general, future developments are difficult to predict. Will societal pressure be strong as a result of testing practices? We all know of cases of women who feel already 'obligated' to opt for prenatal diagnosis. But threats to reproductive autonomy come, of course, from different sides. All genetic counsellors have seen clients who are pressed by their relatives *not* to prevent the birth of a handicapped child, for instance because of religious objections. I doubt whether the present concern is a valid argument for stopping all reproductive genetic testing and/or the development of new reproductive genetic technologies, like PID. After all, the use of these technologies can (and does) prevent serious suffering in many cases. Furthermore, curtailing the present freedom to opt for genetic testing and for the avoidance of the birth of a seriously handicapped child can hardly be seen as an adequate measure to protect reproductive freedom. At the same time, it is imperative to see how the social risk at issue could be minimised. Of paramount importance is, I think, the availability and easy access to adequate health care: if prospective parents have to decide about reproductive risks in the context of inadequate economic (and social) support for handicapped children and their families, decisions aiming at preventing the conception or birth of a handicapped child can hardly be construed as substantially autonomous. Equally important is the gene-ethical education of doctors, more particularly gynaecologists, obstetricians, and general practitioners. After all, there are strong indications that many doctors tend to counsel prospective parents in a more or less directive way, in favour of 'prevention of handicaps' (Marteau et al. 1994).

A *second* socio-ethical concern relates to the disability rights perspective: reproductive genetic technologies might devalue the lives of the disabled. I seriously question that these technologies as such lead to, or implicitly involve, discrimination against handicapped people. In the Netherlands (and I presume elsewhere), it is widely experienced that parents of a handicapped child who use genetic testing to avoid the birth of a second child with the particular condition love the first child no less. Kitcher has, I think persuasively, argued that what holds at the level of parental attitudes can also hold at a societal level (Kitcher 1996). It is, therefore, unwarranted to construe a conflict between on the one hand the needs and rights of prospective parents who want to decrease their risk of having a handicapped child and on the other hand the interests and rights of disabled people.

In this 'ethics of PID', eight issues will be presented in a more or less chronological order.

Research with pre-embryos

The introduction and further development of PID is closely related to pre-clinical research with human early pre-embryos (i.e. the conceptus from fertilisation to the development of the primitive streak). This research aims at investigating the safety of the various biopsy-strategies and the reliability of the diagnostic techniques (Verlinsky 1991). The ethics of this research is highly controversial. Objections come from two different perspectives, one fetalist, the other feminist (Raymond 1987). 'Fetalists', who focus on the moral status of pre-embryos, object that embryo-research unjustifiably treats pre-embryos solely as a means. The fundamental controversy is as to whether pre-embryos have the same moral status as children or adults, who are to be protected from destructive research. Most ethical theories hold that pre-embryos need not to be respected as persons (Hursthouse 1987). Most of the ethics committees who have studied the current issue conclude that the pre-embryo has a relatively 'low' moral status. One of the arguments in favour of this position concerns the absence of developmental individuation. Until the pre-embryonic cells are differentiated and organised to become the primitive streak, there *is* no individual in any sense of the word, biological, legal, or moral. In view of this position, research with pre-embryos can be justified – of course, within some ethical constraints. Procedural conditions are the informed consent of the 'parents' (the providers of the gametes), and the approval of an ethics committee. Material conditions relate, amongst other things, to the goal of the proposed research – there is a strong consensus that the aim of such research should be to benefit human health, not to seek commercial profit – and to the time limit to be respected – most committees and regulations set a time limit of 14 days after fertilisation.

A major point of controversy remains the origin or source of the pre-embryos to be used in research. The 'Convention on Human Rights and Biomedicine' of the Council of Europe prohibits the creation of pre-embryos solely for research purposes (Council of Europe 1996). One may question, however, whether there is a fundamental moral distinction between on the one hand using spare pre-embryos ('left-overs') in research and on the other hand the generation of pre-embryos for research purposes. Of course, the intention at the moment of fertilisation is different – the creation of pre-embryos for re-search implies their 'instrumentalisation' right from the start. Irrespective of their 'origin', however, pre-embryos have the *same* moral status. So, if one accepts the instrumental use of spare pre-embryos, one can hardly object to the creation of pre-embryos for research purposes on the grounds that in involves instrumental use. From a consequentialist perspective, an absolute prohibition of creating pre-embryos for research is disputable, because it blocks an adequate pre-clinical risk assessment of a number of new techniques, like the cryopreservation of eggs, the in vitro maturation (IVM) of oocytes, and new types of PID.

From a feminist perspective, the issue becomes more complex. Some feminist critics question the acceptability of creating pre-embryos for research out of concern for the autonomy and the interests of the women donating eggs for research. After all, women have to undergo hormone stimulation 'therapy' and invasive medical procedures, which carry a number of known and unknown medical risks. Furthermore, so the argument runs, there is a serious risk of exploitation, in view of the temptation to withhold detailed information on risks for fear of losing 'willing' candidate donors (Gerrand 1993). These feminist concerns are, of course, relevant, but they can hardly justify an absolute ban on creating embryos for research purposes. First, the interests of donors may be sufficiently protected by imposing the material condition that medical risks should be minimised by limiting the numbers of hormone treatments as well as the dosage of hormones given to candidate donors. Of course, a valid informed consent presumes adequate information about potential residual risks. Second, the feminist objection seems to be particularly weak with regard to one specific subgroup of candidate-donors: women who opt for experimental reproductive technologies. These women may be asked to donate eggs for pre-clinical feasibility and risk assessment studies concerning these techniques. In this case, those who carry the burden of donating eggs for research may be among the first who can benefit from new techniques themselves. Third, the feminist objection is not an a priori objection, but a contingent one. After all, the creation of pre-embryos for research purposes does not necessarily involve hormonal treatments and/or invasive interventions in donor-bodies to gain access to the eggs. After all, in clinical IVF/ICSI it may happen that some oocytes have not yet reached the appropriate stage of nuclear maturity. If they mature further after 24-26 hours of in vitro culture, these oocytes cannot be used clinically, but they may be a good source for making research embryos. Furthermore, one could split a spare pre-embryo. And finally, IVM of oocytes might make hormonal treatments (for this purpose) obsolete – it could even imply access to altogether new 'sources' of research eggs, including aborted female fetuses and cadavers (Human Fertilisation & Embryology Authority 1994).

In considering the ethics of research aimed at the further development of PID, a preliminary question is, of course, whether PID as such is acceptable. - Critics have various objections, which need to be scrutinised.

A first objection to (*post*-conception) PID holds that selecting pre-embryos is intrinsically wrong, given the 'sanctity of human life'; the physician has, according to this view, a moral obligation to transfer all pre-embryos available (Iglesias 1990). This objection is highly problematic, for several reasons. First and foremost, the 'sanctity of life'-doctrine is based on shaky premises: it presupposes that the pre-embryo should be respected as a human person, (i.e.) that it has an absolute right to life. A more moderate, and more reasonable, view is that the pre-embryo, in view of its potentiality, deserves some respect, that one should not destroy pre-embryos for trivial reasons. It is widely, and I think rightly, accepted that regular prenatal diagnosis and selective abortion can be morally justified as a means to prevent serious suffering for the future child and/or the parents/family. PID can be justified as well: accepting selective abortion while rejecting a selective transfer would, at least at first sight, be inconsistent.

Furthermore, the 'anti-pre-embryo-selection' ethos may have potentially dangerous consequences for the health of the prospective mother. Indeed, it is 'good medical practice' not to transfer tripronucleate zygotes, which may be the result of two sperms penetrating the oocyte. One of the reasons for this policy is that the maternal pronucleus might be extruded, generating a hydatidiform mole, which may develop into a tumour in the recipient (Fishel 1996). In other words: depending on the consequences, it is not the non-transfer but the transfer of defective zygotes/embryos which is problematic from a moral point of view.

To biopsy or not to biopsy?

Another objection to (invasive, post-conception) PID concerns the preparatory biopsy. At least two versions of the objection can be discerned. The first one ('the argument from totipotency') runs as follows: 'The individual blastomeres of a pre-embryo are totipotent; they have exactly the same developmental potential as a pre-embryo. Therefore, isolating a blastomere involves the creation of a second, duplicate, pre-embryo, which will be destroyed during the diagnostic procedures'. (Primarily) for this reason, post-conceptional PID is prohibited by the German 'Embryo Protection Act' (Gesetz zum Schutz von Embryonen 1990). This objection is, however, weak, for two reasons. First, it is unlikely that an individual blastomere isolated at the six- to ten-cell stage is still totipotent (Geber et al. 1995, McLaren 1997). Second, even if it were proven that (invasive) PID inherently involves the creation of a second preembryo – which will be destroyed during or after the diagnostic procedure – one could still justify this technique, in view of a) the relatively 'low' moral status of a pre-embryo, and b) the 'pros' of PID in comparison with a selective abortion.

A second objection concerning the preparatory biopsy is a slippery slope argument: 'PID represents an opening wedge into the concern about the cloning of human embryos for more sinister purposes. Are the dangers inherent in cloning greater than the benefits obtained through preimplantation genetic analysis?' (Verlinsky et al. 1987). This argument presumes, of course, that the artificial production of monozygotic twins by 'pre-embryo splitting' or 'blastomere separation' is necessarily morally wrong, a presumption which needs close scrutiny. An extensive ethical analysis has been presented by the American National Advisory Board on Ethics in Reproduction (NABER) (National Advisory Board on Ethics in Reproduction 1994). Virtually all NABER members would allow several clinical applications of pre-embryo splitting, e.g. to improve the chances of initiating pregnancy in those individuals undergoing IVF who produce only a limited number of pre-embryos for transfer and implantation. Even if one accepts the premise that 'cloning by pre-embryo splitting' is immoral, the present slippery slope argument against isolating blastomeres for the purpose of PID is not convincing. After all, such biopsy neither logically justifies nor automatically results in the artificial production of monozygotic twins.

Disproportionally burdensome?

In the debate concerning the various types of regular prenatal diagnosis, it is often claimed (or at least implicitly presumed) that early diagnosis, by chorionic villus sampling (CVS), is better than later diagnosis (amniocentesis). This 'the sooner, the better' assumption has, however, been questioned, because the assumption is only valid 'all others things being equal' – which is not the case (Boss 1994). Relevant disadvantages of CVS include, amongst others, a somewhat higher miscarriage rate. A comparison of the respective pros and cons of CVS on the one hand and amniocentesis on the other hand is rather complex, and to a large degree subjective, i.e. dependent on the personal circumstances, biography, and preferences of the individual patient.

The same pitfall should be avoided in the evaluation of PID. Of course, it is a major advantage of PID that it can avoid traumatic (repeated) selective abortions. At the same time, PID carries significant disadvantages. First, PID presupposes ART, more particular by IVF/ICSI, which is not the most pleasant way to 'make' babies, carries various sorts of risk for women (infection, ovarian hyperstimulation syndrome, multifetal pregnancies, XE "multifetal pregnancy" etc.), and has only a moderate 'take baby home rate' (TBHR). Second, PID is still experimental: the reliability of the diagnostic tests as well as the safety of the preparatory biopsy (or combination of biopsies) remains to be proven.

At the same time, a second pitfall should be avoided, namely the paternalistic objection to PID: 'it is too burdensome, whereas there are reasonable alternatives'. Paternalistic critics likewise ignore that balancing the pros and cons of the respective options is highly subjective. For some couples the so-called 'reasonable alternatives', more in particular prenatal diagnosis and selective abortion, are a priori unacceptable. And for *infertile* couples at high risk of conceiving a handicapped child, who opt for IVF/ICSI as an infertility treatment, PID may be far more attractive than a non-selective transfer.

This anti-paternalistic comment underscores the importance of the concept of informed choice: PID requires the free and informed consent of the prospective parents. It is of utmost importance that the couple understands the (practical) pros and cons of PID in comparison with regular prenatal diagnosis.

Indications

As the Human Genome Project continues to unravel our genome, the numbers of tests that can be used in the context of PID will steadily increase. One of the 'classical' questions concerning regular prenatal diagnosis is also relevant with regard to PID: what genetic tests should be performed? Should a line be drawn? And if so, where?

The moral justification for selective abortion as well as a selective transfer is the prevention of severe suffering related to genetic defects and disorders, not just suffering of the future affected child, but also suffering of the parents (family). The question then becomes: how severe does a defect or disorder have to be in order to qualify for prenatal testing or PID?

Some commentators have proposed to make an exhaustive, detailed list containing all the acceptable indications. This approach seems to be highly problematic, for various reasons. First, such a list would need continuous updating, in view of the rapid developments in this field. Furthermore, this approach would do insufficient justice to the personal circumstances and values of the future parents, whereas this aspect cannot be ignored in view of the moral justification of prenatal diagnosis and PID mentioned above.

Even though the subjective point of view of the future parents is ethically important, respect for autonomy is not unqualified. Prenatal testing and PID should not be performed for defects/conditions which cannot reasonably be considered to be a serious threat to the well-being of the future child and/or the family. The question 'Where precisely to draw the line?' is, of course, difficult to answer. I would suggest that three relevant factors should be simultaneously considered:
the severity of the defect/disorder;

the age of onset of the disorder;

the penetrance of the genetic defect (the probability that the genotype will affect the phenotype).

I take it for granted that there is a strong consensus concerning the acceptability of prenatal diagnosis and PID for two categories of diseases:

lethal childhood disorders, such as Duchenne muscular dystrophy, Lesch Nyhan syndrome, and Tay Sachs disease;

severely handicapping *non*-lethal conditions which manifest themselves *early* in life (e.g. Down's syndrome).

The great majority of current applications of prenatal diagnosis and PID belong to these categories.

I will focus on prenatal diagnosis as well as PID for three categories of abnormalities/disorders:

treatable childhood disorders;

untreatable late onset diseases;

(monogenic or multifactorial) late onset disorders which may be succesfully treated, e.g. some hereditary cancers.

Concentrating on these (potential) applications is appropriate for two reasons: they are especially controversial, and there seems to be a significant interest in PID among parents at risk of having a child with any of these disorders (Delanthy and Harper 1997).

Let me first look briefly at the ethics of regular prenatal diagnosis of disorders belonging to each of these categories, and secondly at the ethics of PID.

Treatable childhood disorders

Disorders belonging to this category include hemophilia and phenylketonuria (PKU). Hemophilia has a highly variable expression. For the present ethical reflection, the milder form is especially relevant. Prenatal diagnosis of mild hemophilia is in particular controversial, even among (Dutch) genetic counsellors, because it is perfectly treatable. Nevertheless, even the prospect of having a boy with the milder form can be frightening for (future) parents, for instance when an affected relative has died form 'iatrogenic' AIDS (caused by a transfusion of infected blood), or when parents already have an affected boy.

I would argue that prenatal testing for haemophilia (and selective abortion of an affected fetus) can, at least in some cases, be morally justified. In view of the potentially significant psychosocial and emotional burdens for parents, prevention of treatable childhood disorders is not necessarily too trivial a reason to justify abortion morally. A similar argument may apply to prenatal testing for phenylketonuria PKU (Holtzman 1994).

Huntington's disease (HD) is the paradigm case for this category (even though only a small minority of people at risk for HD opt for prenatal testing). Aborting a fetus carrying the HD-mutation has been most explicitly criticised by the American philosopher Post (1991): the child will have 'many decades of good and unimpaired living. Moreover, the parents of the child are not immediately or even directly affected in the way they would be were the disease of early onset'. Posts' reservations about prenatal testing for HD are based on two 'humanistic' considerations: first, our desire not to bring suffering into the world must be tempered by the recognition that suffering is a part of life, and escapes human prevention to a large degree. Technology may prevent our coming to grips with the basic existential reality of contingency from which we never fully escape. Second, we should acknowledge the moral ambiguity of the quest for 'perfect' babies ('perfectionism'), and resist 'the tyranny of the normal'. People who are different and 'imperfect' teach us about the meaning of equality and commitment. We must, according to Post, be highly circumspect about declaring too imperfect those persons who must endure somewhat earlier in life the very sorts of frailties that eventually assault each one of us.

Do these considerations undermine the morality of prenatal testing for HD (aimed at abortion of a predisposed fetus)? No, they don't. Of course, it would be naive and misguided to fight against all contingencies of human life. The question is, however, whether carriers of HD, who have a high (50 %) risk of transmitting the mutation to their children, have the moral right to prevent this by making use of prenatal diagnosis and selective abortion. In view of the fact that HD is a severe disease, and that the penetrance of the mutation is complete, my answer is: yes. It is insensitive, if not an insult, to (dis)qualify preventive measures as symptomatic of 'genetic perfectionism'. Of course, carriers of HD will be healthy during three to four decades. One needs to recognise, however, that the prospect of their eventual fate often imposes an extremely severe burden. The objection that carriers of HD 'endure just somewhat earlier in life' the frailties that eventually assault each one of us, is misplaced. (This objection might be valid, however, with regard to prenatal testing for the late onset version of Alzheimer's disease, which has a substantially later onset than HD.) Finally, Post completely ignores the perspective of the healthy relatives. Personally, I was deeply impressed by the desperate sigh of the widow of a HD-patient: 'When my husband died after twenty-five years of illness, I felt like a light had finally come on at the end of the tunnel. Now I watch my daughter and see her movements and the light has extinguished' (Wexler 1992).

Relevant examples include hereditary breast/ovarian cancer (HBOC) and familial adenomatose polyposis (FAP). To begin with, it should be noted that members of affected families have until now shown hardly any interest in prenatal testing for these disorders. This should come as no surprise, in view of the clinical experience with prenatal testing for HD. Nevertheless, the ethics of such applications needs debate. Lancaster rightly concludes that prenatal testing for breast cancer gene mutations (BRCA) might be more controversial then prenatal testing for HD, because the penetrance of these mutations is incomplete, and preventive interventions may effectively reduce morbidity and mortality in carriers (Lancaster et al. 1996). But again, we should resist premature conclusions with regard to preventing the birth of (female) fetuses predisposed to HBOC. Morally relevant questions concern a) the effectiveness of available preventive and/or therapeutic measures, and b) the burden imposed by the respective medical interventions. The effectiveness of medical surveillance (mammography) and prophylactic surgery (bilateral mastectomy and oophorectomy) is presumed, but still unproven (Burke et al. 1997). Furthermore, prophylactic surgery is irreversible, and has major implications for women's quality of life.

I would argue that the fear of prospective parents ('at risk') that their future children may inherit a BRCA gene mutation is far from unreasonable, and that prevention of the birth of children strongly predisposed to HBOC is not a trivial concern. One may safely assume that future requests for prenatal diagnosis of BRCA gene mutations will primarily (if not exclusively) come from members of severely affected families. In these cases, the penetrance of the BRCA-gene mutations will be highest, and performing prenatal diagnosis least problematic from a moral point of view.

More restrictive indications for PID?

It is sometimes argued that the indications for PID should be (far) more restrictive than the indications accepted for regular prenatal diagnosis. A Dutch committee, for instance, recommended in 1991 that PID should (for the moment) be performed only for 'severe, untreatable' disorders (Kerncommissie Ethiek Medisch Onderzoek 1993). As a consequence, PID for diseases belonging to category A (and maybe category C) would not be allowed. The Ethics Committee of the German 'Gesellschaft für Humangenetik' – to give a second example – suggested allowing PID in case of a 'serious childhood disorder or developmental defect' ('schwerwiegende kindliche Erkrankung oder Entwicklungsstörung') (Gesellschaft für Humangenetik 1996). Following this guideline, PID should not be performed for disorders belonging to category A, B, and C. (How) can such a restrictive policy be justified?

From an ethical point of view, it would be difficult to justify stricter indications *a priori* for PID than for regular prenatal diagnosis. After all, a pre-embryo does not have a 'higher' moral status than a fetus – accordingly, a selective transfer is not more difficult to justify than a selective abortion. Imposing stricter indications for PID might, however, be justified on the basis of (more or less) *contingent* considerations. Let me briefly review (some of) these arguments:

'PID involves a heavy burden, especially for the woman.' This argument is unjustifiably paternalistic. Furthermore, this argument hardly applies to infertile couples at high genetic risk, who opt for IVF to treat their infertility!

'The reliability of the tests is unproven.' I presume that the underlying fear concerns the (small but real) risk of false-negative test results, resulting in an affected pregnancy or even in the birth of an affected child. Even if the experimental nature of the test should be regarded (for the moment) as a valid reason to 'set limits' (at least some of the tests used are currently highly reliable in experienced hands), the conclusion that PID should be performed only for serious, untreatable disorders is a non sequitur. After all, the potential burden imposed by a false negative result would be less if the condition is mild or treatable.

'The experimental biopsy carries unknown risks to the health of the future child.' Obviously, doctors as well as prospective parents should only take risks if they have a good reason for doing so. But what is a good reason? In any case, this argument has become less convincing as clinical experience until now suggests that the biopsy carries no such risk. A systematic anomaly assessment should provide further data (Simpson and Liebaers 1996).

'PID involves an additional loss of embryos.' One might argue, first, that isolated blastomeres are totipotent, and, therefore, are (or have the same moral status as) embryos. The presumed totipotency of individual blastomeres at the 6 tot 10 cell stage is, however, unlikely. A second version of this argument concerns the unintended loss of embryos as a consequence of 'biopsy-failure'. According to the experts, however, such embryo-loss rarely happens in experienced hands.

In summary, it may be concluded that the arguments in favor of more restrictive indications for PID are either logically incoherent or, in view of the clinical experience, weak. Defects or disorders which are 'serious enough' to qualify for prenatal diagnosis, should also qualify for PID.

Less restrictive indications?

Perhaps the real ethical question is not whether the indications for PID should be *more* restrictive than the indications for regular prenatal diagnosis, but whether the indications for PID could be *less* restrictive. After all, many consider pre-embryos to have a lower moral status than fetuses. Accordingly, one might argue that selection of pre-embryos on the basis of less serious grounds could be justified. The paradigm case is, of course, PID for sex selection for social (non-medical) reasons.

An exponent of this position is Robertson (Robertson 1992). He argues that

> screening out embryos on the basis of gender may be less clearly unethical than initially thought. The ethics of choosing the sex of offspring depends very much on the means employed. Abortion for sex selection is very different from preconception sperm separation selection techniques. Embryo selection on the basis of sex seems much closer to preconception techniques than to abortion.

The ethics of sex selection is highly complex. Some of the objections against PID for sex selection purposes are hardly convincing, at least in western culture. Take, for example, the criticism that such selection is inherently sexist, or that it will result in a serious disturbance of the sex ratio. There are, however, some moral issues which need further consideration. First, even if one agrees that the earlier the selection, the less ethically problematic it is, one could argue that destroying embryos for sex selection purposes is at odds with the value of the embryo. Postconception sex selection (for social reasons) could, according to some of its proponents, take place *without* discarding pre-embryos of the undesired sex by donating these pre-embryos to infertile couples (a strategy called 'gender distribution') (Seibel et al. 1994). I wonder, however, whether such donations wouldn't only add pre-embryos to the large numbers of frozen spare pre-embryos waiting for adoptive parents. A related objection is that, in a case in which the transfer of the pre-embryos of the desired sex does not result in an ongoing pregnancy, one has to start a new IVF treatment while there are still 'healthy' pre-embryos available for transfer. Can such a practice be justified, given the costs and the medical risks of additional IVF and PID? Another, third, objection concerns designing the characteristics of future children. Sex selection for non-medical reasons can set a precedent for 'positive eugenics', i.e. selection for non-disease characteristics (intelligence, body build, etc.) that may confer advantages upon the offspring, more in particular the offspring of the economically advantaged, who can afford the costs of such testing. The American philosopher Strong rightly concludes that we would at least need a greater confidence that the benefits would outweigh the harms before we would be ethically justified in proceeding (Strong 1997).

Carrier pre-embryos: to transfer or not to transfer?

As mutation analysis will increasingly be performed in the context of PID, many pre-embryos will be identified as carrying a *recessive* disorder. What should the transfer-policy be with regard to these (healthy) 'carriers'?

The major reason *not* to transfer healthy carriers, would be the parent's wish to prevent difficult reproductive choices for their prospective child. A child carrying a recessive disorder will, indeed, have a higher risk of having a handicapped child him/herself. The magnitude of this risk depends, of course, on the genetics of the particular disorder: carriers of an *autosomal* recessive disease still have a quite low risk of having an affected, homozygous child – the risk will only become high when the partner carries a mutation in the same gene. Female carriers of an *X-linked* recessive disorder, however, have a high risk: each of their sons will have a 50% risk of getting the disease. In view of these facts, the question 'What to do with (healthy) carrier pre-embryos?' will presumably be most relevant in the context of PID for X-linked recessive disorders.

An adequate answer presumes the weighing up of the pros and cons of *three* different policies:

just ignore information about carrier status, i.e. 'non-selectively' transfer all healthy embryos, non-carriers as well as carriers; after all, carriers will grow into healthy children too;

do not transfer carriers;

first transfer non-carriers ('pre-selection'), and transfer the carriers in a next cycle (a 'step by step' approach).

I have not yet developed a strong opinion on this issue. I assume that one should draw a distinction between pre-embryos carrying *autosomal* recessive disorders on the one hand and (female) pre-embryos carrying *X-linked* recessive disorders on the other hand. With regard to the first category of carriers, option B ('do not transfer carriers') seems to be highly problematic. In view of the (very) low risk that the future carrier will be faced with difficult reproductive decisions, it would be disproportional to discard these (healthy) pre-embryos categorically, and to start a new IVF/PID treatment. Option C ('pre-select' non-carriers), however, would be a reasonable option. With regard to female pre-embryos carrying an X-linked disorder, option A ('ignore the information') seems to be problematic, whereas option C ('pre-select non-carriers') is obviously reasonable. But what about option B? Conceiving a daughter at high risk of having handicapped boys herself seems to be completely unacceptable for at least some women/couples who have seen male relatives succumb to X-linked disorders, like Duchenne muscle dystrophy (pers. communication prof. I. Liebaers). I tend to conclude that, in these cases, even option B might be justified in individual cases.

A related problem is, of course, how to balance the traditional criteria for pre-embryo selection (good morphology, etc.), aiming at preferably transferring the most viable pre-embryos, with selection on the basis of (non-) carrier status: should better viability always have priority, irrespective of (non-) carrier status?

In any case, it is important to discuss the issues concerning the provision of information about carrier status and concerning the transfer policy with regard to carrier pre-embryos during the informed consent process.

Autonomy or heteronomy?

In the context of regular prenatal diagnosis, the principle of respect for autonomy is of utmost importance. This means, first, that prospective parents at higher genetic risk should be free to decide whether or not to make use of prenatal diagnosis – the doctor should not put pressure on them to opt for testing. Second, in case of a 'positive' result of prenatal diagnosis, the prospective parents should be free to decide whether or not to terminate the pregnancy – the doctor should support them, whatever decision they make. When applied to PID, this normative principle would, reasoning analogously, imply a) that doctors should never put pressure on prospective parents to opt for PID, and b) that prospective parents should be free to decide whether or not to accept (potentially) affected embryos for transfer. Clinical PID-practice, however, reveals that respect for autonomy is not unqualified. What, then, is 'good clinical practice'? In order to clarify the present issue, I will first comment on the locus of decision making concerning PID, and second on the locus of decision making concerning the transfer. With regard to the first topic, I will focus on the offering of PID in a specific context, namely the treatment of male subfertility (De Wert 1998).

In view of the higher levels of chromosomal and other genetic anomalies in subfertile males, the availability of genetic counselling and the (routine or selective) offering of genetic testing is a prerequisite for clinical ICSI. Genetic testing can take place before the treatment (pre-conception testing for chromosome aberrations or gene mutations), during treatment (PID) or during pregnancy (mainly karyotyping). Looking more closely, the consensus is only partial. There is, indeed, dissent with regard to the *goal* of such testing. This dissent has potentially major implications for the access to ICSI in individual cases. The offering of genetic testing may have two different objectives. First, it enables the couple to make informed reproductive decisions. If they have a higher risk of having a handicapped child, they may – or may not – opt for preventive measures ('avoidance'). Second, genetic testing enables the doctor to take his *own* responsibility for preventing serious harm to children thus conceived. Sometimes, these goals may conflict. Let me give some examples. If an infertile man refuses to be tested for chromosome aberrations or – in case of congenital bilateral absence of the vas deferens (CBAVD) – for mutations in the cystic fibrosis (CFTR)-gene, at least some clinics will not give access to ICSI. Should the man carry a balanced chromosome translocation involving a high risk for the future child, or should both partners be carriers of CF, then most centres will only offer ICSI if the couple intends to make use of prenatal diagnosis or PID offered for avoidance (Silber 1995). These examples illustrate that, at least in some cases, the offer of (preconception genetic testing and) PID is, in fact, a *'coercive'* offer – an offer patients can hardly refuse in view of the adverse consequences for access to ICSI.

This practice is controversial, for two reasons (Bui and Wramsby 1996, Meschede et al. 1995). First, critics hold that a 'coercive offer' clashes with the traditional ethics of reproductive genetic counselling, more in particular with the principle of non-directiveness. According to this principle, the doctor should respect the values and preferences of his clients and give unconditional support, whatever they may choose. Second, the dominant practice involves, according to its critics, an invasion of the right to reproduce. These objections are not convincing, because they ignore that doctors offering ART have their *own* responsibility to avoid serious harm to the future children. For this reason, most infertility centres refuse to give access to, for example, a HIV-seropositive couple. If we do accept such selection, it cannot be argued consistently that any *'genetic* selection' by doctors involved in assisted reproduction is a priori illegitimate. Those who object that the refusal to give unconditional access to 'high risk' patients amounts to an invasion of their right to reproduce, wrongly interpret this *negative* claim right (or liberty right) as a *positive* claim right. Indeed, people's right to reproduce is the right to procreate without interference from the state or a third party. Infertile patients do not have an unqualified 'positive' right to reproduce, i.e. a right to assistance in reproduction, which would imply an unqualified duty of the physician to provide ART.

The real issue, then, is not *whether* it is acceptable to offer PID 'coercively' to infertile couples at high genetic risk, who apply for ART (i.e. to give access to those couples only *on the condition* that they opt for PID), but *when* this is acceptable, which criteria should be used. In general, the greater the magnitude and probability of predicted harm to the future child, the less morally justifiable it is to conceive children or to assist in reproduction (Arras 1990). Even if we would agree that assistance in procreation is morally unsound when there is a high risk of devastating or serious harm to the future child, this 'harm principle' invites controversy if applied to individual cases. After all, a harm that some parents and doctors might view as excessive, might be perfectly acceptable for others. And a level of risk that some find prohibitive, might be quite tolerable to others.

In any case, with regard to the present issue I tend to conclude that when clients at high risk of conceiving a CF-child apply for ICSI, doctors may justifiably make access dependant upon the couples' willingness to make use of PID (or prenatal diagnosis).

The second issue to be scrutinised is the decision making authority when PID has a 'positive' or inconclusive result. (This issue has, of course, broader relevance than the first one, which relates only to infertile couples at high risk of conceiving a handicapped child, who apply for infertility treatment.) At first sight, this may seem to be a purely theoretical issue, or even a 'non-issue'. One may, after all, safely assume that doctors and prospective parents agree that severely defect pre-embryos should not be transferred. It is important, however, to realise that couples may insist that pre-embryos be transferred in case of an inconclusive result of PID, and/or when they consider the residual genetic risk for the future child to be acceptable – especially when there are no other, 'definitely healthy', pre-embryos available for the transfer (Soussis et al. 1996). Furthermore, doctors and prospective parents may have widely different views regarding the seriousness of specific disorders. It is sometimes argued that, given an adverse prognosis, the choice, whether to have the pre-embryo replaced or not, must lie with the potential mother (Dunstan 1993). In view of the physicians' *own* professional responsibility to prevent serious harm to the prospective child, however, a (partial) shift with regard to the 'locus of decision making' seems to be inevitable. At the same time, this shift raises complex moral questions: what standards should be used in making these decisions, i.e. in overruling the preferences and autonomy of the couple? How to operate in the context of uncertainty with regard to the prognosis of an affected pre-embryo? When would physicians cross the boundary between a legitimate concern for the wellbeing of the prospective child on the one hand and a dubious 'preventive perfectionism' on the other hand?

In view of the potential dissent with regard to (un)acceptable harm/probability ratios, it is, again, imperative that the transfer-policy of the IVF-clinic be discussed with the couple in advance of PID.

While PID has been introduced as an alternative option for couples at very high (25-50 %) risk of transmitting a genetic defect, it could also be routinely applied in the context of regular IVF. Of special interest is the preimplantation genetic screening for aneuploidy (PGS) in embryos of older women.

The potential 'pros and cons' of this screening have been neatly sketched by Reubinoff and Shushan (1997). First, if only chromosomally normal pre-embryos (or at least pre-embryos normal for the tested chromosomes) were to be transferred, there could be a significant increase of the success of IVF. After all, it seems that pre-embryonic chromosomal anomalies are a major cause of IVF failure. Second, such selection could be reassuring, especially for older women. Currently, older women can opt for amniocentesis or CVS. These invasive procedures are associated with 0.5-1 % pregnancy loss. Therefore, it is not uncommon that infertile women are reluctant to jeopardise their 'precious' conception by invasive prenatal testing, and risk the birth of an affected child. In addition, couples with moral or religious objections to pregnancy terminations also avoid prenatal screening. The feasibility and value of PGS for aneuploidy has, however, not yet been established. Reubinoff and Shushan rightly stress that several difficulties must still be addressed before this screening can be routinely applied in women of advanced age opting for IVF, including the following. First, it is currently not known whether embryo biopsy might adversely affect implantation and pregnancy rates. And second, blastomere analysis will, at least in some cases, be not representative of the whole embryo, due to the high frequency of chromosomal mosaicism. Mosaicism could lead to misdiagnosis and to the transfer of abnormal embryos. However, the biological significance of mosaicism is unclear. Some authors have claimed that abnormal cells in the early embryo are subsequently eliminated or diverted to the trophectoderm, and thus do not impair normal development. Therefore, discarding mosaic embryos might lead to the loss of potentially normal embryos.

According to some investigators, the high level of mosaicism makes PGS on the basis of polar body analysis more attractive: 'If polar bodies are analysed, the mosaicism of preembryos would become irrelevant. This would avoid discarding mosaic embryos that may self-correct and be viable and give rise to healthy infants' (Strom 1996). A disadvantage of this approach is, of course, that it is somewhat less informative, as it cannot identify paternally derived chromosome abnormalities.

What about the ethics of PGS for aneuploidy? There are no valid a priori, *categorical*, moral objections to this type of screening; after all, we rightly accept screening for chromosomal abnormalities during pregnancy.

Nevertheless, PGS for aneuploidy raises some ethical (and ethically relevant) issues and questions which need further debate.

First, PGS for aneuploidy is experimental. Vital, unanswered questions concern, amongst other things, the effectiveness of the screening ('does it improve the TBHR of IVF?'), the potential adverse effects of the biopsy on the implantation rate, and the implications of mosaicism (cfr. above). This type of PGS should, therefore, be introduced in the context of a research project, aimed at a systematic evaluation of its presumed pros and potential cons. Participation in this research presumes, of course, a 'free and informed consent'.

Second, what is the optimal timing of this screening: post-, pre-, or 'intra'-conceptional? What are the respective – medical and moral – pros and cons of the various scenarios? Postconception screening for aneuploidy is most informative, but is hampered by the high incidence of mosaicism. Analysis of the (first) polar body would avoid this complication. According to (some of) its proponents, this alternative strategy has a *moral* advantage too: after all, biopsy and diagnosis of the (first) polar body aims at a selective fertilisation of normal oocytes, thus avoiding the pre-embryo-selection and discard inherent in *post*conception analysis. The leading investigators, however, have recently recommended that both the first and the second polar body should be studied (Verlinsky et al. 1996). Although they continue to qualify this strategy as *pre*-conception testing, this combined biopsy implies in fact a shift towards '*intra*'conception PID – after all, the second polar body appears during the fertilisation process. What, then, is the moral status of the oocyte during the fertilisation process? There is no consensus on this point. In view of its potentiality, I would suggest that the oocyte 'in statu fertilisandi' is (the moral equivalent of) a pre-embryo, not (the moral equivalent of) an unfertilised egg.

A point of concern is the safety of polar body biopsy (Medical Research Council 1990). Even though Verlinsky et al. have already introduced this technique in the clinic, there may still be a need for a pre-clinical risk assessment, involving the creation of human pre-embryos for the purpose of research (pers. communication, Prof. A. van Steirteghem).

A third issue concerns the costs, and the cost-effectiveness, of PGS for aneuploidy. The current clinical trials will hopefully deliver relevant data.

A fourth issue concerns, again, the 'locus of decision making'. Who would have decision making authority with regard to, first, the actual use of such screening in individual cases – the doctor or the couple/woman? As long as the screening is experimental, the answer is self-evident: it is for the woman/couple to decide whether or not to participate in the trial. But what if this screening proves to be efficient, cost-effective, and safe? Will it become the professional standard, part of 'good clinical practice' – just like screening for the correct number of pronuclei? And who has decision making authority with regard to the *selection* of the chromosomes that would be included in the 'screening panel'? What are the normative implications of the finding that inclusion of some chromosomes (e.g. no. 16) is highly relevant if one wants to improve the success rate of IVF, but not if one gives priority to preventing the birth of chromosomally abnormal children? (Egozue 1996). What if patients do not want to be informed about mild chromosomal aberrations, like XXY and XYY? And, finally, who has decision making authority concerning the disposal of chromosomally 'abnormal' pre-embryos? What if a couple would insist on transferring a pre-embryo with, for instance, a XXY or XYY karyotype?

Preimplantation genetics: a case for preventive ethics

'Applied preimplantation genetics' is a dynamic field. The first imperative of preventive ethics is the timely discussion of the potential pros and cons of new developments. Let me just give a few examples:

a. Technological break-throughs like primer extension preamplification (PEP) and serial biopsies will allow the performance of different genetic studies at the same time. What are the ethical and psychosocial problems and pitfalls of making a 'genetic profile' of pre-embryos (Handyside 1996)? Would, to mention just a few questions, an informed consent to such testing be possible? Assuming that each of the pre-embryos available may have a 'genetic problem' (e.g. a susceptibility for one of the common late onset multifactorial disorders), will couples be able to make reasonable decisions given the complex trade-offs?

b. PID might be used as a method to select (healthy) pre-embryos which would qualify after birth as a suitable, HLA-matched, 'donor' of bone-marrow (or cord blood) for a seriously ill sibling (Warwick 1997). Relevant examples may include Fanconi Anemia and betha-thalassemia. Is it justified to use PID in order to select HLA-matched pre-embryos, and if yes, on what conditions? How to weigh the interests of the affected child, the parents, and the future donor?

c. At a recent conference, an American expert argued that 'serial nuclear transfer could be benefical in the context of a preimplantation diagnosis program for the propagation of genetically normal embryos' (Wolf 1997). What are the moral and non-moral pros and cons of this type of 'reproductive embryo cloning'? Would this technique be the moral equivalent of pre-embryo-splitting in order to increase the 'take baby home rate' of IVF? Or does the application of embryo cloning in the context of PID raise additional, more complex, issues?

Applied preimplantation genetics may not be reduced to PID and PGS. A technique which needs further ethical analysis is, of course, germline gene therapy. This therapy is currently being studied in various non-human species, and may eventually be technically feasible in the human. Many countries have already banned human germline gene therapy, or have announced to do so. Nevertheless, from an ethical point of view, the wisdom of a categorical ban is by no means self-evident (Walters and Palmer 1997).

It is the challenge for ethics, and the responsibility of researchers, to contribute to a timely, integral, preimplantation technology assessment.

References

Arras, J.D. (1990), 'AIDS and reproductive decisions: having children in fear and trembling', *Milbank Mem. Fund. Q.*, Vol. 68, pp. 353-82.

Boss, J. (1994), 'First trimester prenatal diagnosis: earlier is not necessarily better', *J Med Ethics* Vol. 20, pp. 146-51.

Bui, T.-H., Wramsby, H. (1996), 'Micromanipulative assisted fertilisation – still clinical research', *Hum. Reprod.* Vol. 11, pp. 925-6.

Burke, W., Daly, M., Garber, J., et al. (1997), 'Recommendations for follow-up care of individuals with an inherited predisposition to cancer', *J. Am. Med. Assoc.* Vol. 227, pp. 997-1003.

Council of Europe (1996), *Convention for the protection of human rights and dignity of the human being with regard to the application of biology and medicine: Convention on Human Rights and Biomedicine*, Strasbourg.

Delhanty, J. D. A., Harper, J. (1997), 'Genetic diagnosis before implantation', *Br Med J* Vol. 315, pp. 828-9.

Dunstan, G. (1993), 'Ethics of gamete and embryo micromanipulation', in: Fishel, S., Symonds, M. (eds.), *Gamete and embryo micromanipulation in human reproduction,* Edward Arnold: London, pp. 212-8.

Egozcue, J. (1996), 'Of course not', *Hum. Reprod.* Vol. 11, pp. 2077-8.

Fishel, S. (1996), 'Assisted conception in the human – the embryological view', in: Evans, D. (ed.), *Conceiving the embryo. Ethics, law and practice in human embryology*, Martinus Nijhoff Publishers: The Hague, pp. 13-26.

Geber, S., Winston, R. M. L., Handyside, A. H. (1995), 'Proliferation of blastomeres from biopsied cleavage stage human embryos in vitro: an alternative to blastocyst biopsy for preimplantation diagnosis', *Hum. Reprod.* Vol. 10, pp. 1492-6.

Gerrand, N. (1993), 'Creating embryos for research', *Journal of Applied Philosophy* Vol. 10, 175-7.

Gesellschaft für Humangenetik e.V. (1996), 'Positionspapier', *Med. Genetik* Vol. 8, pp. 125-31.

Gesetz zum Schutz von Embryonen (1990), BGBI.I S.2746.

Handyside, A. H. (1996), 'Commonsense as applied to eugenics: response to Testart and Sele', *Hum. Reprod.* Vol. 11, pp. 707.

Holtzman, N. (1984), 'Ethical issues in the prenatal diagnosis of phenyl-ketonuria', *Pediatrics* Vol. 74, pp. 424-7.

Human Fertilisation & Embryology Authority (1994), *Donated ovarian tissue in embryo research & assisted conception, Report*, London.

Hursthouse, R. (1987), *Beginning lives,* Blackwell: London & Cambridge.

Iglesias, T. (1990), *IVF and justice. Moral, social and legal issues related to human IVF*, The Linacre Centre for Health Care Ethics: London, 1990.

Kerncommissie Ethiek Medisch Onderzoek (1993), *Jaarverslag 1991 en 1992*, Gezondheidsraad: Den Haag.

Kitcher, P. (1996), *The lives to come. The genetic revolution and human possibilities,* Allan Lane, The Penguin Press: London.

Lancaster, J. M., Wiseman, R.W., Berchuck, A. (1996), 'An inevitable dilemma: prenatal testing for mutations in BRCA1 breast-ovarian cancer susceptibility gene', *Obstet. & Gynecol.* Vol. 87, pp. 306-9.

Marteau, Th., Drake, H., Bobrow, M. (1994), 'Counselling following diagnosis of a fetal abnormality: the differing approaches of obstetricians, clinical geneticists, and genetic nurses', *Journal of Medical Genetics* Vol. 31, pp. 864-76.

McLaren, A. (1997), 'A note on 'totipotency'', *Biomedical Ethics. Newsletter of the European Network for Biomedical Ethics* Vol. 2, No.1, p. 7.

Medical Research Council (1990), *Human Fertilisation and Embryology bill. A response to the second reading debate in the House of Lords.*

Meschede, D., De Geyter, C., Nieschlag, E., Horst, J. (1995), 'Genetic risk in micromanipulative assisted reproduction', *Hum. Reprod.* Vol. 10, pp. 2880-6.

National Advisory Board on Ethics in Reproduction (1994), 'Report on human cloning through embryo splitting: an amber light. National Institutes of Health. Final Report of the Human Embryo Research Panel', *Kennedy Institute of Ethics Journal* Vol. 4, pp. 251-82.

Post, S. (1991), 'Selective abortion and gene therapy: reflections on human limits', *Human Gene Therapy* Vol. 2, pp. 229-33.

Raymond, J. (1987), 'Fetalists and feminists: they are not the same', in: Spallone, P., Steinberg, D.L. (eds.), *Made to order: The myth of reproductive and genetic progress*, Pergamon Press: Oxford.

Reubinoff, B., Shushan, A. (1997), 'Preimplantation diagnosis in older patients. To biopsy or not to biopsy?', *Hum.Reprod.* Vol. 11, pp. 2071-78.

Robertson. J. A. (1992), 'Ethical and legal issues in preimplantation genetic screening', *Fertil Steril* Vol. 57, pp. 1-11.

Seibel, M. M., Seibel, S. G., Zilberstein, M.(1994), 'Gender distribution – not sex selection', *Hum Reprod* Vol. 9, pp. 569-70.

Silber, S.J., Nagy, Z., Liu, J., et al. (1995), 'The use of epididymal and testicular spermatozoa for intracytoplasmic sperm injection: the genetic implications for male infertility', *Hum.Reprod.* Vol. 10, 2031-43.

Simpson, J. L., Liebaers, I. (1996), 'Assessing congenital anomalies after preimplantation genetic diagnosis', *J Assist Reprod Genet* Vol. 13, pp. 170-6.

Soussis, I., Harper. J. C., Handyside, A. H., et al. (1996), 'Obstetric outcome of pregnancies resulting from embryos biopsied for preimplantation diagnosis of inherited disease', *Br. J. Obstet. Gynecol.* Vol. 103, pp. 784-8.

Strom, C. M. (1996), 'Mosaicism and aneuploidy in human pre-embryos', *J. Ass. Reprod. Genet.* Vol. 13, pp. 592-3.

Strong, C. (1997), *Ethics in reproductive and perinatal medicine. A new framework*, Yale University Press: New Haven & London.

Verlinsky, Y., Cieslak, J., Ivakhnenko, V., et al. (1996), 'Birth of healthy children after preimplantation diagnosis of common aneuploidies by polar body fluorescent in situ hybridization analysis', *Fertil. Steril.* Vol. 66, pp. 126-9.

Verlinsky, Y., Kuliev, A., (eds.) (1991), *Preimplantation Genetics,* Plenum Press: New York/London.

Verlinsky, Y., Pergament, E., Binor, Z., Rawlins, R. (1987), 'Genetic analysis of human embryos prior to implantation: future applications of in vitro fertilization in the treatment and prevention of human genetic diseases', in: Feichtinger, W., Kemeter, P., (eds.) *Future aspects in human in vitro fertilization.* Springer Verlag: Stuttgart/Heidelbarg, pp. 262-6.

Walters, L., Palmer, J. L. (1997), *The ethics of human gene therapy.* Oxford University Press: New York.

Warwick, R. (1997), 'Collections of cord blood', *Lancet* Vol. 350, pp. 297 (letter).

Wert, G. de (1998), 'Ethics of intracytoplasmic sperm injection: proceed with care', *Hum.Reprod.* Vol. 13, supplement 1, pp. 219-27.

Wexler, N. (1992), 'Clairvoyance and caution', in: Kevles, D., Hood, L., (eds.), *The Code of Codes. Scientific and social issues in the Human Genome Project*, Harvard University Press: Cambridge, pp. 211-44.

Wolf, D.P. (1997), 'Genetic manipulation by nuclear transfer', *Journal of Assisted Reproduction and Genetics* Vol. 14, pp. 415-80, Special Issue: Abstracts from the Second International Symposium on Preimplantation Genetics, see: A 88 (p. 480).

2 Preimplantation diagnosis. A reflection in light of a personalist ethics

Paul Schotsmans

Introduction

The development of reproductive technologies has been one of the major challenges of the last three decades for bio-ethical reflection. The debate is still going on and is far from being concluded: the indications (infertile couples or single women or lesbian couples with a request for a child?), the moral statuts of the embryo and the quality control of Infertility Centers are only a few issues, upon which agreement is not yet possible in the context of pluralistic societies. One further step in this ongoing debate is the possibility of preimplantation diagnosis (PID). We observe the interconnection of infertility treatment and clinical genetics, which is more or less typical for the medical practice: in Belgium e.g. the centers for human genetics are only situated inside Academic Hospitals, where Infertility Treatment Centers are also operating. PID can therefore be expected to become a further factor in the medical setting for the beginning of human life. It does not represent a radically new challenge, but is in itself symbolic for several ethical issues, which have long been in the picture.

I will present in my contribution a personalist-ethical approach to PID. I will also link this to the clinical practice of a large hospital, where IVF and PID seem to be logically connected. Indeed, when a couple needs medical assistance in order to reproduce, PID seems to be a necessary quality improvement of the medical infertility treatment system.

One of the first steps in the ethical reflection is the analysis of the clinical practice (Praktische Moralität). It is therefore worth observing the way in which PID is presented. As Müller (1998, p. 281) observes, PID has a number of obvious advantages: only non-affected embryos are transferred to the woman's uterus; no abortion is needed in the event of a pathological result; and there is no need to begin what amounts to a pregnancy on probation as is the case if the health of the fetus has to be determined by prenatal diagnosis (PND). After a PID examination, a woman can accept her future child from the beginning of the pregnancy. She does not have to hold back her feelings toward it until the 10th or even the 18th week of gestation, when it has been established whether it will be healthy or not, i.e. whether it will be aborted.

PID has also obvious medical drawbacks. It requires a complex and distressing procedure of medically assisted reproduction, namely in IVF with embryo transfer (ET). On the one hand the prospects of a pregnancy after IVF and ET are limited, while on the other hand there is a risk of multiple pregnancies if a number of embryos are simultaneously transferred back into the mother.

One medical point of discussion remains: the indication for PID. The most obvious one is to offer PID to couples who are infertile and have to conceive by IVF and who have a particular inheritable risk of having offspring with a genetic abnormality. From a medical viewpoint it seems clinically logical to offer these couples PID as an element of quality of service, when available in the hospital. Other indications are, however, not so immanent in clinical practice. Müller observes five eventual indications: couples who are infertile and have to conceive by IVF, who do not have a particular inheritable risk of having offspring with a genetic abnormality; some forms of male infertility which are consequences of genetic abnormalities and can result in additional complications; women and couples in a specific genetic risk group who have undergone PND and abortion, but still want a healthy child of their own although they cannot accept a further round of conventional PND; PID for at-risk couples who for ethical reasons will not consider termination of pregnancy under any circumstances; PID on embryos for couples at risk for Huntington's disease, and certain other dominantly inherited disorders: PID would allow the disease to be prevented in their own offspring without disclosure of the parental phenotype (Müller 1998, pp. 284-286).

These eventual indications do require an ethical reflection on the eventual integration of this diagnostic technique. Many ethical approaches are possible; I will present here a personalist reflection, which of course first has to be clarified in its methodology and will then be applied to the specific case of PID.

A personalist ethical framework for reflection

Personalism functions as an ethical frame of reference, so that those who are working in the context of personalism can develop an identical ethical evaluation and structure their human practice in light of this evaluation and their understanding of the implications for concrete human realities. For those who practice this line of reasoning, it provides coherence and offers an integration of several traditions in moral theology and moral philosophy. Personalism suggests that it is essentially important to clarify the development of some anthropological options, which can then be used for the formation and functioning of the human conscience. By virtue of its very being, the human person is multidimensional, open to itself, to another and society. Three basic values are foundational and may realise the humanly desirable (Ricoeur 1975): the values of subjectivity, intersubjectivity and solidarity. These three fundamental value orientations are the framework for the personalist criterion: personalists will classify human decisions and acts as morally good if they promote the humanum, that is, if in truth they are beneficial to the human person adequately considered in all his dimensions and relationships. Because of the historicity of the human person, this criterion suggests that we should constantly reconsider what possibilities we have at our disposal at this point in history to serve the advancement of the human person. This requirement is part of a dynamic ethics which summons us to do that which is better or more according as its actualisation becomes possible. In conjunction with this dimension of historicity, we must – in our acts – respect the originality of every single human being as much as possible (Janssens 1980, p. 14).

Because of this historicity – by which all the essential aspects of the human person are affected – an ethics of responsibility on a personalist basis must indeed necessarily be a dynamic ethics. By virtue of the progress of science and technology, e.g. PID's new possibilities are constantly being opened up for our activity. It is the specific task of ethics to inquire as to how the growing possibilities can be realised to serve the dignity of humankind and how the developing experience of values is to enrich our activity. The promotion of the humanum – that which promotes the human person, adequately considered – becomes a moral obligation insofar as it becomes possible (le souhaitable humain possible, cf. P. Ricoeur). Ethics is indeed fundamentally a way of living and in its own growth must keep step with human life itself as it unfolds throughout history.

The personalist criterion clarifies a morally good disposition: our inner attitude must be such that we are genuinely prepared to place our activity as much as possible at the service of the promotion of the human person (self and others) adequately considered in himself as a subject in corporeality and in his openness to the world, to others, to social groups and God and to respect the originality of each person in our conduct as much as possible. The good disposition is the source and the dynamic principle of our moral life: it is only real and authentic insofar as it leads us to strive toward its realisation and incarnation in concrete acts.

But which actions are appropriate to realise and incarnate our morally good disposition? Every human action is characterised by ambiguity. This is true for two reasons. The first is our temporality. When we, at any given moment, choose to perform a certain action, we must simultaneously neglect all other possibilities (omissio), at least temporarily. The second reason is our spaciality. Our actions as active commerce with material realities with their complex multiplicity of properties and physical laws involve an inseparable connection between negative aspects (disvalues) and positive attributes (values), such that they are simultaneously both detrimental to and beneficial for the human person. Because of the progress of medicine, for example persons who suffer from certain hereditary defects, and who in previous times often died at an early age, have been given a long life (value), but at the same time it becomes possible that they may have children and through that fact the genetic quality of posterity decreases (disvalue).

This example, already discussed in Janssens (1980), leads us immediately to the possibility of PID. An ethical evaluation of PID must answer the question of when there are proportionate reasons (ratio proportionata) to perform an activity in a morally responsible manner which simultaneously results in values and disvalues. Moralists have attempted to answer this question for a long time and we can learn much about it from the Catholic tradition which has always dealt with the question of priorities in its reflection about the order of love and of values (ordo caritatis et bonorum). For us, it may be the guiding principle for our ethical evaluation.

A personalist approach to PID

The consideration of the disadvantages and medical drawbacks, as developed by Müller (1998), is the necessary starting point to deal with the concrete problem of PID in light of an ethics of responsibility on a personalist basis. As has already been mentioned, couples may enter a PID program in different ways. Often, the primary concern will be a genetic disorder (e.g. cystic fibrosis, myotonic dystrophy, thalassemia) that the couple's offspring has a significant risk of inheriting. It seems, however, clinically more indicated to offer PID to those couples who are being treated for a fertility problem and at the same time have serious genetic problems. Here, IVF will need to be carried out in any case, and an embryo biopsy can be performed with relative ease as an additional procedure to safeguard against particular genetic defects in the conceptus (Meschede and Horst 1998, p. 293). This leads to the clinical guideline to offer PID in any case as an element of the medical standard procedure for the treatment of infertility: it would indeed demonstrate a lack of concern for clinical quality if these couples were not to be offered PID, when available.

The ethical problems remain, however, for all indications the same. From a personalist perspective, it is crucial to balance the values and disvalues in order to come to an adequate ethical integration of the procedure.

Macro-ethical concerns

In the context of a societal integration of PID, two conditions need to be fulfilled: first, the possibility of PID should not lead to a social discrimination of people with genetic disorders. It is therefore essential to develop societal initiatives to assure an adequate protection and integration of all those who are handicapped or who are threatened with genetic problems in their offspring. Western societies have in the past created for the most part adequate infrastructures to take care for the handicapped. These initiatives should not be discontinued, but improved to promote the integration of the handicapped.

Another danger of the development of PID would be the exercise of pressure on probable parents to avoid genetic risks as much as possible. It could even lead to one-sided social stimuli in order to force them to conform with the expected behavior, e.g. financial barriers in the social insurance system or rejections of adequate projects for the education of their children. Again, the societal responsibility of all human beings requires that we treat every other human being as equal and that we provide all those in need with adequate possibilities for development and integration.

The macro-ethical challenges transcend of course the possibilities of hospital managers or those who are responsible for Centers of Clinical Genetics. It is a concern for the whole society. This must not be underestimated, but is usually not a part of the daily responsibility of physicians and hospital managers working in hospitals. The social concerns are crucial for political leaders, being responsible for the creation of an attitude of social responsibility in the society. They may also help a legal framework to be established for an adequate social setting for medical practices.

Going back to daily medical activities in hospitals and thus also to clinical reality, it is more crucial to analyse the most important ethical values and disvalues connected with the application of PID for individual patients and couples. Indeed, our basic question remains: when are there proportionate reasons to perform an activity in a morally responsible manner which simultaneously results in values and disvalues?

Micro-ethical analysis

PID is a very ambiguous technique with several values and disvalues which are internally connected. The ethical evaluation can only clarify the different issues involved and see how they can be balanced in order to promote the human person in all his dimensions and relationships.

The moral status of the human embryo

PID cannot be developed without pre-clinical experimentation on human embryos. Although some experts doubt that this is an absolute necessity, this delicate issue can ultimately not be ignored. Of course, it would be preferable to have PID developed on human fibroblasts, on human unfertilised oocytes and human spermatozoa. The development of the technique with mouse embryos is also clearly more indicated from an ethical point of view. I think, however, we must consider PID from the perspective that at least in the final stages of the development of specific diagnostic applications, some human embryos will be needed for the ultimate quality tests of concrete PID applications.

The debate on the moral status of the embryo is almost as old as human history. For those who want to start from the need for an adequate protection of the human embryo, the embryo research involved in the development of PID certainly creates a very delicate ethical dilemma. For the sake of clarity, the adequate protection of the human embryo seems to be a cornerstone of every democratic society, as set out in the recent European Convention on Human Rights and Biomedicine (article 18, part one): 'Where the law allows research on embryos in vitro, it shall ensure adequate protection of the embryo'.

The nature and the moral status of the human embryo is a vast and difficult subject. As described elsewhere (Schotsmans 1998, p. 306), I think it is right to suggest that the Roman Catholic Community, to which I belong, shares an approach which tries to protect the embryo as much as possible. It must, however, be acknowledged that the debate on the moral status of the human embryo inside the Roman Catholic Community remains open. Recently, some Catholic moral theologians, e.g. R.A. McCormick, P. Verspieren and J. Mahoney, have brought more diversity into the Catholic approach to the human embryo. While the offical magisterium still rejects any nuances, R.A. McCormick accepted the distinction between genetic and developmental individualisation. The former is certainly present from the earliest beginnings of life, the latter is not: 'Developmental individualisation is completed only when implantation has been completed, a period of time whose outside time-limits are around fourteen days' (McCormick 1989, p. 345). This implies a more open attitude to integrating not only IVF, but also PID and human gene therapy.

It may, however, be clear that the societal and moral debate about an adequate protection of the human embryo has been and will always remain a point of discussion (cf. Honnefelder 1996). At the same time, it cannot be ignored that the techniques like IVF, ICSI (intracytoplasmic sperm injection) and PID would not have been possible without research on human embryos. Further, once we accept the ethical integration of IVF (Schotsmans 1993, p. 22), techniques such as the cryopreservation of human embryos must also be accepted, in full awareness of the fact that only a certain limited percentage of the frozen embryos will survive the procedure. This has been justified with the proportionate argumentation that the values are more important than the disvalues and that the application of IVF creates the most humanly possible alternative for infertile couples (le souhaitable humain possible).

All these reflections bring us to the conclusion that the ethical concern for the human embryos must be viewed in light of the potential values of PID for couples. When PID seems reasonably indicated, the protection of the human embryo is only one value in the balance with several other values to be realized by PID. The debate on the moral status of the human embryo may in other words not inhibit a serious clarification of other values and disvalues involved. It is clear that there are many other positive outcomes of the implementation of PID, which we should also consider and balance against each other.

Purpose of PID

It cannot be ignored that PID will lead to the transfer of the non-affected embryos, which implies that the affected embryos will not be transferred. This has been seriously criticised as an example of direct selection of the affected embryos. This would not be present in the current practice of prenatal diagnosis. Selection is, however, not the main purpose of PID: in essence, PID may serve the prevention of transmitting serious genetic diseases and early lethal developments and/or the prevention of traumatic prenatal tests, possibly followed by a late abortion. These obvious advantages are helpful for the couple in that they can help them to accept their future child from the beginning of the pregnancy so that they do not have to hold back their feelings until the 10th or the 18th week, as was mentioned earlier (Müller 1998).

These are all values, in comparison with which eventual disvalues must be proportionally balanced. It may have become clear that the proportionate ethical judgment may lead to conscientious decision making for every couple involved. This implies also the need for an individualised approach to the application of PID, which may become clear in the following guidelines.

Practical guidelines for the clinical application of PID

The previous clarification makes us cautious concerning the application of PID: the relative protection of the human embryo remains a serious ethical disvalue, which necessitates limiting PID to very specific and well circumscribed cases. It may for the moment also lead to the requirement that priority should be given to those couples who have also infertility problems, whereby PID could become a medical standard procedure of accurate quality of care. In any case, interdisciplinary guidance of the development of the technique should be guaranteed: not only the clinicians and researchers should be involved, but also psychologists and/or psychiatrists should guarantee adequate clinical guidance of the couple. In the best cases of all, the advisory structure of a well functioning Hospital Ethics Committee seems unavoidable.

In order to illustrate these guidelines, I refer to a concrete model which was developed in a Belgian Hospital Ethics Committee:

- Couples who besides an infertility problem also have a serious inheritable risk of having offspring with a genetic abnormality should be offered PID as an integral medical standard procedure of clinical care.
- PID can – in the case of fertile couples – only be proposed as an option of second order.
- Every case should be presented to an interdisciplinary team, with the members of the PID expert team as central participants. The team should be composed by a gynaecologist, a clinical geneticist, a clinician who has expertise in the specific genetic abnormality, a psychiatrist with special expertise in the counseling of infertile couples and a representative of the Hospital Ethics Committee.

This procedure clearly implies that decisions are not made on a general basis, but are specifically directed to individual indications of couples concerned.

An ethical model for finite (imperfect) conditions

One of our basic questions concerned proportionate reasons to perform an activity in a morally responsible manner which simultaneously results in values and disvalues. It is clear that PID stands symbolically for the integration of several values, but also disvalues. The obvious advantages must be balanced against some disvalues, like the failing protection of the human embryo and the eventual direct selection for genetic abnormalities.

It may be helpful for this debate to refer to the posivitive recommendation of the Hospital Ethics Committee of the K.U. Leuven (Belgium) concerning the cryopreservation of human embryos (Hospital Ethics Committee 1993, p. 83):

These recommendations can be fit in with the need to make a choice between two imperfect conditions: conjugal infertility on the one hand and embryo manipulation on the other hand. The Committee would like to stress more particularly the specific character of medicine often faced with delicate situations calling for a decision. Most of the time, the physician is expected to carefully balance values and disvalues (positive and negative indications). More than often he has to take the responsibility, but is not always able to predict the outcome of his decisions with certainty. As to IVF, this means that the responsible physician, based on an attitude of respect for beginning human life, has to aim for the option which he considers to be the most humanly possible. The human embryo is human life in development and has to be treated with all due respect... So far, the loss of a certain rate of embryos due to cryopreservation has been biologically inevitable, thus creating an ethical problem. Here however, a major ethical criterion is the intention of the action, the fundamental disposition the action is based upon. Therefore, everything should be done to maintain a fundamental attitude of respect for human life. Temporary freezing should only be seen as a means of increasing the chances of developing beginning life.

Similar comments may be made concerning PID: the most important criterion remains the fundamental disposition upon which the choice for PID is made. Essentially this should always be a service to couples who have been confronted with serious genetic risks in their family and want to prevent further problems in the future. Although it is clear that PID creates many ethical problems, it must also be obvious that it offers concrete problem solving for couples confronted with serious risks of genetic abnormalities for their children. A careful balancing of values and disvalues in concrete clinical cases can help to integrate ethically the possibilities of PID in such a way that this integration promotes the humanly possible, even though we know that it remains impossible to realise the humanly desirable.

References

Council of Europe (1996), *Convention for the Protection of Human Rights and Dignity of the Human Being with Regard to the Application of Biology and Medicine: Convention on Human Rights and Biomedicine*, Directorate of Legal Affairs: Strasbourg.
Honnefelder, L. (1996), 'The Nature and Status of the Embryo: Philosophical Aspects', *Third Symposium on Bioethics. Medically-assisted Procreation and the Protection of the Human Embyro*, Strasbourg, November 1996, distributed document.

Hospital Ethics Committee, Faculty of Medicine, K.U Leuven (1993), 'Renewed and Updated Recommendations on In Vitro Fertilization and Embryo Transfer', in: Borghgraef, R. and Schotsmans, P. (eds), *The Technological Advances in Health Sciences and the Moral Theological Implications*, University Press: Leuven, pp. 79-84.

Janssens, L. (1980), 'Artificial Insemination. Ethical Considerations', *Louvain Studies*, Vol. 8, pp. 3-39.

McCormick, R.A. (1989), 'Therapy or Tampering: The Ethics of Reproductive Technologies and the Development of Doctrine', in: idem, *The Critical Calling. Reflections on Moral Dilemmas since Vatican II*, Georgetown University Press: Washington D.C.

Meschede, D. and Horst, J. (1998), 'The Possible Impact of Preimplatation Diagnosis for Infertile Couples', in: Hildt, E. and Mieth, D. (eds), *In Vitro Fertilisation in the 1990s. Towards a Medical, Social and Ethical Evaluation*, Ashgate: Aldershot, pp. 293-5.

Müller, H. (1998), 'Connecting Lines from a Medical Point of View', in: Hildt, E. and Mieth, D. (eds), *In Vitro Fertilisation in the 1990s. Towards a Medical, Social and Ethical Evaluation*, Ashgate: Aldershot., pp. 281-91.

Ricoeur, P. (1975), 'Le problème du fondement de la morale', *Sapienza*, Vol. 28, pp. 313-37.

Schotsmans, P. (1993), 'Bioethics and Human Reproduction. An Ethical Approach of In Vitro Fertilization and Embryo Transfer', in: Borghgraef, R. and Schotsmans, P. (eds), *The Technological Advances in Health Sciences and the Moral Theological Implications*, University Press: Leuven, pp. 15-26.

Schotsmans, P. (1998), 'Connecting Lines from an Ethical Point of View', in: Hildt, E. and Mieth, D. (eds), *In Vitro Fertilisation in the 1990s. Towards a Medical, Social and Ethical Evaluation*, Ashgate: Aldershot, pp. 301-10.

3 Ethical aspects of germline gene therapy

Alexandre Mauron

Abstract

Although it has never been attempted in humans so far, germline gene therapy has been an object of ethical controversy for a long time already. The classical arguments in favour and against germline gene therapy will be briefly reviewed. Much of the vagueness and lack of focus of the debate stems from two conceptual problems:

1. Germline therapy on humans is a technology whose concrete empirical outlines can only be guessed at. Ethical evaluation of a technology which still belongs to a speculative future is beset with epistemological uncertainties, which raise the more general problem of anticipatory evaluation and regulation of 'exotic' biotechnologies.

2. It is not clear what sort of germline interventions would qualify as 'therapy' (straightforward application to humans of today's animal transgenic techniques would almost certainly not). This is an added element of conceptual uncertainty that makes an ethical evaluation difficult.

Nevertheless, I want to propose an ethical framework based on E. Juengst's distinction between phenotypic vs. genotypic prevention, as an alternative to the conventional view that relies heavily on the somatic vs. germline distinction.

Introduction

The ethics of germline gene therapy has acquired the status of a classical topic of bioethics. No textbook, no reader in bioethics would be complete without at least some cursory presentation of this issue. And yet, compared to most classical bioethics issues, it is a very odd topic indeed. There are no juicy case-reports to entice students with, since germline gene therapy has not been attempted in humans. All one can proffer to raise their interest is, at best, a set of anticipations from present knowledge and practices, and at worst, silly science-fiction scenarios. This lack of empirical focus has a definite effect on the ethical discussion, which has had two phases. In the first one, which took place in the eighties, the conceptual framework for the general discussion of gene therapy was laid down. This is based on the distinction between somatic and germline gene therapy on the one hand, and between therapeutic and ameliorative genetic interventions on the other. The result of these early discussions is the classical conventional wisdom according to which, firstly, somatic gene therapy is OK, but intervening in the germline is a no-no; secondly, that gene therapy for healing 'real' diseases is acceptable, but gene therapy that aims at 'improving' human nature by adding novel biological properties not usually found in human persons is eugenic, i.e. immoral by definition, and should not be allowed (see for instance Anderson 1985, Walters 1986).

This conventional wisdom went on to have a rather paradoxical history. It was largely adopted within the 'official' bioethics done by international organisations and law-making bodies, even inspiring a constitutional amendment in Switzerland that solemnly asserts (art.24 novies, §2, Federal Constitution):

> a. Interventions into the genetic material of human gametes and embryos are not acceptable;
> b. non-human germinal and genetic material may neither be transferred to, nor integrated into human germinal material (...).[1]

In scholarly debate however, this view has never met with unanimous assent but continued to invite controversy, often along along the following two lines: the conceptual relevance of these distinctions was challenged (especially the distinction between *bona fide* therapy and 'enhancement'), or the ethical rejection of germline gene therapy and/or genetic enhancement was questioned (Lappé 1991, Mauron and Thévoz 1991, Munson and Davis 1992, Wivel and Walters 1993, Zimmermann 1991, and more recently: Agar 1995, Fletcher and Richter 1996, Holtung 1997). This is, in the main, the substance of the second phase in the debate, that was rather lively in the early nineties but has tapered off since, so that little has been added to the store of arguments *pro* and *contra* germline gene therapy in recent years (good summaries of the arguments are provided by Coutts 1994, de Wachter 1993, and Walters and Palmer 1997, chap. 3-4). In addition, specific protocols that do not fit the established distinctions well were presented as more or less theoretical possibilities (Rubenstein et al. 1995).

Before moving on to a brief recapitulation of the arguments, it should be stressed that the two conceptual distinctions essential to the conventional wisdom outlined above are very different in their inherent solidity and their implications. The therapy vs. enhancement distinction tends to be conceptually fragile, as anyone who has followed the debates in the philosophy of medicine as regards the fuzzy border between the normal and the pathological will recognise (in the French-speaking world, this thread of thought is mostly associated with the work of G. Canguilhem (Canguilhem 1966). I will not delve further into this matter, except by referring to the philosopher Ph. Kitcher, who concludes that '(...) the popular idea of using genetic interventions to restore normal functioning, only normal functioning and nothing but normal functioning, is mistaken' (Kitcher 1996, p.213). The diversity of therapeutic paradigms at work in existing somatic gene therapy protocols already illustrates this point (Mauron 1997). This does not mean that a consensus against *some* forms of genetic enhancement is conceptually impossible, but it does imply that the therapy vs. enhancement border must be considerably refined before it can become a workable and ethically relevant concept (Torres 1997).

On the other hand, the distinction between somatic and germline interventions stands on much firmer ground as it is based on a fundamental empirical fact of higher vertebrates: ever since Weissmann laid the conceptual foundation of the *soma* vs. *germen* distinction in 1885, the notion that the precursor cells giving rise to the gametes are segregated from the somatic cells early in embryonic development has been recognised as basic to the very structure of succeeding generations as it inserts a kind of biological firewall between parents and offspring. It is the reason why there is no Lamarckian inheritance of acquired characteristics and why genetic intervention on somatic and germ cells have radically different consequences. There cannot be any logical slippery slope from somatic gene therapy to germline gene therapy.

The 'classical' arguments

Even before the first clinical trials, it was clear that somatic gene therapy was not basically new in the kinds of ethical issues it raises and by and large, could be dealt with in the same way as any innovative therapeutic experiment, by having established ethics committees (IRBs) review the protection of patient's rights and safety. The added dimension of biological safety as regards third parties, especially for protocols using *in vivo* vectors, fell naturally under the remit of safety-monitoring bodies overseeing genetic engineering in general. This is not to say that somatic gene therapy poses no ethical problems, far from it. But these problems, however important and often troubling they may be, do not differ in kind from those that are inherent in many clinical trials of new and unproved treatments, with perhaps the additional dilemmas caused by the hype and false hopes that have surrounded some early gene therapy trials.

On the other hand, most observers agreed that germline gene therapy was quite another matter. To contemplate gene transfer into the human germline was to place the issue squarely into the realm of transgenerational therapy, with the consequence that the whole genome of certain future people would be envisioned as the object of wilful and targeted modification. I will discuss four types of arguments against germline gene therapy, each of which refers implicitly to a broader conceptual problem.

A first family of arguments opposes germline interventions as 'playing God', and condemns it as an arrogant and illegitimate interventions into the natural order. The basic idea, buttressed by recourse to familiar icons such as the Sorcerer's Apprentice and Drs. Faust and Frankenstein, is that man does not have the wisdom and foresight needed to exert the powers of the Creator (and if he was indeed wise enough, he would abstain from acting above his God-given station in the Universe). There are at least two types of problems with this line of argument. The first arises if the reference to God is taken literally. The quality-control specialists in charge of God-related arguments, called theologians, are not usually enthusiastic about prohibitions on 'playing God', logically invoking the notion that man is called upon by God to be a co-creator, and not merely a passive and subservient caretaker of the Creation. In addition, religious thinkers may have other moral agendas that place this particular issue on the back-burner. For instance, in a visionary statement dating back to 1990, the Catholic Health Association of America (CHA) expressed approval of germinal cell modification to forestall genetic diseases, since this procedure would obviate the need to perform a prenatal diagnosis possibly leading to abortion (CHA 1990). Discussing an explicitly theological content of 'playing God' arguments is rather moot anyway, as they are not usually meant to be taken literally but rather point in a general way to the *hubris* involved in changing human nature. *Homo faber sui*: this is the ultimate perversion of modernity for many conservative thinkers (Bruaire 1978). The problem here is linked to what I have called elsewhere 'genomic metaphysics' i.e. the notion that the genome of a person is ontologically central to that person's nature, whereas all other attributes are more or less peripheral (Mauron 1996). An assumption of this sort is necessary if one is to understand why mankind is permitted to change itself by health care, immunisation, education, social conditioning, ideological brainwashing and so on, but is not allowed to touch the genome. But this essentialist conception of the genome is quite problematic (Mauron 1995, Mauron 1996). Furthermore, it is ironic that the sacralisation of the genome is an ideological move that originated with the eugenic movement (Kevles 1985, chapter 4). It was eugenics that proffered the preservation of human 'germ-plasm' as an overarching goal for public policy. At the end of the day, it is not clear why we should respect the genome more than any other contingent aspects of human nature.

A second style of argumentation against germline interventions is basically prudential. It is sometimes put forward that by removing disease genes from the genome of future persons, one may unwittingly eliminate the hidden collateral benefits that these genes may also have. It is true that some, perhaps many, recessive disease genes have been maintained in human populations by selective pressures favouring heterozygotes. The classical case are the molecular diseases of haemoglobin, which can be devastating for homozygotes having a double dose of the abnormal gene, but where the heterozygote state provides some resistance to malaria (there are hypotheses about the heterozygote resistance for a few other recessive diseases). But this sort of benefit is only relative. Furthermore, it is populational rather than individual, and usually reflects the evolutionary past of human populations rather than its present sanitary conditions. It is implausible to conclude that recessive disease genes should always be preserved for the sake of this hypothetical populational benefit against the interest of actual suffering individuals. In addition, the argument is invalid for dominant disease-causing mutations, where the hidden benefit is excluded by definition. The intuitive appeal of this argument may be linked to what I have called the Panglossian view of the genome (Mauron 1993): Just as Voltaire's Dr. Pangloss thought that all evil is a hidden good, it is seductive to believe in a kind of pre-established genomic harmony, where disease genes are present for some good reason, 'otherwise Nature would not have put them there'. In a sense this is true, but the 'Nature' that put them there is just the sum-total of the blind and opportunistic strivings of natural selection, utterly indifferent to the good of human individuals.

The prudential line of reasoning can however be expanded to consider the fact that germline gene therapy is open-ended in a way that somatic therapy is clearly not. The issue of long-term deleterious effects is therefore more serious in the first case. Everyone who is not opposed to germline therapy at the outset would nevertheless want to see it scrutinised very carefully for its long-term safety. But some would also argue that any treatment that irrevocably modifies the biological constitution of future people – and therefore resonates indefinitely into the future – can never pass muster in terms of safety, because some of its possibly deleterious effects would necessarily lie beyond the horizon of every possible prediction. A more explicitly ethical variant of this reasoning would point to the fact that transgenerational gene therapy would amount to non-consented therapy on not-yet-existing people. Persons belonging to the distant future and affected by germline therapy performed now would be held hostage to what *we* think is good for *them*.

This line of argument is far more complex and I will limit myself to just one aspect. If it implies that medical interventions are only beneficent and ethically acceptable if their consequences are entirely foreseeable and reversible, then this is an impossible standard to uphold for most medical innovations that have large-scale applications. Think of immunisation against polio, or the eradication of smallpox: these public-health measures have changed the world irrevocably. The smallpox virus is gone forever, however much deep ecologists might conceivably lament its demise. Human beings themselves are changed forever. In fact, it is not the same people who populate the earth now than those who would exist if the polio or smallpox vaccines had not been broadly distributed. Most major medical advances not only change our phenotypes but reshuffle the human gene pool itself. The 'small is beautiful' slogan that only accepts technological change if it can be recalled, in the same way as a car manufacturer recalls a defective make of automobile, is deeply mistaken. Any large scale policy choice forces us to choose between causal chains that diverge indefinitely into the unknown and unknowable future. In the words of Isaiah Berlin, 'we cannot legislate for the consequences of consequences of consequences'. And since we cannot do it, we should not be expected to.

Do we want 'genotypic prevention'?

The irreversibility argument outlined in the preceding section contains an important insight however, which forms the basis of the fourth argument, which was formulated by E. Juengst (Juengst 1995). This line of argument starts with an important conceptual distinction, between phenotypic and genotypic prevention. Phenotypic prevention aims at forestalling the pathological manifestations (i.e. disease phenotypes) associated with genetic abnormalities. In contrast, the objective of genotypic prevention is more directly connected with these genetic abnormalities themselves, as it attempts to prevent their transmission to future individuals. Within present medical practice, there is a legitimate place for both kinds of prevention, albeit with different goals and scope. Present examples of both kinds of prevention would be: (1) the special diet for children with phenylketonuria (phenotypic prevention); (2) prenatal diagnosis for Lesch-Nyhan disease, with a view to offering the possibility of interrupting an affected pregnancy. Phenotypic prevention is largely uncontroversial and constitutes an accepted objective at the individual, familial and societal level. On the other hand, genotypic prevention is more limited in scope, at least if we stick to the traditional ethos of genetic counselling. Within this tradition, the acceptable forms of genetic prevention are those which can be understood as an aspect of reproductive liberty. These preventive measures are among the available options to women and couples who exert their reproductive rights. Indeed, preventing the birth of a child affected with a serious pathology falls within the purview of reproductive autonomy of individuals and couples in a free society and constitutes a major dimension of reproductive health. In the words of E. Juengst:

> (...) the geneticist's goals are not so much 'preventive' as directly therapeutic: The reproductive planning problems they address are already fulminant when their clients engage their services, and their treatment consists of giving them information, counselling, and options they need to address their problem in terms of their own values and beliefs (Juengst 1995, p. 1600).

In complete contrast, the sort of genetic prevention that would be explicitly preventive and populational in scope, such as trying to rid the gene pool of certain disease genes, would be radically different and would be eugenic in the classical sense of the word. Eugenics has often been conceived by its proponents as a kind of super-medicine for a super-patient, namely the gene pool itself. This shift in priorities from the individual and familial level to the collective and populational level is what Juengst refuses, correctly in my opinion. The traditional emphasis on personal rather than public interests and values is central both to the intrinsic moral merit of genetic medicine and to its societal acceptance in free societies.

The ethical test proposed here is therefore based on the answer to the following question: is the procedure under scrutiny aimed at fulfilling the reproductive goals of individuals? or is it exclusively or largely populational in its objectives? This test is goal-oriented rather than technique-oriented as is the case for the traditional somatic vs. germline distinction. The question now is whether the application of this test would lead to different ethical evaluations than the conventional wisdom view. This would indeed be the case, because there are conceivable forms of germline therapy that would have to be considered phenotypic prevention. For instance, if it ever became possible to treat gametes by some kind of homologous recombination with a view to replacing a dominant disease gene by a normal gene, that would be a way for an individual to fulfil his or her reproductive goals and would therefore fit into the usual ethical framework for reproductive health. In contrast, germline gene therapy that is broadly-oriented to the collective health of unspecified descendants of the treated person would be outside this framework and considered unacceptable. Generally speaking, germline therapy for purposes other than the reproductive health of the presenting individual or couple would be excluded. In effect, applying the traditional ethos of medical genetics would lead neither to the wholesale rejection of germline gene therapy nor to a general acceptance of it. It would lead to a scrutiny of the goals being pursued rather than to approve or taboo the technique itself.

In conclusion, germline gene therapy that meets the reproductive goals of actual people would be acceptable, even if it has long-term repercussions. These long-term effects would be viewed as secondary effects, much as the genetic effects of anti-tumour radiotherapy are considered side-effects that are potentially deleterious, but that we must take in our stride, lest we infringe the reproductive liberties of cancer patients. Conversely, germline gene therapy for genotypic prevention would be rejected as inimical to the ethos of empowerment and autonomy that is so central to genetic medicine. Of course, this conclusion presupposes that the future would actually bring germline gene therapy protocols that are realistic and acceptable in terms of risks and benefits, which is very much a speculative conclusion. In addition, it may well be that germline gene therapy for genotypic prevention may never become a realistic proposition in purely scientific terms. In fact, it is quite conceivable that it may become an obsolete therapeutic paradigm before ever coming into existence, if it came to be viewed as a speculative offshoot of a naive 'germ theory' of disease genes that is being abandoned by medical genetics itself.

Why the debate lies fallow: the problems of anticipatory regulation

It is quite significant that the debate on germline gene therapy has not been very lively in recent years, ethical commentators restricting themselves to analysing potential border situations such as foetal gene therapy or very special marginal cases such as the correction of gene defects in mitochondria (Rubenstein et al. 1995). This may reflect the inherent limits of anticipatory bioethical debates. There is only so much one can discuss about a technology that only exists as a future dream or nightmare. This suggests that anticipatory debates and also anticipatory regulation of far-fetched technologies have certain limits, as noted by several authors in a series of articles published a few years ago by the Journal of Politics and the Life-Sciences (Bonnicksen 1994, Cook-Deegan 1994). Once – and if – a technology is applied in actuality, the ethical discussion inevitably undergoes major changes that cannot always be anticipated. Some may draw from this state of affairs a pessimistic conclusion about the power of bioethics to make a difference in public debates on the desirability of major technological innovation. They would note that before the technology is implemented, it is too early really to know what the technology is about and what its precise effects will be, so that pre-emptive regulation makes little sense. But once the new technique has become a reality, it is too late to do anything about it: its further progress is dictated by the technological imperative according to which everything that is doable will be done. Those who are critical of the whole bioethical enterprise and who charge that bioethics is basically a strategic device of the scientific-industrial complex to force societal acceptance of controversial technologies may then feel vindicated.

However, there is an alternative, more convincing view of the issue, that leads to the formulation of a more constructive and realistic role for bioethics. Bioethicists should not primarily think of themselves as prophets that foretell future problems by doing more or less enlightened exercises in futurology. Rather, they should be competent and critical observers of biomedical advances in real time, intervening in ethical debates as they emerge from the concrete reality of research and healthcare. Neither second-guessing the future, nor running after past problems, but squarely facing the present as informed, critical and constructive debating partners to researchers, healthcare workers and the public: that is the role that bioethicists can reasonably expect to fulfil. But of course it is less comfortable and less visible than the self-aggrandising posture of Cassandra or of the flamboyant social critic...

Eight years ago, E. Juengst introduced a thematic issue of the Journal of Medicine and Philosophy on gene therapy by proposing that bioethical issue evolve in three stages: romantic, precise and generalising (Juengst 1991). He added that germline interventions still belonged to the initial romantic stage of inquiry where imagination roams free for want of any reality-check provided by concrete experiences. Surprising little has changed since then as regards the ethical debate on germline gene therapy.

Note

1   Author's translation, without official standing.

References

Agar, N. (1995), 'Designing Babies: Morally Permissible Ways to Modify the Human Genome', *Bioethics*, Vol. 9, No. 1, pp. 1-15.

Anderson, W.F. (1985), 'Human Gene Therapy: Scientific and Ethical Considerations', *Journal of Medicine and Philosophy*, Vol. 10, pp. 275-91.

Bonnicksen, A. (1994), 'National and International Approaches to Human Germline Gene Therapy', *Politics and the Life Sciences*, Vol. 13, No.1, pp. 39-49.

Bruaire, C. (1978), *Une éthique pour la médecine*, Fayard: Paris.

Canguilhem, G. (1966), *Le normal et le pathologique*, PUF: Paris.

CHA (1990), 'Ethical Issues in Genetic Testing, Counseling and Therapy', *Catholic Health Association of the United States*, MO: St. Louis.

Cook-Deegan, R.M. et. al. (1994), 'Symposium on Human Germline Gene Therapy', *Politics and the Life Sciences*, Vol. 13, No. 2, pp. 217-48.

Coutts, M.C. (1994), 'Scope Note 24: Human Gene Therapy', *Kennedy Institute of Ethics Journal*, Vol. 4, No. 1, pp. 63-83.

Fletcher, J.C., and Richter, G. (1996), 'Ethical Issues of Perinatal Human Gene Therapy', *J. Matern. Fetal Med.*, Vol. 5, No. 5, pp. 232-44.

Holtung, N. (1997), 'Altering Humans – The Case For and Against Human Gene Therapy', *Cambridge Quarterly of Healthcare Ethics*, Vol. 6, No. 2, pp. 157-74.

Juengst, E.T. (1991), 'Human Germline Engineering: Back to Basics', *Journal of Medicine and Philosophy*, Vol, 16, pp. 587-592.

Juengst, E. T.(1995), '«Prevention» and the Goals of Genetic Medicine', *Human Gene Therapy*, Vol. 6, No. 12, pp. 1595-1605.

Kevles, D.J. (1985), *In the Name of Eugenics: Genetics and the Uses of Human Heredity*, Knopf: New York.

Kitcher, P. (1996), *The Lives to Come: The Genetic Revolution and Human Possibilities.*, Simon and Schuster, New York.

Lappé, M. (1991), 'Ethical Issues in Manipulating the Human Germline', *Journal of Medicine and Philosophy*, Vol. 16, No. 6, pp. 621-39.

Mauron, A. (1993), 'La génétique humaine et le souci des générations futures', *Folia Bioethica*, Vol. 14, pp. 1-28.

Mauron, A. (1995), 'HGP: Holy Genome Project? An Answer to the Questionnaire Concerning the UNESCO Declaration on Protection of the Human Genome, September 1995', *Eubios Journal of Asian and International Bioethics*, Vol. 5, pp. 117-9.

Mauron, A. (1996), 'The Human Embryo and the Relativity of Biological Individuality', in Evans, D. and Pickering, N. (eds) *Conceiving the Embryo: Ethics, Law and Practice in Human Embryology*, Martinus Nijhoff, The Hague, pp. 55-74.

Mauron A (1997), 'La thérapie génique sous l'angle de l'éthique et du droit', *Médecine et Hygiène*, Vol. 55, pp. 1552-4.

Mauron, A. and Thévoz, J.-M. (1991), 'Germline Engineering: A Few European Voices', *Journal of Medicine and Philosophy*, Vol. 16, pp. 649-66.

Munson, R. and Davis, L. (1992), 'Germline Gene Therapy and the Medical Imperative', *Kennedy Institute of Ethics Journal*, Vol. 2, No. 2, pp. 137-58.

Rubenstein, D.S., Thomasma, D.C., Schon, E.A. and Zinaman, M.J. (1995), 'Germline Therapy to Cure Mitochondrial Disease: Protocol and Ethics of *in vitro* Ovum Nuclear Transplantation', *Cambridge Quarterly of Healthcare Ethics*, Vol. 4, No. 3, pp.316-39.

Torres, J.M. (1997), 'On the Limits of Enhancement in Human Gene Transfer: Drawing the Line', *Journal of Medicine and Philosophy*, Vol. 22, No. 1, pp. 43-53.

de Wachter, M.A.M. (1993), 'Ethical Aspects of Human Germline Gene Therapy', *Bioethics*, Vol. 7, No. 2/3, pp. 166-77.

Walters, L. (1986),'The Ethics of Gene Therapy', *Nature*, Vol. 320, pp. 225-7.

Walters, L. and Palmer, J. G. (1997), *The Ethics of Human Gene Therapy*, Oxford University Press: New York, Oxford.

Wivel, N.A. and Walters, L. (1993), 'Germline Gene Modification and Disease Prevention: Some Medical and Ethical Perspectives', *Science*, Vol. 262, No. 5133, pp. 533-8.

Zimmermann, B.K. (1991), 'Human Germline Therapy: The Case for Its Development and Use', *Journal of Medicine and Philosophy*, Vol. 16, No. 6, pp. 596-8.

4 'Quality control' in reproduction – what can it mean, what should it mean?

Dieter Birnbacher

As a philosopher, I take the liberty of beginning with a commonplace remark. It is the dialectics of any extension of our practical knowledge and technology that some old problems are solved and some new problems are generated. Adding to our possibilities of explanation, prediction and control means that the mastery of nature is pushed one step further. It also means that we are confronted with new problems of decision-making and with the problem of giving these decisions a sound ethical foundation. Ethics has to take over where nature is no longer sovereign. With any increase in the number of choices we can make, there is also an increase in accountability, and once we can change the course of nature, it is inevitable that non-intervention stands in need of justification no less than intervention. We are no longer on the safe side, ethically, by 'letting nature take her course'.

The pressure to accept responsibility not only for purposeful interventions but also for 'letting nature take her course' is more keenly felt and more resolutely rejected in human reproduction than in other fields in which medical technology has been successful in altering the course of nature. 'Responsible parenthood' is widely felt to be a deeply *ambivalent* notion, and for good reasons. Sexuality, pregnancy and birth are among the last spheres of human life in which natural forces still largely act *on* us rather than being acted on *by* us, and many people feel that this is as it should be, that in these spheres human domination of nature should have limits. By being subjected to the pressures of technological rationality, the very essence of sexuality and reproduction, their freedom, spontaneity and 'naturalness', seem to be threatened.

This, I think, is one reason for the emotional ambivalence likely to accompany the term 'quality control' in its application to human reproduction. Another, more specific reason is that 'quality' can be given more than one interpretation, and that not all of these interpretations are equally acceptable

So far as I see, 'quality' can have *three* meanings in the sphere of human reproduction: a *preferential* meaning, a *moral* meaning, and what might be called an *axiological* meaning.

In its *preferential* meaning, 'quality' refers to the contingent preferences of the parents concerned, to their own personal standards. Taken in this sense, 'quality' is a thoroughly subjective notion, devoid of any normative force. It is an expression of taste rather than the enunciation of a standard that claims universal acceptance. Exercising reproductive quality control in this sense means that parents exercise their own personal choices in making use of reproductive, diagnostic and therapeutic techniques, thus realising their own preferences in regard to their future children. 'Quality control' in this subjective sense is a logical extension of planned parenthood in the sense of control of the number and timing of pregnancies and births in accordance with the parents' personal wishes. It is a logical extension in so far as not only *quantitative* characteristics of offspring like number and timing but *qualitative* characteristics such as sex, probable health status and possible handicaps are made the objects of deliberate selection.

What has ethics to say to this kind of selection? I think that there is a strong prima facie case in favour of quality control *qua* extension of parental choice. One relevant consideration is that to some extent, choice of the characteristics of offspring is the choice of the course of one's *own* life for at least twenty years to come in which there will be close symbiosis between parents and children. If we agree that freedom of choice is an important good in respect of marriage partners, freedom of choice should be even more important in the choice of children, given the irreversibility of parenthood. Another consideration is that empirical surveys show that parents generally (though by no means universally) have in fact a strong preference for *Wunschkinder*, i. e. for children with certain desired, or without certain undesired characteristics. These preferences are, in the most cases, of the personal kind discussed here and not of an altruistic, moral or axiological kind. I. e. if one does not want to have a child of a certain description, this is not primarily for the child's own sake, or for moral reasons or because the potential child is thought to be less valuable than another child but because one does not want it for personal reasons (cf. Hennen et al. 1996, p. 117). In so far as quality control in human reproduction is an extension of reproductive freedom, there is no reason why it should not go ahead.

Why, then, is reproductive selection, and the medical techniques that make it possible (such as preimplantation diagnosis and prenatal diagnosis) so often the object of moral censure, at least of moral reservations? What is morally objectionable in extending one's freedom of choice to the qualitative nature of offspring? The question has to be put so bluntly because it seems that selection cannot be wrong *in itself,* simply as interference with the 'course of nature'. Medicine is an interference with the course of nature anyway. Nature cannot be sacrosanct. It might even be said that it is man's very nature to interfere with nature. So it cannot be wrong on *that* account to modify the course of reproduction at will.

The negative overtones of reproductive selection seem to a large extent to be the result of what might be called the *projective identification* of the *methods* of selection with their *aims*. Control of the quality of offspring would be regarded as much more 'innocent' than it is if selection did not involve, in most cases, the intentional destruction or discarding of human embryos and fetuses. If we suppose for the moment that selection of offspring were practised by no other technique than the intentional timing of conception or by gamete selection (like sex selection by centrifuging sperm), it would in all probability seem as 'innocent' to morally sensitive observers as the Knaus-Ogino method of birth control seems to the Vatican. Of course, there would still remain some matters for concern, for example the psychological effects a widespread practice of reproductive selection has on the bearers of the characteristics rejected by all or most of those making the selective decisions, such as the female sex in India or people with Down's syndrome in Europe. But even a widespread practice of selective decisions against a certain unwanted characteristic would, I presume, have much less impact on the self-respect of the bearers of these characteristics if its instrumental aspect did not involve the destruction or discarding of a potential human being and would bear less resemblance, on a symbolic level, to an act of selective euthanasia in the Nazi sense of the term.

As matters stand, selection of offspring continues to be effected predominantly by such ethically controversial practices as selective abortion and selective discarding of embryos. Whoever thinks these practices morally indefensible or at least objectionable will have to balance the moral gains of advancing parental freedom of choice against the moral damage done by intentionally destroying human embryos and fetuses. The exact result of this moral balancing depends on the assumed strength of the right to life ascribed to embryos and fetuses. If an absolute deontological verdict on killing human life is upheld, selection of offspring by these methods is never defensible. A deontological consequentialism, on the other hand, which allows a calculation of consequences but makes consequences count in proportion to their intrinsic moral rightness or wrongness, might come to a different conclusion, depending on whether a practice of selective abortion or implantation raises or reduces the sum total of killings. Seen from such a perspective, a practice of highly *selective abortion* might seem preferable if a practice of *indiscriminate abortion* would involve even more violations of the embryo's right to life.

My own view is that there are no rational arguments against the practices of selectively discarding or aborting embryos as such, independently of the physical and psychological effects these practices have on parents and the symbolic effects they have on third parties. The arguments by which abortion is commonly rejected as immoral (the *potentiality*, the *identity*, the *continuity argument* etc.) do not seem to me to carry much conviction and do not seem to be universalisable in the sense of being acceptable to everyone independently from his or her cultural and religious background (see Birnbacher 1995).

This is not to say that there are no moral risks in a potentially widespread practice of reproductive control. There are, first, some social and some biological risks. If selective choices should become the rule rather than the exception, the preparedness to accept children with imperfections might be seriously weakened. Giving parents the liberty to choose the sex of the child might, moreover, result in an unwelcome imbalance of the sex ratio. Biologically, the overall variety in the gene-pool might be significantly, and possibly irreversibly reduced.

There are, second, some *psychological* risks to consider, both for the children resulting from parental reproductive choices and for others. The self-image of children may be profoundly changed by the knowledge that they are in some respect *chosen*. They may feel, rightly or wrongly, that something is expected from them that would not be expected from children resulting from the free play of 'reproductive roulette'. It may prove difficult, moreover, to safeguard their individual right not to know about their own genetic dispositions, given that these were the criterion by which they were selected by their parents. The adverse psychological effects on third parties are, however, more serious. If selection according to widely shared criteria becomes an established practice this must be felt as an offence by all those who in fact have the unwanted characteristics. Of course, the primary source of feelings of stigmatisation would not be the practice of selection itself but rather the attitudes underlying it which become manifest not only in reproductive choices but in many other spheres of private and social life. And it seems plausible to assume that the extent to which reproductive selection is felt as an offence would be roughly proportional to the stigmatisation felt in these other spheres. In this respect, the rejection of prenatal diagnosis and selective abortion by organisations for the protection of the handicapped like the 'Lebenshilfe' in Germany seem to me to be misguided. These practices are symptoms rather than causes of social discrimination of the mentally handicapped. It seems illusory to change attitudes by rejecting the practices in which they manifest themselves.

All these risks certainly carry moral weight. I doubt, however, that they are weighty enough to tilt the balance against reproductive control and to justify restrictions in reproductive choices. Certainly, reproductive freedom is no absolute value. But unless one of these risks turns out to have really dramatic dimensions, reproductive freedom is, in my view at least, the axiologically more important value.

The prima facie case for a moral *obligation* to make selective decisions in respect of offspring is much weaker than the prima facie case for a moral *permission* to such choices. If the term 'quality' is interpreted in a *moral* rather than a preferential sense, 'quality control' looks much less promising. The main problem with 'quality control' in the moral sense is that there are good reasons to be wary of subjecting reproduction to the pressures of moral criticism and other social sanctions. This is not to say that it is always wrong to blame parents for taking the risk of having children which they know will have a very unhappy life. 'Responsible parenthood' is not an altogether empty notion. But in view of the high value of reproductive freedom and the fact that reproductive decisions belong to the innermost circle of the private sphere, the threshold for legitimate moral criticism should be high. Moral criticism should be in order only of the life of the future child is very miserable indeed and the probability of this occurring substantial. In Germany, Kielstein and Sass (1992) have recently given examples of situations in which the quality of life prospects of a potential child seem in fact so gloomy that genetic counsellors should be forgiven if they deviate from the customary and on the whole beneficent principle of non-directiveness.

The idea of a 'quality control' of offspring in the moral sense is sometimes rejected by arguing that having a very unhappy child cannot be blameworthy because nobody is *harmed*. Even a very unhappy child will find its life worth living and will not think of preferring its non-existence to its existence. After all, without the 'harm' involved in its very existence it would not live at all. It is indeed a *conceptual* truth that nobody can be harmed who does not already exist. But that does not settle the moral question. In fact, it seems doubtful why there can be a moral difference at all between the act of (case 1) first producing A and then harming it so that A is in a deplorable state S, and (case 2) producing B under conditions in which it is certain, or highly likely, that B will be in S. Though B is not harmed in case 2, the moral situation does not seem radically different from that in case 1. Even if B does not *ex post* want *not* to be born, the production of B can be an object of legitimate moral criticism *ex ante* to the extent that there were other options open to the parents, such as the production of C who would live without the quasi-harm S from which B suffers, or the decision not to have any genetically related children. Although B, once he is born, has no alternative acceptable to him, his parents possibly had such an alternative.

An indication for 'quality control' in the moral sense will seem to exist in all cases in which the existence of the (potentially, probably) unhappy child is a result of *assisted reproduction*. 'Quality control' in this sense seems a plausible argument for setting limits to such risky techniques as *cloning* or *germline therapy*. 'Quality control' will seem much less plausible in cases in which the existence of the unhappy child is the result of the deliberate *non-use* of reproductive and diagnostic techniques. Again, the moral distinction operative here is not that between an act of commission and an act of omission (begetting children is an act of commission), but the distinction between an area in which high moral standards should prevail (as in the controlled and rational sphere of assisted reproduction) and an area (the private sphere) in which morality should not be allowed to stifle the spontaneous expression of one's most natural, and often deepest, emotions.

The most promising candidate as a measure of 'quality' in quality control in the moral sense is the prospective quality of life of the child, where *'quality of life'* is understood in a strictly *subjectivist* way. Ascribing a very low quality of life to a future person is not to *devalue* his or her life (or to *devalue* the subject of this life as a person), but to describe or prognosticate how he or she will evaluate his or her own life. Quality of life judgements, thus conceived, are judgements from the hypothetical subject's own perspective. Being purely *descriptive* judgements, they should not be confused with evaluative or normative judgements about whether someone should live or is 'worthy' to live. It is true that quality of life judgements are often given a role in evaluative and normative contexts, such as in the allocation of scarce medical resources. But this does not mean that they must be conceived as evaluative judgements about the value or disvalue of a life, or as normative judgements about whether one should create or preserve a life. Instead, they should be conceived as judgements about how a person *experiences* his own life. This deliberately subjectivst interpretation of quality of life is in accordance with the way the concept is understood in other medical contexts. What interests us in inquiring into the quality of life of an actual or future person is not his *objective* state of health but the way he himself *perceives* and *evaluates* this state, and how this state affects his personal *well-being*. Therefore, subjective indicators are more relevant than objective ones. It should be added, however, that physicians are often misled by judging the quality of life of their patients by objective health factors. They tend to consider their quality of life to be more massively affected by health problems than the patients themselves, especially when a worsening of symptoms is to be expected. On the other hand, there is a complementary tendency to overrate the increase in subjective quality of life that can be effectuated by medical treatment.

Since the same objective health conditions can be very differently perceived and evaluated by different subjects in different circumstances, judgements about the quality of life prospects of potential future persons are highly uncertain. This uncertainty does not differ dramatically, however, from that confronting the physician in making treatment decisions vis-à-vis actual patients whose future quality of life will be affected by the treatment received. In deciding whether to propose surgery to a cancer patient, for example, a surgeon must not only make up his mind about the consequences of a potential treatment on the patient's physical state but also on the impact of this physical state on his psychological state and on the patient's own evaluation of this psychological state, taking into account such factors as the patient's level of aspiration, his capacity to cope with untoward states, and his tolerance of side effects (cf. Trede 1994, p. 35). I doubt whether quality of life prognostications with respect to the life of a potential child are of a higher order of difficulty. The uncertainty of the prospects of the future person does not in general seem so overwhelming as to make a potential moral obligation not to reproduce, given certain circumstances, strictly pointless.

The third interpretation of 'quality control', the *axiological* one, is much more problematical than the two interpretations so far considered. In the axiological interpretation, 'quality' is something more objective than in the preferential sense, and at the same time something less moralistic than the moral standard of prospective subjective quality of life. Candidates for 'quality' in the axiological sense are objective functionings like health, physical and mental capacities and what in philosophy has been discussed as a 'good life'. Such a standard differs from a pure preference (even a considered preference) in claiming universal acceptance, without, however, making a moral claim. It does not tell us what we should do or not do, but what is desirable and undesirable.

What seems problematic in the axiological sense of 'quality control' in the domain of reproduction is the presupposition that there can be an objective standard of quality apart from either the preferences of the parents or the presumed preferences of the potential child. Would, for example, 'health' be desirable even if nobody wanted to be healthy (or wanted *others* to be healthy)? There does not seem to be much sense in such an idea. My preliminary conclusion, then, is that 'quality of control' in the service of some assumed axiological quality beyond parents' actual and their offspring's potential preferences rightly deserves all the distrust the concept of 'quality control' spontaneously evokes. This may seem a rather harsh verdict. But it should be remembered that it leaves untouched the two other interpretations (the preferential and the moral one) discussed earlier and found acceptable within limits.

5 Does gene therapy have ethically problematic effects on identity?

Ingmar Persson

I shall discuss whether germline gene therapy and other genetic techniques applied at the preimplantation stage – in contrast to e.g. ordinary somatic therapy – affect our identity and, if so, whether this is ethically significant. So, I will not examine all the ethical questions these therapies raise. I will put aside such worries as: might not such therapies have unpredictable repercussions on the genepool? Might they not provide powerful weapons that political leaders might put to disastrous misuse?

What I will attempt to do is to map the territory, to sketch on overall picture of the identity-related questions posed by these techniques and of plausible or possible answers to them. This approach will leave but little space for detailing my own answers to what I take to be the most interesting questions.[1] I propose to start with the following question:

- (Q1) Are we identical with the kinds of entities on which germline gene therapy and other preimplantation techniques are practised, i.e. entities of the kind gamete, conceptus or zygote?

That is, (Q1) asks whether we, the referents of our personal pronouns, like 'I', have once been entities of these kinds or whether they are something distinct from us out of which we have developed. The identity at stake is not qualitative identity or similarity, as it is in cases of, e.g., cloning, where the clone is (more or less) qualitatively identical with the original. It is so-called numerical identity, such as is employed when we talk about the same individual persisting through time and undergoing qualitative changes, e.g., the ones involved in ageing. We are identical with certain individuals existing, say, last week and the week before. The question is whether this identity of ours extends backwards in time all the way to the pre-implantative stage.

To reply to this question, we have to turn to theories of our nature or identity. For our purposes, these can be divided into two kinds, depending on whether they view us as identical with

- animal organisms of the species *homo sapiens* (the biological theory) or
- beings with some degree of mind or consciousness (the psychological theory).

(This distinction can be traced back to the seventeenth century philosopher John Locke, who distinguished between 'man' and 'person', where 'man' is the male chauvinist term for an individual of the human species.) To illustrate the difference between these theories, consider an irreversibly comatose human being, in whom the areas of the brain supporting consciousness have been irreparably destroyed. On the biological theory, this individual would be one of us: it might be me or you lying in this state. On the psychological view, this could not be the case, since we essentially have minds or consciousnesses, and this individual lacks this precious equipment.

I shall not attempt to adjudicate between these theories, but merely examine their implications for (Q1). On the psychological theory, it is obvious that the answer must be no: it is impossible that we existed at the pre-implantative stage because the entities existing at this stage certainly lack all forms of consciousness. Adherents of the psychological theory will insist that we cannot begin to exist any earlier than sometime in the middle of pregnancy or when the signs of consciousness start to appear.

On the biological theory, it is less obvious what the answer to (Q1) is. It might be thought that an animal organism belonging to the human species comes into existence as soon as fertilisation is completed. If so, this account of our identity implies a positive answer. However, the possibility of monozygotic twinning (among other things) creates problems for this view. If one of us exists before the twinning occurs, what happens to this individual when it occurs? It seems that there could be no reason for saying that it is identical with one rather than the other of the two resulting twins. But it is absurd to hold that it is identical to both, since they are evidently distinct.

So, the original individual presumably disappears or ceases to exist due to the division. But it seems counter-intuitive to think that one of us ceases to exist at this early stage. There is a further difficulty if we believe, as many of those who hold that our existence commences at conception do, that we acquire a right to life as soon as we begin to exist. It would then appear to follow that we have a moral reason to prevent the twinning from occuring, since it destroys a being with a right to life! Therefore, the answer to (Q1) is probably negative, regardless of whether we accept the biological or the psychological theory of our nature and identity.

Nonetheless, let us be generous and examine the consequences not only of the negative answer to (Q1), but also of the positive one. On a positive answer, the next question is:

- (Q2) Does germline gene therapy (etc.) disrupt our identity, so that one of us, who already exists, is replaced by another one of us?
- The corresponding question, given the more plausible negative answer, is: (Q3) Does this therapy cause another one of us to begin to exist than the one who would otherwise begin to exist?

In contrast to (Q2), this question does not imply that one of us already exists as the organism to which the therapy is applied. If the answer to (Q2) and (Q3) is no, germline gene therapy does not disrupt our identity. Consequently, the issue of the ethical significance of such a disruption – which is the ethical issue of sole concern here – would not arise. Now, in realistic cases, genetic manipulations do seem to replace such small portions of the genetic material of the organisms on which they are performed that their identity is unaffected. (Compare: replacement of a small part of an organism, e.g., a heart, does not produce a new organism.) It follows that there is no effect on our identity, even if these organisms are something out of which we develop rather than something with which we are identical, since (as I argue in the papers cited in the note) our identity, even if it is the identity of something mental, is not affected if the identity of that out of which it develops is not. Still, since genetic manipulations that would affect identity cannot be excluded – for instance, the choice of one rather than another pair of gametes will have this effect – let us imagine that positive answers are given to (Q2) and (Q3).

This raises a new pair of questions:

- (Q4) Is it of ethical significance that germline therapy affects our identity by bringing one of us into existence by interrupting the existence of another one of us (already in existence)?
- (Q5) Is it of ethical significance that germline therapy affects our identify by bringing one of us into existence by preventing another one of us from beginning to exist?

At first blush, it might appear that a positive reply to (Q4) is plausible, for surely it is ethically significant if the existence of one of us is interrupted? But, to begin with, we must keep in mind that we are now considering ourselves in our most undeveloped form, not in the more or less fully developed form, with consciousness and so forth, that we know from everyday experience. If indeed we are considering ourselves at all, for it should also be remembered that (Q4) arises only on the less plausible route via a yes to (Q2): the more plausible route via a yes to (Q3) raises (Q5).

With this in mind, let us line up all imaginable therapeutic interferences along a continuum at the one end of which we have minimal interferences which plainly leave the identity of the organism acted upon intact, and at the other end of which we have maximal interferences which clearly disrupt its identity. Since this is a continuum, it is hard to believe that somewhere along it there occurs – either abruptly or, more likely, gradually – a shift (from identity to distinctness) having an ethical significance not found elsewhere in the continuum.

This argument holds good irrespective of whether we are identical with the preimplantation organisms on which the interferences are performed. So, it supports a negative reply to both (Q4) and (Q5). However, there are also reasons for positive replies to these questions. Consider a stronger and a weaker reply. The stronger one is:

- (S) Yes, it is of ethical significance because it is morally *wrong* to let one of us rather than another exist – say, because sorting out some of us is incompatible with all of us being equals or of equal value.

The weaker reply is:

- (W) Yes, it is of ethical significance because (although it is not wrong) there is *less* of a moral reason – no person-regarding reason – to let one of us who has the capacity to lead a better life exist in place of *another one* of us who has only the capacity to lead a worse life than there is to give (e.g., by medical treatment) the same one of us the capacity to lead a better life.

That is, an improvement matters more morally if it is enjoyed by the same individual who would otherwise be in the worse condition than if it is enjoyed by another one replacing someone who would otherwise lead a worse life.

Consider (S), is it incompatible with all of us being equals to select one of us rather than another for life? First, it should be realised that some selection of those who will live is unavoidable. For not all human beings who could possibly exist could actually exist because the larger number of humans who are brought to exist, the larger the number of possible ones they could produce. It may be suggested that the most egalitarian thing we could do is to let chance, or the course of nature, determine who will exist and enjoy the goods of living and who will not, as it has done in the past. But the most egalitarian thing we could do is to let nobody exist, since then nobody will be privileged with the benefits of living!

It is in fact considerations not of equality, but of utility, which exhort us to create new beings who will lead worthwhile lives, for this is a way of maximising the sum of valuable life. But then if, as seems to be the case, some pre-human organisms are so genetically defective that it is likely that they will develop into human persons leading lives that are worse for them than lives would be for human persons developing from other organisms, it appears that we should let the latter develop.

Equality enters the picture only at the stage at which human persons or conscious human beings have developed. It demands that we should see to it that these beings lead lives whose value for them is as equal as possible. For even if we do not implant those pre-human organisms that we have found to be seriously genetically defective, great differences in the welfare of human individuals will tend to result because we have probably missed some hereditary defects and because environmental factors also influence the quality of life. Therefore, the ideal of equality will be far from realised even with genetic control at the pre-implantative stage.

Furthermore, both (S) and (W) are really up against the stiff opposition of an idea central to many ethical traditions, namely the idea that *identity is morally irrelevant*. Consider the Christian Golden Rule that you should treat others as you yourself would want to be treated (were you in their situation). This implies that it is morally irrelevant that others are *others*, i.e., not identical with you. The same idea is echoed in Kant's Categorical Imperative that you should act only on maxims that you can at the same time will to be universal laws. To will that a maxim be universal law is to will that it holds irrespective of the identity of the individuals to whom it is applied. The same idea of the universality of morality is also entailed by the utilitarian principle that you should act in the way that maximises the total sum of happiness, whatever the identity of those being happy. Although the matter certainly deserves closer scrutiny, it is hard to see how this well-entrenched universality can be reconciled with the implication of (S) and (W) that the identity of the beneficiary is significant.

I think that (W) derives intuitive appeal from factors that, strictly speaking, are inessential to the comparison made. If the condition of someone who exists and/or will exist is not improved, there will be someone who may learn of this and feel consequent frustration. This frustration is a morally relevant fact which would be absent in the situation where the improvement would be effected by replacement. Thus, if forced to make a choice, we may have a reason to cause a certain improvement by preserving the identity of somebody already in existence rather than to cause it elsewhere by replacement. But this reason is provided by something that is not an essential ingredient of a choice between an identity-preserving and an identity-changing improvement. For a variety of reasons, it may be that the individuals who miss the improvement are not frustrated (because they are unable to conceive of this improvement, are not self-interested, etc.). Thus, tentatively I conclude that, if we succeed in keeping extrinsic features at bay, we will arrive at the opinion that it is irrelevant in itself whether identity is preserved or disrupted.

It is however not part of my present purpose to give a definite answer to (Q4) and (Q5). But I would like to claim that (Q5) provides a more reasonable formulation than (Q4) of the identity-related ethical problem that germline gene therapy and other genetic techniques applied at the preimplantation stage raise. I would also like to stress that it is far from obvious that they do raise this problem, for the negative answer to (Q3) may well be correct. My tentative conclusions are then:

1   Germline gene therapy is not performed on organisms with which we are identical, i.e., we are not identical with organisms existing at the preimplantation stage;
2   In realistic cases, this therapy changes such a small portion of the genetic material that our identity is not affected:
3   Even if it were to affect our identity, by causing another one of us to exist than would otherwise exist, this would not in itself be ethically significant.

However, the aim has not been to defend these conclusions, but to chart a terrain by means of the questions (Q1) – (Q5).

Note

1   Fuller answers are found in my 'Genetic Therapy, Identity and Person-regarding Reasons', Bioethics, Vol. 9, No. 1, January 1995, and 'Genetic Therapy, Person-regarding Reasons and the Determination of Identity – A Reply to Robert Elliot', Bioethics, Vol. 11, No. 2, April 1997.

Part Three
MORAL RIGHTS AND DUTIES

1 Does PID solve the moral problems of prenatal diagnosis? A rights analysis

Deryck Beyleveld

Introduction

Preimplantation diagnosis (PID) and prenatal diagnosis (PD) can both be used to prevent the birth of a child with a genetically inherited condition or defect. When used for such a purpose, the chief moral advantage generally claimed for PID over PD (where PID is possible and practicable) is that PID does not involve terminating a pregnancy.

This will not impress those who believe that a biologically human being has an inviolable 'right' to life from conception, but it does recommend PID to those who believe that the embryo achieves this status only at the moment of implantation. And, even for those who believe that the fetus is owed no protection for its own sake at any stage, it recommends PID on the ground that deliberate abortion should be avoided because of the trauma and risks to the life and health of the mother involved.

Are we to conclude that PID is an ethical advance over PD? We need to be cautious. The permissibility of abortion is not the only moral issue raised by PID or PD. In general, genetic selection in reproductive choice raises the central issue of eugenics, viz., 'What are permissible grounds (if any) on which to select for or against genetic characteristics?'; and against PID there is widespread suspicion that, even if PID is preferable to PD on anti-abortion grounds, PID is more suspect than PD on the issue of eugenics.

Opposition to PID (vs. PD) on the issue of eugenics seems to rest on the conjunction of two claims (or sets of claims):

I PID will (more than PD) facilitate or even encourage selection for or against genetic characteristics that are irrelevant to the possession of moral status.

II To select for or against genetic characteristics that are irrelevant to possession of moral status is immoral.

Whether or not Claim I is true is an empirical question, and in this paper I will restrict my attention to Claim II (which is equally relevant to germline gene therapy), and I will try to assess it within the context of the Principle of Generic Consistency *(PGC)*.

The *PGC* grants rights explicitly to the generic features of (or capacities for) agency to all agents and prospective purposive agents (PPAs). A conceptus is before birth (and, indeed, for some time thereafter) not a PPA, but at most a potential PPA. The *PGC* does not grant *generic* rights to potential PPAs[1] and it is contentious to suggest that it imposes any duties on PPAs not to harm potential PPAs *just because* they are potential PPAs. The entire matter of duties owed to potential PPAs is complex, and for present purposes I shall just assert that there are at least some cases in which it is morally permissible to prevent the further development of a conceptus (whether already impregnated or not). More specifically, I would argue that there are two unproblematic grounds on which the development of a conceptus may be prevented or ended.

For the reason that the conceptus is incapable of developing into a PPA;

For the reason that the conceptus has known properties that mean that either at the unborn stage or after birth it will compromise the generic capacities for agency of the parents (and especially the mother) against their will.

In addition, presuming that the *PGC* does not grant protection to potential PPAs *as such,* there is scope for arguing that there is third permissible ground for preventing or ending the further development of a conceptus: viz.,

For the reason that the mother (in the case of an implanted conceptus) or the parents (in the case of a not yet implanted conceptus) simply does not wish to have *a* child.

In the context of the *PGC* (and other theories that make agency the central property for the possession of full moral status, i.e., of rights), II maintains

II' (All things being equal) it is morally impermissible to select for or against PPA irrelevant characteristics (characteristics that are neither necessary nor sufficient for a being to acquire or maintain the status of a PPA).

II', in turn, entails that it is (all things being equal) impermissible to prevent or end the further development of a conceptus.

For no reason other than that the mother (in the case of an implanted conceptus), or the parents (in the case of a not yet implanted conceptus), does not want to have a child with (or lacking) particular characteristics X, i.e., does not want to have a child having characteristics Z – where possession of Z is compatible with a child having the status of a PPA (the genetic characteristics of the conceptus being such that they will, or are likely to, result in a child with characteristics Z).

Is II' a valid derivation from the PGC?

There are, in principle, two kinds of arguments that can be used to derive II' from the *PGC.*

A Those that attempt to establish that assent to the *PGC logically entails* assent to II'.

B Those that attempt to establish that selection for or against PPA irrelevant characteristics *tends to facilitate or encourage PGC* violating circumstances.

Arguments of type A

If the *PGC* imposes at least a prima facie duty on PPAs not to kill *potential* PPAs *as such,* then II' will be a valid derivation from the *PGC.* In such a case, PPAs will owe such a duty to a potential PPA simply by virtue of the potential PPA being a potential PPA, because to select against a conceptus simply for the reason that it has (or lacks) characteristics irrelevant to its ability to become a PPA will be to deny that being a potential PPA is sufficient to impose a duty of protection on PPAs.

However, I am not persuaded that the *PGC* grants such prima facie protection to potential PPAs as such. If this presumption is correct, then, if II' is to be derived logically from the *PGC,* this form of argument must show that to select for or against PPA irrelevant characteristics is to deny *PGC* protected rights of *full* PPAs *as such.*

How about the following argument? A potential parent who wishes to select against a child having (or lacking) PPA irrelevant characteristics X (i.e., having Z characteristics), in effect claims

(a) 'I do no wrong by selecting against a conceptus with Z characteristics.' Therefore,

(b) 'My *PGC* protected autonomy is violated if I am compelled to become a parent of a PPA with Z characteristics (when this can be prevented).' Therefore,

(c) 'The mere existence of PPAs with Z characteristics against the choice of their parents (irrespective of how they behave) – whose existence could have been prevented – violates the generic rights of their parents.'[2] Therefore,

(d) 'The mere existence of a PPA can violate the generic rights of another PPA.'

137

(e) The *PGC,* however, grants equal rights to all PPAs, reciprocal to which it places equal duties on all PPAs. Thereby, it implies that any rights violation can be prevented by the observance of a duty, which (in turn) implies that the mere existence of a PPA cannot be a violation of the generic rights of another PPA.

(f) However, (d) contradicts (e).

(g) Therefore, selection against Z characteristics violates the *PGC.*

How sound is this? If a type A argument can be made out, I believe it will have to proceed along something like these lines. This particular example, however, is invalid. The valid interpretation of '*the mere existence of a PPA cannot* be a violation of the generic rights of another PPA' in (e) is '*a PPA cannot by its mere existence* violate the generic rights of another PPA'. On the other hand, the valid interpretation of '*the mere existence of a PPA cannot* be a violation of the generic rights of another PPA' in (d) is '*PPAs who do not permit PPAs* to select against Z characteristics violate the generic rights of those PPAs'. So interpreted, there is no contradiction between (d) and (e). For there to be a genuine contradiction, it must be read into (d) that it is *those PPAs who have Z characteristics* who are, merely by having Z characteristics, violating the generic rights of their parents. But (d), so interpreted, is not a valid derivation.

And, of course, there is the converse possibility of arguing that the logical entailment strategy *must* fail. For example, the following case might be presented. Are not would be parents, in effect, trying to select for (or against) PPA irrelevant characteristics simply by choosing particular partners to mate with? The only difference between selection by traditional mating choice and selection through PID or PD is the inefficiency of the former. If so, unless we suppose that mating should be at random, it cannot be intrinsically immoral to select for or against PPA irrelevant characteristics.

This, however, is also fallacious. The *effect* of mating partner selection is, indeed, genetic selection for or against various PPA irrelevant traits. But, while mating choices cannot be illegitimate just because they have such an effect (it is, after all, impossible for there not to be such an effect), it begs the question to maintain that to mate with someone *specifically in order* to produce children with specific PPA irrelevant characteristics is legitimate.

Arguments of type B

Whether or not it is possible to produce a valid argument of type A, arguments depending on contingencies are also available. I will cite just two examples.

1 Although the presumed permissibility of selecting against Z characteristics may not logically imply that PPAs with Z characteristics are of lower moral status than PPAs without them, imagine a child with Z characteristics who knows that its parents would have selected against these characteristics if

they had been able to do so. Imagine, further, that it is now possible *and accepted as legitimate* for the parents to select against Z characteristics. And suppose, as well, that the parents have now had another child whom they have ensured will not have Z characteristics after genetic diagnosis. Will this not be deeply damaging to the self esteem of the child with Z characteristics, in a way that the *PGC* will not permit? In addition, will not acceptance of the legitimacy of selection against Z characteristics tend to produce a sense of grievance in parents who, for whatever reason, are unable to avail themselves of new selection technologies against Z characteristics – thereby tending to cause (albeit irrational) resentment against those of their children with the offending Z characteristics, and thereby resulting in such children being treated with less *PGC* required respect than they would have been treated with had they not had these characteristics?

2 Z characteristics are, in themselves, neutral under the *PGC,* which is to say that no intrinsic rights benefit is to be gained by selecting for or against them. However, fashions can develop for such characteristics. Many such fashions are harmless in themselves. However, if they come to be regarded as conditions meriting medical intervention, they cease to be so. Witness the example of the desire for perfectly shaped teeth that has swept the United States, resulting in children whose parents are unable to afford the treatment that can correct 'imperfections' that are now perceived of as deformities, suffering deep traumas as a result. By extension, it may be argued that permitting selection against Z characteristics, even if this is (ex hypothesi) not intrinsically prohibited by the *PGC,* is likely to produce a culture in which the possession of *PGC* neutral characteristics becomes generically harmful to those who possess them.

Many at least prima facie plausible arguments of this kind can, I am sure, be produced. I would caution only that they point to a need for empirical research, which must be carried out if rational evaluation rather than dogma is our aim.

Conclusion

Although all of this is very tentative, I suspect that no intrinsic argument against selection directed at PPA irrelevant characteristics can be constructed. Thus, the force of rights based arguments against such selection practices (whether in the context of PID or PD – or germline gene therapy for that matter) will necessarily be contingent, being of the form that such and such practices are likely to produce situations more generically harmful to PPAs than the absence of such practices.

On the other hand, on the basis of such arguments against selection practices that are directed at PPA irrelevant characteristics, the question of whether PID is to be preferred to PD (assuming that, as a means to genetic selection, PD's involving killing a fetus, does not constitute an overriding objection against it) is a matter of whether or not PID is more likely than PD to promote such selection. And then, even if PID proves to be more problematic than PD on such grounds, PID will still only be the more problematic *all things considered* if, amongst other things, the eugenic advantages (as measured by the *PGC*) of PD over PID are greater than the advantages of the avoidance of abortion in relation to the disadvantages involved in the traumas of in vitro fertilisation.

All of this is very complex indeed. Apart from deep analysis of the weightings to be accorded various consequences by the *PGC*, much of such an assessment requires empirical research. Such analysis and research will, however, have to be performed if a fully reasoned *PGC* inspired analysis is to be provided.

Notes

1 Simply because these are claim rights, which require the rights bearer to be able to waive their benefits, which presupposes that the rights bearer is a PPA.

2 The possession of some PPA irrelevant characteristics in their children (such as having cystic fibrosis, or Down's Syndrome) might (and does) place greater burdens on parents. As such, would be parents can claim that they have a right to select against these characteristics. Not to do so will interfere with their generic rights when they are not willing to bear these burdens. However, these burdens are contingent, in that they could be avoided or considerably lessened by a supportive state and culture. The *PGC* relevant negative consequences for the parents are not functions of their children possessing the PPA irrelevant characteristics alone.

2   Ethics of Research on Human Embryos

Reiner Wimmer

In my conviction the fundamentals of ethics have their roots in the biological and intercultural conditions of human life and its self-understanding.

Therefore I will start with a brief analysis of the way we understand ourselves and one another in everyday life and in our scientific endeavours. Such an experiental analysis needs neither metaphysical concepts on the one hand nor scientific concepts on the other, neither explicitly nor implicitly. On the contrary, all possible (in the sense of rationally founded) metaphysics and all possible sciences and humanities presuppose conceptually such a self-understanding which is implicit in all human practice, insofar as it first of all refers to truth and to the ability of free consent to truth (or what is believed to be the truth of this or that particular case).

I think that the most succinct, concentrated, forceful formula of such a (of course necessarily to be extended) analysis (which cannot be carried out on a few pages) is the following: The human being is a being which is able to behave towards itself as its own accountable and responsible origin. Obviously, such behaviour towards oneself is a reflective relationship with two aspects: the first one which may be called in the broadest sense 'theoretical' involves perceiving and recognising all sorts of things: living beings, states of affairs, events, one's own acts including (self-reflectively) one's own awareness or consciousness of such perceiving; the other aspect which may be understood in a broad sense as 'practical' includes all sorts of evaluative and, in particular, critical assessment referring to other people's behaviour as well as to one's own and its underlying intentions and aims. In both respects, the human being thinks of him- or herself with conceptual necessity as an accountable and responsible subject which is inevitably driven by and adjusted to the unconditional claims of truth and (not yet to be morally understood) rightness.

To view to oneself or others as beings which are able to perform such theoretical and practical acts is to attribute to oneself and to others the status of a person. In what follows I use the term 'person' in its primary sense as shorthand for the above mentioned basic formula of an experientially oriented anthropology. At the same time, I believe that this formula (or a conceptually equivalent one) adequately represents the nucleus of the concept of person in the Stoic, the Jewish-Christian, and the Kantian tradition as well as the modern conception of unconditional and unrestrained human rights and dignity pertaining to all human beings and which form the basis of the constitutions of the present democratic states. This philosophical and legal conception of the human being as an inviolable person is, as indicated, rooted in our everyday discourse and understanding of ourselves and our fellow men and women.

Today there is a tendency to treat the concept of person not as an experiential concept in the above indicated sense but as an empirical one in the sense of the sciences: the status of person allows grades, somebody is more or less of a person, what he or she as a person is is measurable by degrees so that we consider ourselves to be able to identify higher and lower levels of personhood and consequently to attribute different values to different developmental states of human beings and to weigh them up in situations of conflict. The traditional view according to which all humans are persons in the same way ought to be differentiated – according at least to the opinion of some bioethicists –; otherwise we would have to ignore the obvious fact that there is a large, morally relevant difference between a human fetus and a healthy adult with respect to their personhood and their status as a person. I think that the very point of the classical conception of personhood is not to allow of any gradation so that the real differences synchronically between individuals or diachronically between various states of one and the same individual are irrelevant concerning the *ascription* of personhood; they are highly relevant concerning the *treatment* of a person namely in accordance with his or her needs in a particular situation.

I would like to make a further conceptual remark: I think neither the classical nor the experiential approach to personhood need to be restricted to human beings only. In fact, the traditional position was not that 'being a human' and 'being a person' are intentionally and extensionally equivalent (i.e. that these expressions have the same meaning and refer to the same individuals). Neither was 'being a human' defined via 'being a person' or vice versa, so as to make sure that both expressions meant the same. However, personhood was seen as a necessary, though not sufficient, condition of being a human, and being a human was a sufficient, though not necessary criterion of personhood. Thus, all human beings were to be treated as persons, but not all persons had to be humans. The idea was to account for the personhood of God and of incorporeal spirits.

Of course, the conceptual difference between being a human and being a person opens up not only the possibility to speak of God and of incorporeal spirits as persons but also the possibility of speaking of humans which are neither persons nor are invested with the status of persons as well as of other living and corporeal beings which are persons insofar as they possess the above mentioned abilities characteristic of a person; so it cannot be excluded on conceptual grounds only that there might be genera or species of animals whose members are at the same time persons.

The concept of person and the relation of human persons to themselves or to one another discussed so far exhibit the following features: First, the person is conceived of as the same throughout time, as identical in all varieties and during all variations of properties which can be attributed to him or her as long as he or she possesses the above mentioned abilities characteristic of personhood. Second, the status of person or the attribution of this status does not depend on the degree of development of the bodily, intellectual or emotional abilities of an individual or on the quality of them; there is no more or less of personhood, only all or nothing of it. Third, there is a way of ascribing the status of person to a human being in sense independent of its ability or inability to act characteristically for a person, for instance, when people are talking about their own or other people's beginning in the womb (or perhaps in vitro) or when they are talking about themselves or other people as being or having been in a coma; they say for instance: 'Those were happy days when I felt you the first time under my heart' or 'My mother told me that she conceived me on a nice May day in the first year of World War II' and 'As early as in the fifth month of my existence, before I was even born, I got that terrible disease because of my mother's heavy smoking and drinking'.

These sayings illustrate: we think not only in terms of the continuity of history of a living being but also in terms of the persistence of personal identity during all stages of development, the beginning of which is the event or perhaps better expressed the process of conception as the beginning of a whole though not yet totally individualised being as embryology tells us. The phase- or event-ontology of human beings presented for instance by Derek Parfit and Peter Singer neglects this aspect of identity consciousness and is therefore in discord with our self-understanding and self-assessment.

In my opinion the last mentioned ascription of the status of person can be justified not only by the self-understanding of an adult in retrospect but also by reference to the assumption that a human being without the prerequisite abilities of a person – I am speaking of a human embryo, fetus and newborn –

has in normal circumstances (i.e., if all developmental conditions are fulfilled) the capacity or the capability of becoming a person in the sense of acquiring and executing the relevant abilities. The attribution of the status of person in this third respect is, theoretically speaking, a contrafactual imputation because the genetic and physiological outfit alone is not sufficient for becoming a person, but a practically effective because practice-controlling presupposition without which there would be no human persons: human parents have to treat their newborns as persons (as if they were already persons) in order that their children become persons. But, of course, they do not understand their loving educational behaviour as based on a strategic fiction (that would not be a treatment of human beings as real persons). In so doing they are not only pragmatically correct but also right in the sense that human beings (fetuses, embryos, newborns) usually occupy the status of persons on account of their identity throughout all stages of their development, which identity is at any rate only perceptible from the inside of the grown-up person him- or herself and only in retrospect; seen from the outside they are not yet persons but insofar as they are capable of becoming persons in the sense of behaving as such there is a real foundation for attributing the status of person to them from the outside as well.

But how should we treat human beings of whom we are sure that they do not possess even the capability of becoming a person (as anencephalics) or that they have lost such capability for all times (as people whose brain is irrevocably destroyed)? The very last part of this question I may leave aside because my mandate covers only the moral questions concerning research on embryos.

The moral consequences resulting from the above argued-for and explained position are obvious, so at least I hope. Since human beings during all stages of their prenatal or postnatal existence and development occupy the status of persons as far as these beings are per se capable of developing the abilities characteristic of personhood and since I am unable to see any moral difference between such human beings which are already persons and such which are not already persons but are capable of becoming persons all acts which do harm them such that they loose that capability or which terminate their life are morally forbidden; likewise any research or experimentation on human beings which hold that status but have not given their informed consent or are unable to do it. Of course, embryos are not in a situation to be able to do so. This moral prohibition does not allow any gradation because neither personhood nor the status of person gives any license for it. And since the status of person is the highest moral status due to human beings it cannot be weighed against other impersonal and therefore lower goods. Only in cases where life-claims of human beings occupying the status of persons enter into immediate competition with one another is a weighing up of factors other than their own person-status morally legitimate (for instance, when a fetus endangers the life of its mother). I stress the word 'immediate'; there are no justifiable legal claims which can be made on human beings who would have prevented others from dying or being chronically disabled by donating vital parts, they had consented. For similar reasons it cannot be morally justified that during the totipotent state of its cells an embryo is divided up in order to use the one or the other of its cells for diagnosing the genetic health of the other parts of the embryo whereby the used-up cell by this manipulation is destroyed. A genetical diagnosis which causes no such damage may be morally innocuous, but the aims it serves might not be so. Equally, it is morally inadmissible to experiment with supernumerary embryos after embryo transfer. Because of the unresolved problem of supernumerary embryos it seems to me that IVF is morally highly dubious. Experimentation with and research on embryos seems morally permissible only in cases where diagnostics on embryos are so far developed that they can be diagnosed as incapable of becoming persons without reasonable doubt (for instance, in cases of anencephalics).

In Germany experiments with embryos are legally forbidden. I think that this law is consonant with our deep-rooted morality concerning persons and those beings which are capable of becoming persons. Therefore, our endeavours should aim at institutionalising similarly restrictive legal regulations all over the European Union and ultimately all over the world. Of course, I am not so naive as to think that this aim is realistic under the present circumstances. Political compromises are necessarily called for. But it is not for the ethicist to anticipate them: that is not his or her task. He or she has to think on principle, not pragmatically. Therefore I think that research on human embryos is morally permissible only if their rights which follow from their status as persons are not violated. Therefore, it cannot be morally legitimate to produce 'spare' embryos or embryos only for the benefit of other persons. Consequently, legal authorisation of and regulations for producing 'spare' embryos (for instance, during IVF) or for doing research on them without respect for their rights are equally morally illegitimate, but can be tolerated if no other, morally better legal regulations are available. But it may be morally unquestionable to produce foetal tissue or foetal bodies which are per se not capable of becoming persons if they lack the genetic disposition for evolving a brain. But these questions I leave to moral casuistry.

3 Categorical arguments – Pro life versus pro choice?

Maureen Junker-Kenny

The title 'Categorical arguments – Pro life versus pro choice?', is in itself worthy of analysis. It combines two different levels of moral judgment: the level of moral discourse based on arguments, and the level of basic ethical moral attitudes, expressed in the slogans of two ethico-political movements, 'pro life' over against 'pro choice'. While they highlight the fact that societies are bitterly divided on the matter of the status and rights of embryos, and thus show the relevance and urgency of proper ethical analysis, the danger of this level is that it gets caught in a clash of world views (Mieth 1999) and therefore never reaches the point of critically assessing the ethical reasons behind the respective stances.

I shall start out by explaining what philosophical ethics understands by 'categorical arguments' and then discuss two opposing views on whether these can be applied to embryos. Finally, I shall reflect on how pragmatic and categorical arguments relate to each other in this area.

'Categorical arguments' in philosophical ethics

The following definition of the distinction between the two kinds of ethical arguments, taken from the Enquête-Committee of the German Parliament, shows how closely the use of the term categorical is related to Kant's practical philosophy.

Categorical arguments are concerned with the nature of the interventions themselves. They are valid in every case and cannot be rendered invalid by weighing up advantages and disadvantages. – Pragmatic arguments, however, are based on exactly this kind of weighing process. They consider the benefit and the dangers of the intervention in question, i.e. consequences and side effects and can lead to different judgments in modified circumstances (Enquête-Kommission des Deutschen Bundestages 1987, p. 189).

In order to establish the fundamental principle of his ethics, Immanuel Kant distinguishes 'categorical' from 'hypothetical' imperatives. 'Hypothetical' imperatives have an 'If . . ., so' structure, e.g.: If you want to learn a foreign language well, go abroad. They depend on pragmatic goals and are only valid in relation to them.

The Categorical Imperative, however, is an unconditional principle. Its so-called humanistic formulation goes: 'Act in such a way that you always treat humanity, whether in your own person or in the person of any other, never simply as a means, but always at the same time as an end'. Kant adds: 'This principle of humanity, and in general of every rational agent, as an end in itself . . . is the supreme limiting condition of every man's freedom of action' (GMS, BA 66.69-70. ET 96.98). No 'if', no qualifications, exemptions or deliberations on benefits and risks are allowed here.

What is the basis of this fundamental principle of the priority of the rational human being as an end in herself or himself? Kant does not presuppose its evidence but argues for it from the idea of human dignity which in turn is based on autonomy in the sense of the human capacity to govern oneself by reason.

> Morality is the only condition under which a rational being can be an end in himself . . . Therefore morality, and humanity insofar as it is capable of morality, is the only thing which has dignity . . . Autonomy is therefore the ground of the dignity of human nature and of every rational nature (GMS, BA 77.79. ET 102-3).

To summarise Kant's categorical argumentation: The unconditional recognition of the other which establishes her unalienable rights as the 'supreme limiting condition' for other people's desires and goals, is based on our capacity to move our will through reason, instead of personal wishes and whims. Whether this capacity has to be actualised or whether it can be potential, is one of the important points of debate on the moral status of the embryo. If it can be ascribed the status of a person, questions such as the ethical permissibility of preimplantation diagnosis have to be debated at the categorical, not just the pragmatic level of argumentation.

Can embryos figure in categorical argumentations?

Here, I shall question two different categorical argumentations, one following Alan Gewirth's 'Principle of Generic Consistency' (PGC) which Deryck Beyleveld and Klaus Steigleder have analysed and applied to the case of embryos; and the approach which Ludger Honnefelder takes to show that the embryo is a person and therefore enjoys rights equal to anyone else, born or unborn, autonomous or dependent.

Dignity based on moral agency

The question whether it is sufficient to be destined towards freedom in order to be attributed the dignity of personhood is answered negatively by this approach. Only actualised freedom, autonomy in performance, fulfills the requirements for personal dignity. In his explanation of Alan Gewirth's foundation of human rights on the mutual recognition of subjects with intentions for agency, Steigleder shows that for Gewirth the reason for personal dignity is the actual capacity for agency which at the same time claims the recognition of the other. How can this argumentation be applied to beings who are only potentially capable of agency?

> The basis of dignity is that the agent inevitably *has* purposes she wants to fulfill . . . because agents must attribute to themselves and to each other dignity they must, in different ways, regard human non-persons as connected to their dignity and therefore must confer, in different ways, moral status upon them (Steigleder 1997, pp. 241.239).

The reason for their derived moral status is their potential agency.

> (H)uman beings who are not yet agents must possess moral significance for agents for the sufficient reason that they possess the potentiality to become agents . . . They do not possess the same moral status as agents for they do not possess dignity (Steigleder 1997, p. 241).

Yet their status gives them extensive rights at least in principle:

> The general normative implication of the moral status of human embryos and fetuses as potential agents is a general prescription to preserve, protect and foster them. This implies the general prohibition of harming and killing them (Steigleder 1997, p. 244).

In a way similar to Steigleder, Beyleveld both underlines the differences in moral status between persons and embryos and establishes rights to protection on their potentiality. He argues above all with the principle of caution in favour of beings with uncertain status. However, he also suggests the possibility to found a direct moral status of the embryo on the idea that it represents a necessary condition for agency since it is a necessary condition for the development of an agent.

> (U)ncertain agents are to be treated (as far as possible) as agents. While there can be no reasonable uncertainty about whether human embryos are or are not agents (they clearly are not) the precautionary principle can be applied to uncertainty about their status as *potential* agents . . . There is the thought, too, . . . that being an embryo is a necessary stage for becoming an agent . . . and something can made be made of the idea that being an embryo is thus a necessary condition of agency in being a necessary condition for becoming an agent (Beyleveld 1997, pp. 251).

However, the duty to protect embryos as potential agents according to Steigleder does not apply to the stage of the so-called 'pre-embryo'. He does not recognise any categorical reasons against their being used in wasting research. While he pointed out before the features shared by agents in the full sense, by embryos and by pre-embryos, such as corporeal constitution and historicity, in this most recent argumentation he distinguishes between two potentialities with different normative implications. The

> above argument from potentiality refers to the embryo in the strict sense and not to the so-called 'pre-embryo'. By this term is usually meant the fertilised human egg (zygote) and the further stages of its development during roughly the first two weeks . . . The pre-embryo has the 'potentiality *to produce*', for instance, the embryo. The embryo itself has the 'potentiality *to become*' an agent. It was this last kind of potentiality which figured in the argument from potentiality. Thus, the moral status of the human pre-embryo is different and much weaker than that of the human embryo. It is difficult to see how the status of the pre-embryo as such could justify a categorical prohibition of its use for research. On the other hand, the question is to be considered to what extent and with what consequences we have to attribute to the human pre-embryo symbolic significance (Steigleder 1997, p. 245).

Whatever one may think about situating the fertilised egg closer to the gametes before fertilisation than to the embryo after its differentiation, about the continuity of the zygote with the implanting embryo and about assigning the activities of 'producing' to the 'pre-embryo' and of 'becoming' to the 'embryo', the interesting point here is how the value of the anthropological presuppositions for agency are revised. Instead of postulating discontinuity, in an earlier article Steigleder had attributed higher moral significance to the dimensions of corporeality and temporality. Apart from the potency for agency he had stated them as 'further significant aspects'. Especially the element of historicity

> undermines the possibility of an agent to measure consistently the limits of dignity in an abstract 'Either' (agent) – 'Or' (non-agent). It points to the lines of development and continuities beyond agency and does not permit any 'neutrality' with regard to the neediness given with corporeality (Steigleder 1993, p. 119).

This earlier and the later positions come to similar conclusions in which embryos cannot figure in categorical argumentations. However, the earlier version takes something into account the lack of which can later be seen as the principal weakness of an ethical approach which attributes dignity only to moral agents: its neglect of the need to base one's ethics on a theory of the human being, instead of narrowing it down to problems of justification and then drawing applications from this lean foundation. 'Lines of development and continuities beyond agency' need to be explored first in order not to succumb to an 'ethicistic fallacy' (D. Mieth 1998, pp. 51.56-59).

Dignity based on ontology

The second approach I want to discuss seems to fulfill all the demands for an anthropological reflection which also takes into account natural features, inclinations, and basic 'givens' of human subjectivity. Honnefelder wants to show

> that it is the inner context of two aspects which one can call the 'person principle' and the 'nature principle' which are at the core of the ethos of human rights and furnish the foundation of a consensus of modern society (Honnefelder 1996a, p. 215).

In his attempt to ground an 'absolute' over against a 'relative' entitlement for embryos to be protected (Honnefelder 1996b), he claims Kant for his interpretation that a substantive ontology has to be postulated.

> Kant decides without hesitation in favour of regarding personhood and human nature as co-extensive (*deckungsgleich*). At the same time, however, he has to claim a unity of both which according to his premises theoretical reason cannot know and has to claim a concept of substance in the practical sphere which cannot be demonstrated in the theoretical sphere (Honnefelder 1996a, p. 238).

151

Apart from the question whether his quotes from Kant are indeed as central and as straightforward in their claims to a natural basis for personhood as Honnefelder takes them to be, two critical points have to be raised.

One decisive distinction is obscured in the following argumentation: 'Person principle and nature principle are indissolubly linked. The capability (*Vermögen*) stated in the concept of the person to be a subject has to be considered as the *ground* for the attribution of human dignity, as the *criterion* for the attribution of the property stated in the concept of the human being, to be a living being of a certain nature' (Honnefelder 1996, pp. 260-261). What Honnefelder calls a 'criterion', the feature of being a bodily human being, only refers to the problem of knowing and is not the criterion of validity (*Geltungskriterium*). If it was, then corporeality would be a normative reason for human dignity. This empirical 'criterion' only answers the question of knowability (*Erkennbarkeit*) who is a free human subject, namely whoever has human shape, but is not a criterion in the normative sense.

The second problematic step is his extension of the two interlinked principles of person and nature to embryos who do not have a recognisable human shape. This extension is based on a doubtful explanation of the 'continuity' between the zygote and the future person in terms of substance metaphysics. While Steigleder minimised the continuity between the 'pre-embryo' and the implanted embryo and ignored the fact that it does not only 'produce' the embryo but that part of it 'becomes' the embryo (and another part the placenta), Honnefelder neglects this differentiation and sees the relation between the zygote and the future person as a substantial, rather than a temporal and historical continuity.

Therefore, it can be questioned whether Honnefelder's attempt to combine the 'person principle (being a moral subject)' with the 'nature principle (belonging to the human species)' is successful. His terms are essentialist:

> The embryo is a person because it is a human being, and the human being includes the development form of the subject . . . Human beings are entitled to person status because by nature they possess the capability to be subjects (Honnefelder 1996b, p. 10).

Honnefelder's ultimately naturalistic concept of the person cannot do justice to the evidence that embryos have to develop into free moral subjects. The tradition of substance metaphysics seems to be particularly badly equipped to conceptualise a life whose being – to quote a famous theological title, Eberhard Jüngel's *Gottes Sein ist im Werden* – consists in becoming. Honnefelder's attempt to mediate between the Kantian foundation of dignity on the capability to be a moral subject and an Aristotelian natural teleology comes down on the side of natural law essentialism. The 'naturalism' of the teleological-natural law type of categorical argumentation which Wimmer criticises can also be seen at work in Honnefelder's position (Wimmer 1989, p. 199).

A third approach: Dignity based on being destined towards freedom

Between the ethicistic position of founding human dignity on agency and the ontologising approach based on the potentiality of nature, a third kind of categorical argumentation seems possible which avoids the pitfalls of the other two. It bases human dignity neither on actual performance nor on a given human nature but on the destination for freedom (cf. Junker-Kenny 1998). Kant's concept of human dignity based on the capability to be moral can be extended to human beings who are presently not yet or no longer able to give evidence of their moral capacity. This attempt to base a categorical argumentation on the human destination for freedom even if it is not actually given can also be justified with a view to everyday ethical praxis. Freedom only comes into existence if it is recognised in advance. It has to be anticipated in order to become real. The recognition of the other fundamentally has an innovative and anticipatory dimension and often enough has to be vicarious even among equally able agents. Once the basically advocatory nature of everyday ethical praxis is made clear, it is only a question of gradation not of principle to include humans who are not yet or no longer agents. Everybody's freedom needs the free recognition of others to be mediated to itself (Pröpper, 1995). Thus, it is possible to maintain that the capability for being a moral subject is the normative ground for personal dignity, yet not to use this criterion for excluding those forms of human life from protection which factually, cannot (yet) meet this claim. Whoever has the potential to be a free subject, is included in the categorical imperative of recognising the other as the supreme limit to my interests.

Do pragmatic arguments imply categorical arguments?

Do categorical and relative arguments exclude each other, or can one argue that the latter imply the former for their justification? First, categorical reasoning is not weakened by the fact that there might be important considerations on a relative level as well. But I would argue that, rather than being able to stand on their own, they receive their force in conjunction with categorical judgments. For example, the argument that the unique identity of persons is not to be interfered with, gains its validity from the categorical principle of non-instrumentalisation.

With regard to the ethical permissibility of preimplantation diagnosis it is clear that no measures should be allowed to be planned that do not include the rights of the embryo. Since preimplantation diagnosis is a technique that is geared to selection, that is non-implantation without an alternative, it represents a clear case of a third party disposing over another's possibility for existence as well as over its specificity.

The task is to examine the possibility of a categorical argumentation which is neither essentialist nor reductionist. I have tried to argue that being destined towards freedom or being capable of morality – over against being a fully-fledged moral agent – is a sufficient reason for attributing human dignity to the zygote. This line of reasoning needs to be further justified and compared in its foundation and application with other approaches to applied philosophical and theological ethics with and without categorical reasons – different kinds of Kantian argumentations, natural law, feminist, as well as Utilitarian and Communitarian ethical positions. How do they differ with regard to the role they allow for anthropology, including the bodily constitution, temporality and historicity of humans? How are the tasks of the justification and the application of ethics seen to differ, and how are they seen to interact? How do they apply the principle of non-instrumentalisation to concrete conflicts, e.g. pregnancy after rape, lethal and non-lethal genetic defects?

Pragmatic arguments alert us to specific points: the balance of gains and risks, real or imaginary slippery slopes, or justice issues in resource allocation which have to be debated concretely. Categorical arguments remind us that there is a 'supreme limiting condition' to the objects and projects of our will: the dignity which the capability to be moral confers on us who, according to the Conclusion of Kant's Critique of Practical Reason, are finite beings on a planet which itself is a 'mere speck of dust in the Universe'. A thought suitable for reminding ethicists neither to ontologise freedom nor to take the cosmological and anthropological presuppositions of agency for granted.

Note

Wimmer identifies a categorical argumentation with a deontological understanding of ethics, and a pragmatic one with a teleological-consequentialist orientation.

References

Beyleveld, D. (1997), 'The moral and legal status of the human embryo' in Hildt, E. and Mieth, D. (eds), *In Vitro Fertilization in the 1990s – Towards a medical, social and ethical evaluation*, Aldershot: Ashgate, pp. 239-246.

Enquête-Kommission des Deutschen Bundestages, 'Chancen und Risiken der Gentechnologie', (1987), in *Gentechnologie – Chancen und Risiken Bd. 12*, München: J. Schweitzer, quoted in Wimmer, R., (1989), 'Kategorische Argumente gegen die Keimbahn-Therapie', in Wils, J.-P. and Mieth, D. (eds), *Ethik ohne Chance? Erkundungen im technologischen Zeitalter*, Tübingen: Attempto Verlag, pp. 182-209.

Honnefelder, L. (1993), 'Der Streit um die Person in der Ethik' in *PhJ*, 100, 246-265.

Honnefelder, L. (1996a), 'Person und Menschenwürde' in Honnefelder, L. and Krieger, G., (eds), *Philosophische Propädeutik, Bd. 2: Ethik*, Paderborn: UTB.

Honnefelder, L. (1996b), *Nature and Status of the Embryo: Philosophical Aspects*, Unpublished manuscript for the Council of Europe's Third Symposion of Bioethics, 'Medically assisted procreation and the protection of the human embryo', Strasbourg, Dec 15-18, 1996.

Junker-Kenny, M. (1998), 'Der moralische Status des Embryos im Kontext der Reproduktionsmedizin' in Düwell, M. and Mieth, D. (eds), *Ethik in der Humangenetik*, Tübingen: Francke, 302-324.

Kant, Immanuel (1786), Grundlegung zur Metaphysik der Sitten (= GMS), BA 66.69f. ET: Groundwork of the Metaphysic of Morals, trans. and analyzed by H.J. Paton, New York: Harper, 1964, 96.98.

Mieth, D. (1998), *Moral und Erfahrung II. Entfaltung einer theologisch-ethischen Hermeneutik*, Freiburg i.Ue.: Universitätsverlag.

Mieth, D., (1999), 'Ethische Probleme der Humangenetik – eine Überprüfung üblicher Argumentationsformen', in Engels, E.-M. (ed), *Ethik in der Biomedizin*, Stuttgart.

Pröpper, T. (1995), 'Autonomie und Solidarität. Begründungsprobleme sozialethischer Verpflichtung' in Arens, E. (ed), *Anerkennung der Anderen*, Freiburg: Herder.

Steigleder, K. (1993), 'Menschenwürde – Zu den Orientierungsleistungen eines Fundamentalbegriffs normativer Ethik' in Wils, J.-P. (ed), *Orientierung durch Ethik? Eine Zwischenbilanz*, Paderborn: Schöningh.

Steigleder, K. (1997), 'The moral significance of potential persons' in Hildt, E. and Mieth, D. (eds), Aldershot: Ashgate.

4 Selection through prenatal diagnosis and preimplantation diagnosis

Hille Haker

Selection in PND and PID

In the context of biomedicine the term 'selection' is understood to refer to a decision for or against one or more human beings, namely for quantitative reasons in connection with surplus embryos or multiple pregnancies, or for qualitative reasons in connection with prenatal diagnosis (PND) and preimplantation diagnosis (PID). The qualitative reasons for selective actions can again be divided into medical and non-medical reasons.

Another distinction on the qualitative level is to be made between a negative decision against, and a positive decision in favour of a human being. Whereas PND usually involves a negative decision, PID involves both a negative and a positive decision (Testart 1995). Therefore, it is more precise, in this case, to speak of a *choice between* several embryos.

Selective actions differ according to the context in which they take place, to their aims, the subjects who are involved and the beings who are affected by the actions. For the moral evaluation, the conditions and types of actions are decicive. I will therefore examine some of the differences between PND and PID.

Selective decisions in PND and PID

To speak of a selective decision a pregnant woman makes after PND is not the same as to speak of a selective decision a biologist or physician, with the consent of the woman or couple, makes after PID. But in what way do the decisions and, finally, the actions involved in PND and PID differ?

The agent of selective abortion after PND is a woman who has originally wanted to bear a child (Kolker 1994). However, after having been confronted with diagnostic results, she has come to realise that she cannot bear to continue the pregnancy and give birth to a child that will be adversely affected in his or her health. In most European countries, we leave the decision to continue or terminate the pregnancy in this case to the pregnant women themselves. This is by no means a matter of course, as the practice in China might prove. However, in those European countries that allow termination of pregnancy this is the 'free choice' of the woman.[1]

The process of this decision-making, possibly resulting in the termination of pregnancy, is a heavy strain on the woman. The alternative options clearly show a dilemma: a situation of moral conflict which is not deliberately provoked and where two conflicting duties cannot be resolved by a clear preponderance of one or the other duty.

The option to continue the pregnancy means to make a decision in favour of a child that will lead a life that is considered not to be normal in our society. He or she will not only temporarily, but possibly constantly be dependent on other persons. However, the closest persons concerned will be the parents, and often enough it is primarily the mother who will have to take over the responsibility for her child. Not knowing how the 'defect' will affect her child, and not knowing what kind of life her child will have, the woman is very much dependent on the medical prognoses, on the sensitivity of her counselors (if there are any), on the expected individual and social support, and on her own experience and subjective estimation of what she can bear. Taking all this, she still must decide what is in the child's best interest and morally right. To decide in favour of the child, clearly deserves all respect and credit by others. On the other hand, termination of pregnancy must be tolerated, if it is the result of a thorough decision-making process.

For the option for selective abortion also means that the woman's life-plan is disrupted, at least as far as this particular child is concerned. Above that, it questions her implicit or explicit moral *ideals* of having and caring for a child of her own – a motive that usually accompanies the wish for a child. In deciding in favour of a selective abortion, the alleged biographical and social consequences for the child *and* herself lead a woman to the conclusion that she cannot bear the alleged strain. The consequences for her own life will probably be a much more significant motivation for the termination than the selective choice itself. In abortions after PND, therefore, selection is more a secondary, not directly intended *effect* than a primary and directly intended purpose. Nevertheless, the action has a selective effect, since the decision to terminate a pregnancy cannot exclude so-called qualitative reasons concerning the fetus.

Although it is often stated that PID has the advantage to avoid such dilemmas for the woman, it still causes problems for the ethical evaluation. In PID the decision to select an embryo is made before the pregnancy has begun. Therefore, the agent who decides is not or is not necessarily the woman alone. The decision is taken by a couple (presupposing that in vitro fertilisation [IVF] is open for couples only, so excluding single women), and a professional is much more involved than in a decision on an abortion. In what way does this constellation change the type of action?

First, there is a shift from attachment to detachment or non-attachment which is morally relevant in so far as it may encourage an objectivisaton of human embryos in the context of clinical research. Whereas during a pregnancy the emotional attachment of the woman to her child grows steadily, this process is already delayed through prenatal diagnosis. PID, however, connects the attachment to the child with qualitative criteria from the beginning, since selection already takes place when several embryos (or pre-embryos) are available, although no pregnancy has started so far. This qualitative criterion for the acceptance of a child might, depending on the kinds of PID-clients, be even more obvious to the male partner, since he does not have to bear strain of the IVF-procedure.

Furthermore, the attachment of parents to prospective offspring is influenced by perceptual factors. An embryo at the 4-8-cell-stage does not necessarily suggest a human being to be protected, whereas ultrasound pictures and published photographs of a fetus about the 14th week onwards clearly have changed not only our knowledge, but also our perception of the progress of development in this stage.

Finally, the expert who has no personal interest in the human embryo is interested in achieving a 'good' result of his/her work, namely a successful transfer and a healthy baby-take-home-rate (Lieberman, 1998, p. 318).

The non-attachment to a specific embryo or number of embryos on the part of the professional as well as on the part of the women or couples who wish for a child may lead to a shift in the decision-making. It could be that the professionals rather than the women or couples themselves decide what is bearable and what not, what is desirable, what not. Selective actions will at least partly be influenced by the professionals who with the consent of the women select the embryos according to guidelines set up by medical, political or ethical commissions.

Whether such a shift in decision-making is really taking place is an empirical question. However, the moral priority of female decision-making which holds for selective abortion after PND, might not be justified in the same way after PID.[2]

Second, another difference to PND becomes even more obvious when we take into consideration that the selective decision after PID is made for the purpose of selective choice only. While in selective abortions the presumed biographical and social consequences lead to the possibly tragic conflict of interests between the rights of the woman and those of the fetus, no moral dilemma of this kind is involved when the situation of embryo selection is deliberately provoked and intended. Of course, it is desirable and perhaps even morally demanded to help women to avoid the dilemma situation of selective abortion. Nevertheless, PID might not be the appropriate way to do so. In fact, it might be irresponsible and therefore morally wrong to bring about a situation where decision-making involves the violation and destruction of a form of human life.

Therefore, the shift from attachment to non-attachment with the consequences for the dominant agents, together with the change of purpose, lead to a different moral evaluation than is presupposed in the introduction of PID: tragic conflicts with regard to the termination of pregnancy may not be able to be exluded in praxis, even though the role of public support could (and should) change (Haker 1993) and although the *moral* justification of selective abortions is restricted to borderline cases (Haker 1997). Embryo selection after PID, however, is not the result of a moral conflict like abortion, but based on a positive decision made already with the introduction and application of PID. As a practice, this cannot be morally justified, if the 'production' of surplus embryos and thus the situation of choice between embryos could be avoided. Opponents of PID state that exactly this is the case, since nobody has a right to an own child, if this includes the destruction of another human being.

Nevertheless, such moral evaluation is based on the presupposition that embryos share rights and human dignity with all other stages of human life. But are the beings to be selected human beings whose rights outweigh the parental wish for, interest in or possibly right to a healthy child?

Selection of human embryos

Does it make a difference for moral reasoning with respect to selection whether the selected human being is an embryo or a fetus? To mention only a few of the arguments which are raised by the discussion: the abortion of a human being which is capable of suffering and even viable with the support of intensive care is an action that needs very strong justification to be permissible, if at all. On the other hand, only those who are responsible in that situation can estimate the borderline at which it becomes unbearable for them to care for a handicapped child. It is assumed that the woman who originally wanted the child will act in the child's best interest, but that the law, too, has to define borderlines. This is achieved by the formulation of indications, as for example the medical indication in the German law. Nothing is said about the moral status of the fetus in this law, and therefore the overall protection of human beings is presupposed. Only the physical and psychological health of the mother *threatened by the detected disease of the fetus* legally justifies termination beyond the 12th week of pregnancy. Thus, the German law avoids any statement on the fetus itself but protects the woman, whose health may not be endangered by her child. Still, this is a dissatisfying solution of the law, for mostly not the actual but the future health of the woman is threatened. This, however, cannot be stated scientific terms as it depends on the estimation of the physician and the woman herself. Furthermore, if somebody else would care for the child, the woman would not necessarily have the alleged health problems.

Compared to PND, in PID the moral status of the embryo becomes the central issue in the discussion. Usually it is argued that the human being in question is not yet an individual and definitely not capable of suffering. Therefore, it is maintained that PID should be preferred to PND on moral grounds, specifically with regard to the developmental stage of the being and the the possible avoidance of personal tragedies by selective abortions.

Although this line of argument seems at first glance to be consistent, the element of selection that has to be morally judged connects PND and PID tightly in the following respect: by the destruction of 'affected' embryos as well as by the abortion of 'affected' fetuses human beings are excluded from the community of 'desired beings' on account of their quality, characteristics or disease. Whereas in PND this criterion of quality must be regarded as part of a complex decision, with PID, it becomes decisive for the first time. If this is so, then the moral question is not so much and not only whether it is preferable to avoid an abortion by PID but whether selection for qualitative reasons can be justified. Morality demands to treat all people equal in so far as fundamental respect is concerned. Up to the present, this has been true for all stages of human life although the subjects of respect do not in all cases and not in all phases of their lives fulfill the criterion of being a moral agent or person in a strict sense. Thus, even abortion is not to be seen as a mere choice of a pregnant woman but rather as a solution of a dilemmatic conflict which must be tolerated but which should be avoided. Embryo selection, on the other hand, divides human beings in those who deserve respect and those who do not. The current biomedical praxis is a good example of this shift.

For quite a time now the borderline has been drawn between those embryos which are transferred to the woman and eventually developed further, and those which are not meant to being transferred at all, but used for embryo experimentation or for other, so-called non-reproductive diagnostic measures

(HERP 1994, Khushf 1997, GAEIB on Cloning 1997, Mieth 1997). Embryo selection after PID is a further case which underlines that the embryo *as such* is not considered to have rights at all or rights which are insurmountable if other interests must be weighed against his or her protection.

However, can this biomedical practice which is based on explicit policies and, as in some countries, legal regulations, be morally justified? Are there moral arguments which allow us to draw a normative line between human beings either of different stages of development or even of the same developmental stage?

This problem, hidden already in the selective abortions after PND, is radicalised when unveiled in selective actions in connection with PID. Admittedly, I do not see an argument for restricting human dignity to those beings who are meant to be born. One and the same moral standard must be applied to those cases that can be considered equal. The destiny of a human being does not determine his or her current moral status. On the contrary, the moral status determines what may be done to this human being, and what may not be done. The often stated argument that the 'natural loss' of embryos is fairly high in the first weeks of pregnancy, certainly is not valid as moral argument, since 'nature' is nor moral agent, while persons are indeed responsible for their actions.

Neither do I see an argument that would allow such a division of human dignity for genetic reasons. Again the opposite is the case: morality is meant to protect human beings from being discriminated on the grounds of their biological constitution.

Only if moral rights were completely denied to pre-embryos or embryos no moral problem does arise, because in this case neither the unaffected nor the affected embryo must be protected. On the other hand, if the basic rights of all human beings from conception onwards are considered to be equal, there is no balancing necessary either. In all other lines of argument, the question of how to balance the embryos' rights against possibly existing rights of others is put up for discussion. In everyday thinking, we very well make a difference between an adult person and an embryo, and this is not only empirical but also normative relevant. Therefore, if morality demands recognition of human beings regardless of their actual biological status this differentiation must be interpreted *within* this paradigm. The only way to achieve this will be to balance conflicting interests of two parties who *as such* have no different moral status but whose concrete rights and thus the claims on others still differ.

But even though it could well be that there is no *categorical* argument for embryo protection, since the concept of unique human dignity is more a tradition of thought than a rationally justifiable, there might be a basic misunderstanding of the moral situation we are dealing with, when it is concluded from this that in the cases of embryo research, assisted procreaton and PID the embryo's protection can be put aside. For if one holds that overruling the right or interest of an embryo may be justified in certain cases, these cases must still be considered thoroughly. To state that a human embryo has not the same moral status as a person, does not mean that the embryo has no moral status as such. To determine the embryo's protection right within the concept of human dignity would mean that the conflicting rights of other persons must be taking so serious that balancing is unavoidable. This is exactly the case in PND.

PID implies, as I have argued, selection as direct purpose of an action. A moral right to selection would only exist if two premises concerning conflicting rights were morally right. First, that there is a positive right to assisted procreation of a child of one's own, and a right to a genetically unaffected child in particular; second, that it is morally not forbidden to 'produce' embryos which are not directly intended to be transferred to a woman's womb. I certainly cannot argue the matter here fully, but both premises to me appear to be morally doubtful.

First, how can there be a positive right to a genetically unaffected child, if no medical diagnosis can guarantee this which is to say: nobody can possibly meet this claim? A right presupposes a duty of somebody else. However, this specific duty cannot be fulfilled, since no diagnosis can make a statement on the overall health condition of the future child. Furthermore and with respect to the would-be selective right: there is no moral ground for the right of one person to be based on the discrimination of another. Even though a pre-embryo is not a person in the strict sense of the word, there is no need to refuse him or her the protection we associate with the term of human being, ultimately based on our understanding of dignity. A couple which knows before conception (or fertilisation) and thus *before* the woman is pregnant that they will not be able to bear the strain of a genetically affected child, might misunderstand the potential responsibility that is implied with parenthood and child-rearing. Here, the best interests standard for the child has its appropriate place (Kopelman 1997).[3]

Second, a society which upholds different understandings of human dignity with respect to genetically affected and unaffected human beings might misunderstand the concept of universal respect as well as the concept of tolerance. European societies which tolerate selective abortions after PND (although they should only tolerate it in restricted cases), should not tolerate the promotion of selective actions by professionals of corporate bodies, since these touch the cornerstones of unique respect for human beings stated in all kinds of conventions on human rights. They should also not publicly support the understandable parental wish for, but unjustified interest in a healthy child, since even to meet this interest partly, it would imply the production and destruction of human beings for the purpose of selection.

Moral respect demands the respect for the other as an other, no matter what his or her biological constitution may be. In the gray area of gradual development and graduality of moral rights there must at least be a moral dilemma situation that forces us to weigh up rights (Gewirth 1978). If a moral conflict can be solved without disrespecting justified interests or even rights of the persons or beings affected, this solution must be preferred. This still might not be a perfect solution for either side, but sometimes it might be the only one that is acceptable for all beings affected.

Notes

1 There is social pressure involved with this question, as the stories of women who have had an abortion after PND report. But it is very difficult to prove this empirically, cf. E. Beck-Gernsheim (1997).
2 It might well be that there are indirect reasons that still justify a priority: these would be initially the physical strain of IVF, its low success-rate and the health risk that is connected with it.
3 Kopelman defends the best interest standard, but distinguishes between its employment as a threshold for intervention and judgment, as an ideal for establishing prima facie duties and policies, and as a standard of reasonableness.

References

Beck-Gernsheim, E. (1997), 'Wer heilt, hat Recht?', in Elstner, M. (ed.), *Gentechnik, Ethik und Gesellschaft*, Springer: Berlin et al., pp. 81-96.

Gewirth, A. (1978), *Reason and Morality*, Chicago University Press: Chicago.

Group of Advisors on the Ethical Implications of Biotechnology of the European Commission (1997), *Opinion of the Group of Advisors on the Ethical Implications of Biotechnology to the European Commission: Ethical Aspects of Cloning Techniques*, 28.2.1997.

Haker, H. (1993), 'Human Genome Analysis and Eugenics', in Haker, H., Steigleder, K. and Hearn, R. (eds), *Ethics of Human Genome Analysis. European Perspectives*, Attempto: Tübingen, pp. 290-323.

Haker, H. (1997), 'Ethical Responsibility in Prenatal Genetic Diagnosis', *Biomedical Ethics*, Vol. 2, No. 3, pp. 78-85.

Handyside, A.H. and Delhanty, J.D.A. (1997), 'Preimplantation Genetic Diagnosis: Strategies and Surprises', *Trends in Genetics*, Vol. 13, No. 7, pp. 270-5.

Health Council of the Netherlands: Standing Committee on Medical ethics and health law (1995), *Sex Selection for Non-medical Reasons*, 1995/11.

Human Embryo Research Panel (HERP) (1994), *Report of the Human Embryo Research Panel*, National Institutes of Health, Bethseda.

Jonsen, A. (1995), 'Reproduction and Rationality', *Cambridge Quarterly,* No. 4, pp. 263-7.

Khushf, G. (1997), 'Embryo Research: The Ethical Geography of the Debate', *Journal of Medicine and Philosophy,* Vol. 22, pp. 495-519.

Kolker, A. and Burke, B.M. (1994), *Prenatal Testing. A Sociological Perspective*, Bergin and Garvey: Westport et al.

Kopelman, L. (1995), 'The Best-interests Standard as Threshold, Idea, and Standard of Reasonableness', *Journal of Medicine and Philosophy*, Vol. 22, pp. 271-89.

Lieberman, B.A. (1998), 'Limits of Reproductive Technology', Hildt, E. and Mieth, D. (eds), *In Vitro Fertilisation in the 1990s. Towards a Medical, Social and Ethical Evaluation*, Ashgate: Aldershot, pp. 317-24.

Michaelis, M. and Buckle, S. (1990), 'Screening for Genetic Disorders: Therapeutic Abortion and IVF', *Journal of Medical Ethics*, Vol. 16, pp. 43-7.

Mieth, D. (1998), 'Probleme der Ethik in der Biomedizin. Das Beispiel der Klonierungsdebatte', *Orientierung*, Vol. 62, pp. 41-6.

Testart, J. (1995), 'The New Eugenics and Medicalized Reproduction', *Cambridge Quarterly of Healthcare Ethics*, No. 4, pp. 304-12.

Part Four
SOCIAL CONCEPTS AND MORAL IMPLICATIONS

1 Eugenics comes back with medically assisted procreation

Bernard Sèle and Jacques Testart

The considerable improvements achieved in mapping the human genome should not give rise to false ideas: today's medical genetics still remains a medicine in its infancy. This medicine is neither curative nor palliative because it does not have any therapeutic tool. It is not a preventive medicine either because the occurrence of a genetic accident is a completely unpredictable event. The improvements achieved in the knowledge of the human genome make it a descriptive medicine. Its single objective is to recognise and identify the accident, and then to avoid the worst, which is its reoccurrence.

It would be pointless to base our hopes on gene therapy on germinal cells for two reasons: first, even if it was efficient enough to treat individual embryos, it would only be performed after the accident had occured once, so that the abnormality to be cured would have been identified, second, it will not be useful since the genetic sorting of the embryos will allow the selection of unaffected embryos.

Reproductive medicine has several aspects. First, fertility was neutralised and sterilisation campaigns with openly eugenic objectives were set up in democratic countries at the beginning of this century. Later contraception arose and is characterised by its reversibility. Then medicine took care of infertility. Because of its lack of therapeutic tools it actually bypasses (rather than solves) the problem by trying to satisfy the desire of a child without treating the handicap (which persists after the birth of a child). Reproductive medicine started 30 years ago in the area of male infertility. The practice of AID (or artificial insemination with donors) was taken out of the realm of secrecy and profit. But this practice is only a substitute for a treatment because it distorts the parental project by introducing alongside the couple a third person as the sperm donor. Later the first palliative treatment for female infertility appeared with in vitro fertilisation (IVF). More recently male infertility also benefited from a palliative medicine with the development of assisted fertilisation by intracytoplasmic sperm injection (ICSI) (microinjection of one sperm into the oocyte).

Today's ethical considerations should take into account the joint evolution of genetics and reproductive medicine, and especially their conjunction which results in preimplantation diagnosis (PID) of an embryo obtained by IVF. We will concentrate on showing how the evolutions of these approaches were based on the same ideology. To illustrate our purpose we will successively look at:

– the evolution in the practice of artificial insemination with donor sperm;
– the arguments usually used against the practice of sperm injection into the oocyte (or ICSI);
– the future of PID.

The practice of artificial insemination with donor sperm

Sperm banks were first constituted with anonymous donors. When samples were delivered, only ethnic types and blood groups were taken into account, in order to mimic compatibility (even if today this kind of pairing is totally inadequate because of genetic printing technologies).

A consensus then appeared to analyse the donors' chromosomes systematically, so that carriers of balanced chromosomal abnormalities would be eliminated, because of the higher risk for their offspring of being born with a handicap. However, the donors' population is biased because for psychological reasons only men who have had children are recruited. So this population is different from the infertile male population in that the incidence of balanced chromosomal abnormality is lower, and the fact they have fathered healthy children minimises the risk even more. It is now also known that, unlike genetic diseases, most chromosomal abnormalities (such as trisomy 21) are not inherited from parental abnormalities. They arise by accident, and on top of that, they are more often of maternal origin. Finally most of these abnormalities are eliminated by spontaneous abortions. Under these conditions the systematic analysis of the chromosomes of sperm donors seems unnecessary and unable to reduce the genetic risk. It could even be considered harmful because it engenders a false feeling of security in those who advocate the least risk. This practice of the genetic identification of the donors went even further with family genetic inquiries. These inquiries are the same as those used in medical genetics when a genetic disease is diagnosed in a family.

The method for investigation is the same: it uses genealogy (family tree study) to estimate the likelihood that the donor is an unknown carrier of genes known to be deleterious. As a result of this inquiry, three situations can arise: 1) the donor is considered to be free from any genetic risk (this is the rare situation), 2) the donor has a high risk of carrying a dominant deleterious gene and is therefore rejected (this is equally a rare situation), 3) the donor has a high probability of carrying some recessive deleterious genes or polygenic unfavourable characteristics (and this is the most frequent situation). The donor is then accepted, but his sperm samples will not be given to a woman in whose family the same unfavourable factors have been identified. Indeed, in theory these genes are only dangerous when they are associated through fertilisation with mutations of the same nature from the partner. So gradually a policy of genetic pairing between donors and inseminated women was set up. The choice could have been made to respect the random character of natural procreation. Genetic pairing has been prefered with the legitimate excuse of preventing genetic handicaps.

However this handicap prevention is virtually impossible (since it targets the parental phenotype). Even if the handicap prevention were efficacious, this logic goes beyond the request of the infertile couple which is, in fact, not to conceive a child of better 'quality' than is allowed by natural procreation.

The child to be born is therefore invested with the false idea of least defect, and here we enter into an attitude that promotes the rejection of the deviants from the norm.

Arguments against ICSI

This more recently developed technique was the first to allow an effective response to male infertility. It consists of injecting one sperm directly into the oocyte. As with previously developed techniques, there were questions about the innocuity of ICSI. This time the criticisms were louder than ever, and the practice was explicitly compared to experiments on human beings sanctioned by the Nuremberg laws. After several thousands of births by ICSI it appears that in fact this technique is safe for public health. However alarmist comments continue to spread. But these are about genetic risk and even praise the advantage of insemination with genetically checked (controlled) sperm donors. In fact for the first time the question is raised of sterile men's offspring. There was concern that a sperm which was unable to fertilise would contribute to the genetic constitution of the fertilised egg. It is genetically assumed that an individual sperm, unable to fertilise, would be more likely to have an abnormal genetic constitution. According to this assumption, sterility would then be a natural protection against the handicap. The same principle would also apply to the ejaculate of a fertile man: the spermatozoa would compete to fertilise the oocyte and the highest chance of transmitting a good 'quality' genetic constitution would be given to those more able to fertilise. However numerous scientific arguments seem to support the opposite hypothesis, that there is no correlation between fertility and the genetic content of a sperm, except if a sperm has grossly abnormal morphology. Therefore an infertile male would have no greater risk of transmitting an impaired genetic constitution than a fertile male. This notion is also supported by the observation of several thousands of children born after ICSI. By the way, it is worth noticing here that the treatment of dysovulation in women has never raised the same questions, although ovulation problems are sometimes related to genetic disorders.

However in some male infertilities a genetic origin is now proven or suspected. In these cases, all the somatic cells and high proportions (if not all) of the sperm carry the same genetic abnormality that is responsible for the infertility. In this specific context, the child conceived despite sterility is at risk of inheriting the problem. Some argue that ICSI should not be used if there is a risk of perpetuating sterility. One can oppose this argument with the fact that, because of ICSI, male infertility cannot be considered as a major handicap anymore, even when it is of genetic origin. Otherwise medical treatment for infertility should be refused to any patient with diabetes, or short sight, or obesity etc.

Therefore some criticisms which are opposed to ICSI seem to be questioning its genetic innocuity but are in fact of eugenic nature (and would naturally lead to preference for a genetically selected sperm donor, or for a PID of the embryos conceived by ICSI).

The future of PID

PID is the result of the conjunction of technologies used in reproductive medicine and molecular genetics. Indeed, it is based on the genetic identification of eggs obtained by IVF. It is often presented as an improvement of prenatal diagnosis (PND) and is offered today to couples exposed to a high risk of a severe genetic disease. The abnormality that has to be detected should be known before, and the use of the diagnosis is a consequence of genetic counselling. Although the couples usually do not have a fertility problem, IVF is required for PID. PID is often presented as an interesting alternative to PND because it avoids medical abortion which is the outcome of an unfavourable PND. PID technologies are gradually being set up for various genetic diseases in several laboratories, but it is worth noting that most published cases involve infertile couples. Therefore a drift is already being observed in the applications. It is as if infertility is becoming more important than genetic reasons, and that infertility in practice provides the opportunity to perform genetic diagnosis. However, the infertile candidate population for IVF is much larger than the population of fertile couples exposed to a genetic risk who are candidates for PID. One can therefore expect a change in the nature of PID requirements with a level of expectations different from the couples exposed to a known severe genetic risk. For instance, in the US PID is already offered to women over 38 years of age and candidates for IVF.

PID should not be seen as an improvement of PND because it is fundamentally different. Specific samplings, (e.g. trophoblast or amniotic fluid ponction) are only performed for prenatal diagnosis. This diagnosis is performed on one fetus only, which is eliminated in the case of a genetic handicap. On the other hand, PID requires an IVF which is also performed in a context of treatment of infertility. PID is performed on several fertilised eggs and possibly on high numbers of embryos, if several IVFs are performed in a short period of time. It therefore provides a real opportunity for genetic sorting of the embryos, which PND on one fetus cannot offer. The future of PID is already recognisable in the drift in application noted above, which is due to the fact that its procedure allows the medical doctor to detect too much and then make choices. What is unacceptable in the PID is not the first choice of the embryos unaffected by the genetic disease, but the subsequent choice of embryos corresponding to any particular wish of parents under social pressure. Given such power, it is unlikely that medical science will resist the temptation to satisfy parents' wishes in offering them a child not only unaffected by the genetic disease that was the purpose of the diagnosis, but also the brother that is missing in a girl's family, and gradually other, more utopic options. This is how PID could lead to a painless rejection of potential children through the control of numerous fertilised eggs, many more at each attempt than all the fetuses that could possibly be submitted to PND in an entire life time. Compared with the genetic selection of sperm donors, PID is a better method for scientific eugenics because its target is the fertilised egg in which genetic constitution is completed. And since PID is a much more efficient eugenic alternative than PND, it will make higher standards in the estimation of what is tolerable and/or acceptable in society. Because PID offers incomparable possibilities of choice, the way will be open to look for risk factors with no limits, especially when our knowledge of the human genome is continuously expanding. We will be far then from the basic eugenics of PND which is the only acceptable one, since it only allows the avoidance of the worst and the rejection of some too painful lives. Today's concern is therefore to decide about boundaries within which the eugenics which follows the evolution of medicine can be contained.

How to guard against eugenics

Let us suppose that only the couple should define genetic standards for their children. Given the conformity of individual desires to collective models, if only parental desire was to be respected, there would be no reason to be opposed to other possibilities offered by artificial reproduction, such as cloning or parthenogenesis. The notion of a child's quality brings up too many real or imagined interests for social institutions to be able to rely on such a spontaneous regulation. For example, sperm banks could have put official limits on their responsibilities, by giving up genetic control in the recruitment of sperm donors. The social conditions under which donor recruitment takes place, as well as elementary sanitary precautions in terms of public health, would have been sufficient to guarantee good practice. Eugenic ambitions have to be slowed down so that they do not become unlimited phantasies. Since it is not possible to define the difference between a severe disease and a light handicap, nor to establish a limited list of impediments which would be relevant for PID, this practice has potentially unlimited fields of application. This is why there is no alternative to being against PID, even when it is justified at a human and individual level. This extreme position should be maintained until society has had sufficient time to make clear and informed decisions. Much determination will be needed to resist the ideology will of molecular medicine and its eugenic inspiration. It will even be more difficult since these new options are connected to considerable professionable and industrial interests. They also fulfil phantasies from time immemorial which make them attractive to users.

References

Testart, J. and Sèle, B. (1995), 'Towards an Efficient Medical Eugenics: Is the Desirable Always the Feasible?', *Human Reproduction*, Vol. 10, pp. 3086-90.

Testart, J. and Sèle, B. (1996), 'Le diagnostic préimplantatoire n'est pas un diagnostic prénatal précoce', *Méd Sci*, pp. 1398-401.

2 Germline gene 'therapy': Public opinions with regard to eugenics

Sigrid Graumann

Scientists and ethicists often lament the emotionality and irrationality of the various positions maintained by critics of germline gene 'therapy'[1] in political discussion and in the media. This is particularly the case with respect to positions which rely on a characterisation of germline gene 'therapy' as eugenic (Fletcher 1995). The role of applied ethics in this context is primarily viewed as that of contributing to the rationality and objectivity of the discussion. The public is to be informed.[2] I want to advance the hypothesis that the bioethical discussion up until now has not achieved this and has not been able to achieve it, because under the notion of eugenics quite different things are understood. According to position and context, the notion of eugenics is given a biological, historical or socio-cultural interpretation. I will briefly sketch these three different interpretations, which incidentally are not always separable, so that I can afterwards show which positions and arguments are to be located on which level of interpretation. I want to argue that it is possible to reconstruct rationally a core of the positions which rely on a socio-cultural understanding of eugenics and that this core provides a good argument against germline gene 'therapy'. First however I want to address the positions which are maintained in the public.

The discussion of germline gene 'therapy' in the German media

When germline gene 'therapy' is referred to in the German media it is generally handled like a hot potato and treated with considerable reserve. For the most part, it is rejected 'on account of the intentional transmission of altered germ-cells'.[3] When negative consequences are pointed out, alongside incalculable risks, 'eugenic consequences'[4] play a particular role:

> Whoever allows this kind of therapy accepts the next step to the intentional direction of genetic material, to eugenics, as well.[5]

Nevertheless, one can in no sense speak of uniform rejection or ban on discussion of germline gene 'therapy' in the German media. Future 'help for suffering human beings'[6] or the possibility that 'the frequency of serious inherited diseases can be cut down' is also discussed.[7] The various attitudes in the media demonstrate, however, the controversial nature of germline gene 'therapy' in public debate and witness the fact that germline interventions are associated with 'eugenic consequences' which are in general rejected.

What does 'eugenics' mean?

Francis Galton introduced the notion of eugenics in 1883. By this term he understood the applied science of human genetics with the goal of limiting the distribution of genes with disadvantageous effects in human populations on the one hand (negative eugenics), and of maintaining or even increasing desired gene-constellations on the other (positive eugenics).[8]

This means that the biological definition of 'eugenics' in modern scientific discourse is the improvement of the human genome. In this context the issue is not the genome of an individual human being, but rather the gene pool, which is defined as the genes of *the* or *a* human population as a whole. It is also important that although 'eugenics' is a scientific notion, it nevertheless, due to its aim of 'improving the human gene pool', contains an unambiguously normative presupposition. If therefore one speaks in the context of germline gene 'therapy' of eugenics in a biological sense, a genetic manipulation of the human germ-cell with the goal of the genetic improvement of the human species (or of a particular community of human beings, for example a 'race') and therefore a *material* change is meant.[9]

Eugenics received its historical significance through its political application in Europe and North America in the first half of this century, and here particularly due to its connections to the crimes which were carried out in the name of eugenics during the Third Reich.[10] In Germany, the 'Law for the Prevention of Genetically Ill Progeny' was enacted in 1933, as a consequence of which hundreds of thousands of allegedly 'genetically damaged' people were sterilised. In 1939, the bureaucratic preparation of the eugenically motivated euthanasia programme began. By the time public discontent led to the official discontinuation of the euthanasia programme in 1941, more than 70,000 patients had been killed (Schmuhl 1987, p. 220 ff.).[11] After the end of the Second World War, the full extent of the crimes which in the name of eugenics had been committed against sick and handicapped in Germany was made internationally public.

In the years after World War II, eugenics became a dirty word (Reich 1995).

From the perspective of historical investigation, eugenics is to be understood as a social project, in which eugenics as a scientific discipline – and it was acknowledged and established as such in contemporary scientific community – admittedly plays a decisive role, however, it is not limited to this. The clear interweaving of science, ideology, research and demographic politics in the notion of the 'improvement of the human race' is evidence of this. If reference is made in the context of germline gene 'therapy' to the historical experience of the crimes which have been perpetrated in the name of eugenics, this is going beyond the historical facts. The continuity of eugenic goals in science and politics is being asserted and a warning is being given about new violations of human rights of which science and politics are considered to be capable on account of historical experience (Meyer-Seethaler 1997, p. 311).

The socio-cultural perspective concentrates, thus overriding the historical experience of the crimes of eugenically motivated politics and the danger of a 'relapse', on the interrelationship between science, politics and mass consciousness in the contemporary world. Eugenics is described as a socio-cultural phenomenon which develops not by means of laws, repression and violence, but rather through the 'regulation' of mass consciousness. There is talk in connection with prenatal diagnosis of 'mothers under the pressure of private eugenics'[12] or of the preparation of a 'eugenic thinking'.[13] Positions against germline gene 'therapy' which refer to a socio-cultural understanding of eugenics of this sort fear that due to the interconnection of science, politics and mass consciousness, social norms and pressures become established which make free and responsible decisions with respect to an offer of germline gene 'therapy' impossible. In the words of Elisabeth Beck-Gernsheim, the profile of demand for parents would change – the 'quality child' would become a 'social duty' (Beck-Gernsheim 1991, p. 56).[14]

177

Bio-ethical answers to the fear of a 'new eugenics'

In the (international) ethical discussion of germline gene 'therapy', a whole row of controversial positions have been maintained which are clearly based on a purely biological but nevertheless normative understanding of eugenics (a reduced understanding for analytical purposes) which has in that form scarcely played any role in the public debate (in the German media). For example, it is argued that through the elimination of monogenetic defects, future suffering could be avoided, or that there can be no objection to improving the human genetic constitution with a view to reducing suffering (Zimmerman 1991). It is stated that there can be no objection to germline gene 'therapy' as a form of positive eugenics, since we already intervene in the human genetic constitution in prenatal genetic diagnosis. (The comparison with established practices, however, says absolutely nothing per se about the moral legitimacy of such practices.) Opposing voices fear a loss of genetic diversity in the human gene pool which could offer possibilities for adapting to changing environmental conditions. Against all these 'evolution arguments', Davis objects that 'principles of population genetics offer no support for this hope'. Given that most homozygous genes which can lead to a monogenetic disease are recessive and therefore occur unnoticed in the population, and that dominant inherited defects in most cases arise through new mutations, germline gene 'therapy' cannot achieve 'the theoretical ideal of purifying the gene pool' at all (Davis 1992). This is certainly a valid and important argument: it does not, however, banish the fear that eugenic goals are held to despite this, so to speak 'irrationally'.

Various concrete arguments have also been criticised in the ethical discussion of germline gene 'therapy' which have been maintained in the political sphere and in the media. Among these positions are arguments to the effect that we should not play God (Rifkin 1986), and the rejection of intervention in the germline with reference to nature or to a right to the randomness of the genetic origin of the human genome (Catenhusen et al. 1987). The fact, however, that a situation up to now has been physically unchangeable is not in and of itself a good reason for its morally unchangeable, even when the burden of proof resides with those who want to alter the existing circumstances (Wimmer 1989). These kinds of arguments for or against germline gene 'therapy' appear in general to regard the human genome as a 'collective soul of mankind, the human essence, in which we all participate' (Mauron 1993). From the perspective of a socio-cultural understanding of eugenics, one can accuse all of these positions not only of not being maintainable, but even of promoting 'eugenic thinking'.

From the perspective of a deontological conception of ethics, a genetic improvement with eugenic goals is not compatible with our understanding of human rights, the dignity of the human being, the nature of the person as a good in and of him- or herself and her or his resulting freedom of self-determination (Wimmer 1989). That is in my opinion the most important argument against germline gene 'therapy' with a eugenic purpose. If, however, eugenics today is indirectly expressed as a socio-cultural phenomenon by means of social norms and pressures – and this is obviously a major concern in the public debate – then this position does not address the entire problem.

The discussion of so called 'slippery slope' arguments in the ethical discussion of germline gene 'therapy' can be understood as a reflex to those fears in the public debate which refer to a reoccurance of historical experiences with eugenics. Here the decisive question is seen as being whether in a democratic society in contrary to a totalitary regime a boundary line can be drawn between therapeutic and non-therapeutic uses of germline gene 'therapy' by means of moral and legal regulations. In this sense it is suggested, for example, that the distinction between 'maladies' and 'non-maladies' be the boundary line. Suffering is only then to be described as a 'malady' when it is connected with 'death, pain, disability, loss of freedom and pleasure.' In such cases, a 'general interest of avoiding these evils' can be reckoned with. Germline gene 'therapy' is to be limited to maladies because borderline conditions contain the danger of a slippery slope, (Berger and Gert 1991). Against such attempts at drawing boundary lines because of the danger of sliding down the slope, Gardner argues that 'the relevant moral distinction will not adequately influence our choices', for the reason that genetic enhancement 'will be undermined by the dynamics of competition among parents and among nations' (Gardner 1995). As further factors which could facilitate a slippery slope development, the alleged prevalence of the perception of eugenics in society (McGleenan 1995) and 'the force of scientific interests' are mentioned. I doubt, however, that here the concerns of the public about the development of a 'new eugenics' are really being addressed. From the historical perspective one would have to say that eugenically motivated sterilisations and murders were carried out on genuinely sick and handicapped individuals without them being any the less morally reprehensible. For this reason even the basic distinction between 'enhancement' and 'therapy' in this context does not seem to be valid. Beyond this, most of these attempts to draw boundary lines imply at least the 'life worth living' predication of 'eugenic thinking' as well.

The socio-cultural phenomenon 'eugenics' as an argument against germline gene 'therapy'

According to an understanding of 'eugenics' as a socio-cultural phenomenon, however, it is precisely in this 'life worth living' predication, along with the availability of the new medical techniques, that the problem lies. Viewed from a sociological perspective, the standards against which actions are evaluated begin to shift as soon as changes start to take place in the scope for action (Beck-Gernsheim 1991, p. 41). To use Foucault's word, the biopower is here at work. 'Biopower' is directed at individuals as well as at the population as a whole. It intends monitoring, control and increase of the physical efficiency of individual bodies as well as the regulation of the population (Foucault 1983, p. 61 ff.). This modern form of power is not something which is outside society and affects it from outside, but rather a phenomenon which permeates society itself.[15]

> We find ourselves accordingly inside a power which has taken control of the body and of life, or which [...] has occupied life with the poles of the body on one side and the population on the other (Foucault 1983, p. 40).

The relationship between the individual and the social dimension of germline gene 'therapy' can be understood with Foucault as a phenomenon of the 'society of normalisation' in which the norm of the disciplining of the body and the norm of the regulation of the population are bound together (Foucault 1983, p. 40). This means that the norms which are produced in the 'truth discourse' of the medical community and the norms which are reproduced in other discourses in, for example, the media which relate the question of what is to be considered as sick and healthy, or rather desirable and undesirable, are aimed, together with the new medical techniques (the future availability of germ line gene 'therapy' and the already available prenatal genetic diagnosis), at the disciplining of individuals with respect to their decisions about reproduction and at the regulation of the quality of the gene pool. And precisely this is eugenics as a socio-cultural project which is carried out by means of supposedly 'autonomous' individual decisions. The controversial and emotionally loaded discussion of germline gene 'therapy' and of gene- and biotechnology in general can be interpreted as an expression of the fact that the issue has to do with a hotly contested field of the 'biopower' or rather of 'biopolitics': as Foucault points out, power and resistance against power always occur together. The 'emotional' voices in the public debate which argue against germline gene 'therapy' with recourse to its 'eugenic character' would in this case be reflexes of resistance to an indirect heteronomy in decisions regarding reproduction. The development of germline gene 'therapy' would undermine the right to make free decisions with respect to future parenthood.[16] Given that freedom is the prerequisite for moral actions and that the availability of germline gene 'therapy' would be connected with serious moral problems, there are a number of things which from a socio-ethical point of view speak against the development of germline gene 'therapy'. Perhaps

Foucault can be interpreted in this sense when he advocates that we give ourselves 'the legal rules, the leadership techniques and also the morals, the ethos, the praxis of the self, which make it possible to play within the power games at the cost of a minimum of dominance' (Foucault 1993, p. 25).

Notes

1 The term therapy is consequently set in signs of quotation, because it is not clear at all if there could be a therapeutic option of germline genetic engineering.

2 Not only in the popular media, but also in medical and ethical publications authors work with the expected emotional response of the reader. This takes place, for example, in case-descriptions, when the probable future deterioration of a child with a particular genetic disease is movingly described. In the example which has been analysed by Tod Chambers with respect to the rhetoric of case-descriptions (in a different clinical context), the role of emotional responses becomes particularly clear (Chambers 1996).

3 From an analysis of the Frankfurter Rundschau, Jäger et al. 1997, p. 123.

4 From an analysis of the ZEIT, Jäger et al. 1997, p. 183.

5 From: 'Darf man in Keimzellen eingreifen?' ZEIT 24, 6. 1994, cited according to Jäger et al. 1997, p. 183.

6 From an analysis of the ZEIT, Jäger et al. 1997, p. 183.

7 From an analysis of Focus, Jäger et al. 1997, p. 218.

8 This is expressed in newer terms; Galton did not use the word gene, because this expression for a unit of inheritage was later introduced by Johnson.

9 It is asserted in this context that the germline gene 'therapy' – to the extent that it could be applied successfully in the future – would make an entirely new quality of positive eugenics possible, because with it eugenics not only needs to be carried out by means of selection of the parents who engage in reproduction, but can instead be effected through direct intervention in the genetic constitution of the progeny.

10 I dicuss here only the German history of eugenics, which however does not mean that eugenics can be reduced to this: there were laws in force in almost all US federal states until the 1930s which made the sterilisation of the psychologically ill, criminals and the homeless compulsory. As criticism arose, the eugenic policies of the 30s were stopped in most states (Reich 1995). Research policy however, in particular that of the Rockefeller programme, continued nevertheless to pursue eugenic ideals (Kay 1993).

11 With the stopping of the T4-Action in 1941, the mass killing of the sick and handicapped was by no means at an end. It was more or less secretly continued (Schmuhl, 1987, p. 220 ff.).

12 From an analysis of the TAZ, Jäger et al. 1997, p. 107.

13 From an analysis of the Frankfurter Rundschau, Jäger et al. 1997, p. 125.

14 It is of course not being maintained that eugenics as a socio-culural phenomenon originally arises because of germline gene 'therapy'. On the contrary, given the selection of fetuses (prenatal diagnosis) and embryons (preimplantation diagnosis) as a result of gene diagnosis, social pressure to make use of this new technologies are viewed as already existing.

15 According to Foucault, power is more exercised than possessed and operates primarily productively (Sawicki 1991, p. 21).

16 This is ultimately the case when the power relationships are no longer dynamic but instead have hardended into dominance.

'It seems to me one has to distinguish between power relationships as strategic games between freedoms (that is, games in which one group tries to determine the behaviour of another, and the other responds with the attempt not to allow itself to be determined or on their part to determine the behaviour of the first group) and conditions of dominance, that is, what one usually calls power' (Foucault 1993, p. 25).

References

Beck-Gernsheim, E. (1991), *Technik, Markt und Moral. Über Reproduktionsmedizin und Gentechnologie*, Frankfurt a.M.

Berger, E.M., Gert, B.M. (1991), 'Genetic Disorders and the Ethical Status of Germline Gene Therapy', *The Journal of Medicine and Philosophy* Vol. 16, pp. 667-83.

Catenhusen, W.-M. and Neumeister, H. (eds) (1990), *Chancen und Risiken der Gentechnologie. Dokumentation des Berichts an den Deutschen Bundestag*, Campus: Frankfurt a.M.

Chambers, T. (1996), 'Dax Redacted: The Economics of Truth in Bioethics', *The Journal of Medicine and Philosophy*, Vol. 21, pp. 287-302.

Davis, B.D. (1992), 'Germline Therapy: Evolutionary and Moral Considerations', *Human Gene Therapy*, Vol. 3, pp 361-3.

Fletcher, J.C. (1994), 'Germline Gene Therapy: The Costs of Premature Ultimates', *Politics and the Life Sciences*, Vol. 13, No. 2, pp. 225-7.

Foucault, M. (1983), *Der Wille zum Wissen. Sexualität und Wahrheit 1,* Suhrkamp: Frankfurt a.M.

Foucault, M. (1993), *Freiheit und Selbstsorge. Interview 1984 und Vorlesung 1982*, Frankfurt.

Gardner, W. (1995), 'Can Human Genetic Enhancement Be Prohibited?', *The Journal of Medicine and Philosophy* Vol. 20, pp. 65-84.

Jäger, M., Jäger, S., Ruth, I., Schulte-Holtey, E. and Wichert, F. (1997), *Biomacht und Medien. Wege in die Bio-Gesellschaft*, DISS-Verlag: Duisburg.

Jahn, I., Löther, R. and Senglaub, K. (1985), *Geschichte der Biologie*, Fischer Verlag: Jena.

Jungk, R. and Mundt, H.J. (1988), *Das umstrittene Experiment: Der Mensch. Dokumentation des Ciba-Symposiums 1962 'Man and his Future'*, J. Schweitzer Verlag: Frankfurt a. M., München.

Kay, L.E. (1993), *The Molecular Vision of Life. Caltech, the Rockefeller Foundation, and the Rise of the New Biology*, Oxford University Press: Oxford.

Lappe, M. (1991), 'Ethical Issues in Manipulating the Human Germ Line', *The Journal of Medicine and Philosophy* Vol. 16, pp. 621-39.

Mauron, A. (1993), *Genetics and Intergenerational Concerns. Yearbook of the Societas Ethica*, Utrecht.

Mayr, E. (1984), *Die Entwicklung der biologischen Gedankenwelt*, Springer-Verlag: Berlin.

McGleenan, T. (1995), 'Human Gene Therapy and Slippery Slope Arguments', *Journal of Medical Ethics* Vol. 21, pp. 350-5.

Meier-Seethaler, C. (1997), *Gefühl und Urteilskraft – ein Plädoyer für die emotionale Vernunft*, CH Beck: München.

Olby, R.C. (1990), *Companion to the History of Modern Science*, Routledge: London.

Pauly, P.J. (1987), *Controlling Life. Jacques Loeb and the Engineering Ideal in Biology*, Oxford University Press: New York, Oxford.

Peters, T. (1995), '«Playing God» and Germline Intervention', *The Journal of Medicine and Philosophy*, Vol. 20, pp. 365-86.

Reich, W.T. (1995), *Encyclopedia of Bioethics*, MacMillan: New York.

Rifkin, J. (1986), *Genesis zwei. Biotechnik – Schöpfung nach Maß*, Hamburg.

Sawicki, J. (1991), *Disciplining Foucault. Feminism, Power, and the Body*, Routledge: New York.

Schmuhl, H.-W. (1987), *Rassenhygiene, Nationalsozialismus, Euthanasie. Von der Verhütung zur Vernichtung 'lebensunwerten Lebens'*, Vandenhoeck & Ruprecht: Göttingen.

Wimmer, R. (1989): '«Kategorische Argumente» gegen die Keimbahn-Gentherapie?', in Wils, J. P. and Mieth, D. (eds.), *Ethik ohne Chance? Erkundungen im technologischen Zeitalter*, Attempto-Verlag: Tübingen, pp. 182-209.

Zimmerman, B.K. (1991), 'Human Germline Therapy: The Case for its Development and Use', *The Journal of Medicine and Philosophy*, Vol. 16, pp. 593-612.

3 Predictive genetic medicine – a new concept of disease

Lene Koch

When the EU-Commission first proposed the Genome mapping project in 1988, the title of the proposal was 'Predictive Medicine'. The initial paragraph of the proposal, the 'Reasons for proposal', went like this:

Fifty years ago the principal cause of morbidity and mortality was infectious disease but with the discovery of antibiotics, and improvements in hygiene and pest control, it is now a minor one in industrialised countries. Apart from the consequences of accident or war, much disease today has a genetic component which may be of greater or lesser importance. Over the past few years a great deal has been learned about those diseaeses which are due to the inheritance of a single defective gene, though in most cases we are still far from a remedy. However when it comes to the common diseases such as coronary heart disease, diabetes, cancer, autoimmune diseases, the major psychoses and other important diseases of Western society, the major position is far less clear. These conditions have a strong environmental component, and although genetic factors are undoubtedly involved, they do not follow any clear cut pattern of inheritance. Put another way, the disease results from the exposure of genetically susceptible individuals or populations to environmental causes; prevention will depend on reducing the levels of exposure, or more probably, those of susceptible individuals. As it is most unlikely that we will be able to remove completely the environmental risk factors, it is important that we learn as much as possible about the genetically determined predisposing factors and hence identify high risk individuals. In summary, predictive medicine seeks to protect individuals from the kinds of illnesses to which they are genetically most vulnerable and, where appropriate, to prevent the transmission of genetic susceptibilities to the next generation.

As the original argumentation and legitimation for the EU genome mapping project, these paragraphs constitute the presentation of a new medical paradigm based on a new concept of disease. It calls itself predictive medicine, and its basis is a concept of disease which understands disease in genetic terms.

When we discuss the concept of disease involved in the genetic techniques of preimplantation diagonsis (PID), germline gene therapy (GLGT) and also the method of therapeutic nuclear transfer (TNT) it seems important to remember the whole genetification process that preceded theses techniques and which paved the way for their application. These technical options – one in use, the two others perhaps on their way – are all made possible through the development of the human genome project, and represent a genetified concept of disease. In the following I shall do two things: first I shall try to place the concept of predictive genetic medicine in a medical historical context, second I shall illustrate how the three technical options represent a new medical paradigm and a new genetified concept of disease, and how these changes affect the patient-doctor relationship.

The bacteriological revolution

In the history of medicine it is recognised that a number of different medical paradigms have existed, one evolving from another. I shall try to illustrate very briefly how the dominant paradigms of medicine were also accompanied by different concepts of disease – ending up with what I call a genetic concept of disease.

The great breakthrough in modern medicine took place with the discovery of the role of bacteria and vira in infectious diseases and the possibility of preventing and treating them with vaccine and antibiotics (penicillin). The bacteriological revolution marks the advent of a concept of medicine we may call laboratory medicine. The discoveries of e.g. Pasteur and Koch were followed by a change in the corpus of knowledge employed by medicine as such as well as a whole new relationship between doctor and patient.

Medicine left the bed side and entered the world of sciences, and employed scientific results and thus obtained an autonomous status as a science in its own right. It became possible for doctors to construct their own professional concept of medicine, based on the new scientific knowledge. The symptoms of the patient remained important of course, but their interpretation and treatment became more dependent on the scientific microorganic analysis by the doctor. As a result, the doctor came to possess exclusive access to the interpretation of the symptoms and to the treatment to be recommended. The concept of disease was being scientised, therapeutic nihilism abandoned but within a paternalistic authoritarian medical system. The doctor became the active expert, the patient passivised.

Preventive medicine

The paradigm of bacteriology gradually became challenged by a change in the spectrum of diseases. When infectious disesases began to decrease in numbers and severity, others like chronic diseases began to take up more attention: coronary artery disease, cancer, diabetes were diseases which somatic medicine had not been able to counter. Genetic diseases also took up a greater proportion of the total spectrum of diseases than earlier, though their heyday came somewhat later. As psychology and social medicine assisted by epidemiology began to address the common chronic diseases, the interest in environmental and other risk factors began to grow. The concept of risk factor actually originated from a study of coronary heart disease in the USA in the 1950s (the Framingham study). The patient-doctor relationship also underwent radical change. Prevention of risk factors and the marketing of preventive strategies placed the patient in the center of medicine. In this paradigm risk is calculated by the individual's group-relations. Risk factors might be environmental but just as well psychological, behavioural and most often related to the life style of the individual (e.g. smoking). Preventive medicine is characterised by concepts different from those dominant in laboratory medicine: multifactorial causes and probabilities but no certainties that disease will occur, and thus prevention and reduction of risk factors – the more the better – is the medical recommendation. Medicine becomes an institution where risks are calculated. The patient is no longer just the person with symptoms, factually ill, but rather a member of the group of persons vulnerable to the risks inherent in his environment. In this paradigm the concept of patient is changed, since the patient is not (yet) sick; also the role of the patient changes radically and the authority of medicine is threatened because of the strong need for patient compliance with medical recommendations. Sometimes the difference between the layman's and the expert's perception of the substances and behaviours deemed risky by statistical methods and controlled clinical trials is so huge that medicine looses credibility because the aetiological factor is so small or the time perspective so long that the medical recommendation becomes abstract and unrealistic or directly opposed to the life-experience of the patient.

187

Predictive medicine

Predictive genetic medicine – as it was presented by the EU – may be seen as a natural successor to preventive medicine. As genetics plays a more and more important role in medicine, it has been proposed that we are entering a new medical paradigm where medicine is genetified or geneticised (Lippmann 1991, p. 15-50).

The concept of genetification deserves to be more precisely defined.[1] Recently coined as a result of the development of molecular genetics but also borrowing meaning to a great extent from classical genetic theory (including less scientific ideas of determinism, hereditarianism and biologism), it comprises important aspects of modern medicine: the increasing use of methods and practices (e.g. experimental, diagnostic, pharmaceutical) generated by molecular genetics as well as the mode of explaining and understanding disease characteristic of Mendelian genetics. Instances of genetification are found at different levels of medicine: 1) at the level of the concept of disease, 2) at the level of medical practice including both diagnosis and therapy, 3) at the level of medical and health policy. This third use of the concept is amply illustrated by the retorics of the previously quoted EU proposal. Theoretically the meaning of genetification at these levels may differ. One important issue is the relationship between predictive and genetified medicine. The model of predictive medicine introduced in the EU proposal is of course not identical with a genetified model of medicine. Predictive medicine is a concept focusing on only one aspect of genetified medicine, namely the precise identification of risk individuals and prediction of future disease – but is still a concept that implies important changes in medical practices and in the structure of medical services. One major instrument for the implementation of these functions is genetic diagnosis, which again relies heavily on the advances of molecular medicine. In this context one might add that genetics is increasingly becoming molecularly based and that much medicine for this reason may be understood as molecular medicine. Thus the concepts introduced here are to some extent interchangeable, and at any rate very closely linked. A more complete study of their relationship is beyond the scope of this paper. It should be mentioned however, that predictive medicine also encompasses non-genetic biomedicine – e.g. measuring levels of various cellular components in the body. Genetic diagnosis on a probabalistic or biochemical basis also predates the recent development of molecular medicine.

Medicine is undergoing a major change under the influence of the developments in molecular genetics, in particular genome mapping and the genetic technologies generated by this project. This change may be compared to a differentiated inavasion, since different areas of medicine are influenced with different strength and speed. When I speak of the genetification of medicine I do not of course imply that a genetic paradigm replaces other medical paradigms from one day to the next. New and old paradigms coexist side by side, only their respective importance and influence fluctuate. Interaction between paradigms also takes place. Rather, the proposition that medicine is becoming genetified means that the ideas and models of explanation known and becoming known in human genetics are becoming more and more powerful, are gaining influence in more and more medical disciplines and practices that were previously unrelated to genetics. A good example is oncology, where a whole new discipline of cancer genetics is emerging – and an interesting process of integration and competition between the genetic and oncological traditions is taking place (Stemerding et al. 1997, pp. 25-30). The concept of disease is of course a crucial point and the focus of this paper. What constitutes disease and the modes of explaining disease are fundamental issues in any medical paradigm because they are the means of deciding who is sick and who is not and of deciding what is the cause of disease and its rational treatment is. It follows from this that the concept of disease is not irrelevant for the structure of the medical system, nor for the relation between doctor and patient nor for the concept of patient as such. With the introduction of the concept of predictive genetic medicine the concept of disease – and what it entails – is being reconstructed. This was illustrated in my short historical flashback.

The persuasive power of genetics and probably also the reason for its tremendous success is – among other factors the convincing simplicity of the genetic model of explaining disease – a simplicity which is often characteristic of the media's representation of the new genetics: disease is caused by defective genes. And genes, we are told, constitute the blueprint of the organism. Correct the blueprint and presumably the whole organism is corrected. This line of thought is closely linked with medical essentialism, a belief held by medical doctors in earlier centuries, that disease was caused by 'something' inside the sick person (Wulff et al. 1986). Essentialism was driven by the hope of finding an objective explantation for disease, a quest which has always met with the difficulty of individual and cultural differences in patients' behaviour and subjective experience of disease. The genetic concept of disease is often referred to as building on a deterministic and monocausal model of disease, though what is really the case is that in predictive medicine the importance given to the genetic components of a given pattern of disease is increasing. Only in a rather limited number of monogenetic Mendelian diseases may we speak of genetic determination and even here, the actual expression of disease may vary.

In preventive medicine, as I have just described it, the healthy person's life is medicalised through attempts to reduce relevant risk factors. The ideal is the internalisation of an ever present awareness of risk factors throughout the life of the potential patient. This impossible demand has no doubt produced a contradiction between medical and lay constructions of health and disease, and in this respect the genetic concept of disease in predictive medicine does not seem to offer much improvement. Only in specific cases such as rare monogenic diseases with a Mendelian inheritance do genetic tests give the individual person certain evidence of disease. The information molecular medicine offers about disease is often of a probabilistic nature. In predictive genetic medicine the risk group is constituted by the genes people have in common and predictions thus concern the individual and his family. Their genetic status may be well defined, but the outcome is not. Those who are diagnosed as carrying a disease gene still have to live with uncertainty about their own futures and those of their children.

When we consider the patient-doctor relation, the possibilities for patient control in predictive genetic medicine seem different. Knowledge about one's genetic status may be more difficult to reject and predictive genetic medicine thus holds new potentials for medical and social control over patient behaviour. As in preventive medicine, not the past but the future of the identified gene carrier is medicalised, since those whom predictive genetic medicine identifies as future patients may not have any symptoms of disease. But those identified as risk persons are left with a heavy individual responsibility for compliance, not only concerning themselves but their whole family. This takes on a different character from that which we saw in the preventive era, where everyone in a high risk group was in the same boat, so to speak.

As I have argued, there are very obvious links between predictive and preventive medicine, and actually one might argue that predictive genetic medicine may be the way to ultimate prevention by combining specific knowledge of individual risk with knowledge of external risk factors. This line of thought seems to be implied in the EU proposal from 1988, and the positive association with preventive medicine has actually been a guiding line in much genetic discourse on the place of genetics in health policy even back to the 1960s.

If we look at the developments I have sketched, we find that the concept of disease includes a number of variables: what constitutes disease; what constitutes a patient; which diagnostic and therapeutical interventions are considered relevant; how the structure and services of the health system (the purpose of medicine are affected); how the patient-doctor relation is affected; how disease is detected. I will discuss some of these variables and see how they are actualised in the case of PID and GLGT.

What constitutes a disease

In everyday language, disease usually refers to human subjects but as medical specialisation intensifies, organs, cells or genes may be also considered as sick. In the case of PID, GLGT and TNT the disease is the presence of the unwanted genetic variation and the first medical concern will be to decide which genetic variations to consider unwanted. Since the disease has no manifestations, no as yet visible phenotype and no symptoms, the decision has to be made on a more theoretical basis. It has often been debated whether a concept of seriousness should be applied before genetic diagnosis is considered justified – and whether the finding of e.g. so called normal features such as intelligence, sex, height or behavioural characteristics should be sufficient to justify abortion. This problem is joined by another question taken up already in the EU proposal, i.e. the extension of the number and nature of diseases we may expect to battle by predictive medicine. Whereas genetics was previously considered relevant for only a minor group of diseases, rare and all different, it is now considered relevant in the battle against the major common diseases such as cancer, diabetes and coronary heart disease. Thus the EU proposal outlines a whole new area for medical genetics, namely an expansion of its object of interest from rare monogenetic diseases with a Mendelian inheritance to the common diseases hitherto considered to be outside the scope of genetics. This of course implies a whole new classification of disease, as more and more diseases are now understood as genetic diseases and certainly some of the common diseases may turn out to consist of many minor diseases differentiated by a different aetiology and only similar in their phenotype. I shall illustrate with cancer once more: after the cloning of BRCA1 and 2, it seems relevant to ask whether breast cancer is really one disease, or rather a number of genetically different diseases which should be treated differently, and which have only their phenotype in common?

A genetified concept of disease makes diagnosis of genetic predispositions just as legitimate as diagnosis of rare genetic diseases. And even though PID is as yet only considered for rare genetic diseases of great seriousness such as cystic fibrosis or mental retardation why not consider dispositions for cancer, diabetes, alzheimer, coronary heart disease, and other diseases where genes of importance for the development of the disease have been localised and cloned? If such genetic variation becomes the target of PID the market for this method will increase tremendously, as will the demand for IVF – the prerequisite for PID.

Another aspect of the concept of disease has to do with the fact that we are no longer talking about disease in humans, but in cells. Can cells and genes be sick in the same way as humans can? Since the genes are not yet expressed phenotypically, we can only diagnose, change or select according to more theoretical approaches to the matter, such as averages and probabilities seen in other cells which have been allowed to express themselves.

The concept of the patient

With PID, GLGT and TNT not only the concept of disease is changed, but also the concept of patient is deconstructed. The living human being with certain symptoms is the patient of traditional bedside as well as bacteriological medicine. We left that paradigm with the advent of preventive medicine where well people also became the objects of medical intervention and care. In a medical system where the living are struggling for access to limited health care resources, we now encounter a new patient, the cell, the fertilised egg.

How does this affect other medical principles and practices? Let me illustrate with the example of the purpose of medical services. If the patients are no longer living human beings, but potential human beings, in the shape of cells and nuclei, I see a return to a classical eugenic situation, where the objects of concern are the future generations, rather than those living in the present. Instead of focusing on the health of those living, we intervene in the genetic material of those who are not yet human beings. GLGT is an obvious example, which easily compares with positive eugenics, which unsuccessfully tried to improve the quality of future generations.

This has consequences for the practice of medical ethics. Who is to consent to all this, since the patient is not yet here (and when she does turn up she may arrive in a shape that is genetically different from the one she would have had if not treated and then it is too late to protest since she is no longer what she might have been)? As long as we thought of selective abortions and discarding of eggs in the light of the traditional abortion where the mother was the patient, who did not want to have this particular baby – we could claim that the mother was the patient; she had to consent and no one else needed to know or consent. When eggs become patients, all this changes, as far as I can see. One reason is obvious: we are assisting each other in meddling with the fates of our children or grandchildren, and in principle all future generations. When we treat future generations – as is the case with GLGT – who should consent? No one but the parents are present, and it seems that the established principle of individual autonomy is violated. Unless of course the medical profession considers their role a different one, as the geneticist James Neel did when he conceptualised his role as physican to the gene pool – eugenics again (Neel 1994).[2]

What constitutes therapy

The major problem for the new genetics has been the growing gap between diagnostic and therapeutic capabilities. Perhaps the new interest in PID and the other methods is perceived as a way out of this since selection and rejection of eggs seems more acceptable than abortion. Predictive medicine as it was conceived in the late eighties and early nineties was primarily considered at a limited number of points in the human life cycle. Genetic diagnosis as it has been known till recently has primarily been offered to pregnant women who wanted their fetuses examined, to newborns and adults whose carrier status was doubtful. With PID the scope of genetic diagnosis reaches far beyond this. As IVF has made fertilised eggs accessible in greater numbers, the wish to diagnose the fertilised egg before implantation seems to satisfy many additional needs. The most important is the ethically controversial possibility of selective abortion after traditional diagnosis as we know it – with PID there is no pregnancy to abort until after diagnosis and in case of a diagnosed defect, it seems easier for everyone to throw away the fertilised egg than to perform an abortion on a much older fetus.

With PID predictive medicine is performed on the fertilised egg, the absolutely initial stage of the human life cycle, where the fewest possible human characteristics are recognisable, and this conceals the act that is performed. Not an abortion – and for that reason many people seem to prefer PID to prenatal diagnosis and subsequent abortion – but rather what we might call a 'virtual abortion' where the act of selection is performed without the bloody consequences. In this analysis, to call PID therapy is a euphemism, since the fertilised egg is discarded if not found satisfactory. In GLGT therapy takes place at the genetic level, either by substitution or change – a term like genetic surgery may be used to describe the procedure or perhaps genetic medication.

The patient-doctor relationship

Genetification also affects the patient-doctor relationship in several ways. With the change in the concept of patient, the relationship between the parties is also affected. We have known similar problems in clinical genetics for a while. As the focus on hereditary disease intensifies and the concept of patient changes, so does the concept of integrity and privacy. Genes are shared by families and a host of problems of disclosure of information and testing has arisen as members of families do not have the same views on how to proceed with respect to predictive testing and reproductive behaviour. The doctor experiences dilemmas when one member wants information which necessitates the participation of a family member who does not want to be tested. And should the doctor disclose genetic knowledge relevant for a larger family circle or respect the one patient's confidentiality? These problems have normally been defined as ethical, but the question is whether they should not also be considered social, as predictive genetic medicine also reshapes the social relations between familiy members as well as between doctor and patient. Ethical conduct in genetic counselling, a central aspect of the doctor patient relationship is usually defined as non-directive, and with adherence to patient autonomy. Post-war human genetics made a point of individual autonomy and non-directiveness to shield itself from eugenics, but as it turns out, autonomy is obviously an insufficient problem-solver in a family conflict such as the one mentioned above. The conflicting views of autonomous individuals can only be solved on a more social basis – if at all.

When cells and fetuses become patients it is no longer obvious that the primary decision maker is the woman, pregnant or not yet pregnant. With a genetified concept of disease, the genetic aspects of family relations may be given greater importance, and social aspects diminish in importance. The large array of new actors who are now entering the reproductive scene will inevitably create new social conflicts, as we are now seeing in Denmark where the concept of genetic fatherhood is being introduced into Danish familiy law and may push out the old pater-est principle. Traditionally any child born in marriage is considered the legal child of the woman's husband – the pater-est rule. With the new means of genetic analysis genetic paternity may be determined with great certainty – regardless of the social arrangement of the pater-est role. A new report from the Ministry of Justice on child law proposes that any man who has had sexual intercourse with the mother in the period of conception has a right to have his possible paternity tested. Thus a genetic relation is given precedence over the marriage relation and the pater-est rule which provided stability to the family (Betænkning nr 1350, København 1997).

When the selection process implied an abortion, the final decision belonged to the woman, but with PID the decision to select a diagnosed embryo is being removed from female control. Once the egg is out, the number of parties involved in the decision making process has increased and both genetic and social fathers as well as medical expertise/genetic counsellors may influence the decision. This is an important difference between prenatal diagnosis and PID and the direct consequence of the removal of the selection process to the preimplantation stage.[3] These are examples of how the genetic understanding of social relations is reshaping social power relations – inside and outside medicine, though it remains an open question whether this is creating more equality within the couple.

We may now list a spectrum of patients new and old: the nucleus, the cell, the fertilised egg, the fetus, the individual, the couple, the family, and the population. Strangely enough, the more we focus in on the minute genetic elements affecting health at the request of the individual, the more difficult it becomes to avoid affecting other people.

Conclusion

Genetification has affected the concept of disease, concepts of therapy, the patient-doctor relationship and also the structure of health services. With the new methods of PID, GLGT and TNT an additional number of features become visible, tendencies which previously have only vaguely been discernible. This paper has tried to sketch a number of issues of interest in this process and a more systematic attempt to analyse this development is needed before we can fully appreciate the implications of this development.

Notes

1   The idea of genetification was originally sketched in Lene Koch 1993.
2   James Neel is known for his work with Japanese atomic bomb casualties after World War Two. His most recent book was called 'Physician to the Gene Pool'.
3   See Hille Haker's contribution in this volume.

References

Justitsministeriets Børnelovsudvalg (1997), Betaenkning om børns retsstilling, Betaenkning nr 1350, København.
Koch, L. (1993), 'The genetification of medicine and the concept of disease', *Diskussionspapiere 1*, Hamburger Institut für Sozialforschung: Hamburg.
Lippman, A. (1991), 'Prenatal Genetic Testing and Screening: Constructing Needs and Reeinforcing Inequities', *American Journal of Law and Medicine,* Vol. 17, No.1-2, pp. 15-50.
Neel, J. (1994), *Physician To the Gene Pool*, John Wiley and Sons: New York.
Stemerding, D., Koch, L. and Bourret, P. (1997), 'DNA Diagnosis and the Emergence of Cangergenetic Services in Europe', *European Journal of Human Genetics*, Vol. 5, Suppl. 2, pp. 25-30.
Wulff, H., Pedersen, S.A. and Rosenberg, R. (1986), *Philosophy of Medicine*, Blackwell: London.

4 Animal Models: an anthropologist considers Dolly

Sarah Franklin

Introduction: the Dolly debate

When Dolly the sheep was introduced to the scientific community and the press in February (23, 1997), public debate instantly crystalised around the ethical acceptability of cloning humans. Several scenarios repeated themselves with generic regularity, such as the possible cloning of 'evil' dictators such as Hitler or Saddam Hussein, and the converse possibility of cloning 'geniuses', movie stars, or athletes, or the possibility for wealthy billionaires to clone themselves. The overwhelming opinion expressed by commentators, columnists and scientific journalists around the world was that human cloning is neither a realistic nor a morally defensible option. Dr Ian Wilmut of the Roslin Institute, as well as Dr Ron James of PPL Therapeutics, were both widely quoted expressing their opposition to the attempt to clone humans. President Clinton called for an immediate moratorium on such activities. As the former Archbishop of York, John Habgood, put the matter succinctly: 'I cannot see any morally convincing reason why anybody should want to clone a human being, and some good reasons why they should not' (*The Observer*, 2 March 1997, p. 27).

Not everyone agreed with this assessment. Writing in *The Sunday Times* (2 March 1997, p. 15), Princeton biology professor Lee Silver argued that human cloning could save lives, overcome infertility and provide a wide range of useful medical functions. Such views were, however, rare.

197

Schematically, the Dolly debate aligned along a number of significant axes. A primary division of opinion split off those who favoured the possibility of human cloning from those who did not. A second set of opinions polarised around whether the cloning of sheep or other higher mammals was acceptable in its own right. On this question, a majority of British and American commentators spoke enthusiastically in favour of its medical benefits, and only a minority of voices expressed opposition to the Roslin technique. MP David Alton called for a moratorium on cloning until a committee of inquiry could prepare a report for Parliament. John Habgood suggested that cloning 'might turn out to be biological folly', by reducing biodiversity, and he feared it was also morally degrading:

> To assimilate the world of living things into the mechanical model, and to manipulate it to fit the needs of mechanised production, might on a superficial level seem to promise greater human freedom and prosperity. On the contrary, the more we treat animal life as being manipulable for human convenience, the greater the temptation to think of human life in similar terms. (ibid)

From the Vatican came calls for the establishment of an international committee of inquiry to examine delicate matters of human morality and ethics raised by recent developments in the life sciences, epitomised by the Dolly episode.

In addition to these two axes of divergent views on human and animal cloning were other key lines of division in the Dolly debate at the level of the terms or contexts of argumentation. For example, a consistent effort was made to separate the question of whether humans *should* be cloned from whether this was in fact even possible. Many expert commentators, such as Ian Wilmut himself, emphasised that although the possibility that humans could be successfully cloned was strongly indicated by the Dolly technique, the practical obstacles to so doing were overwhelming. Such objections were primarily founded on technical details: human embryonic stem cells differentiate earlier than those of sheep, too many egg donors would be necessary, it would be illegal under the Human Fertilisation and Embryology Authority even to attempt such an experiment without a license, and so forth. As Robin Mckie, who broke the Dolly story in *The Observer* on 23 February wrote:

> Human cloning, although now close to reality, would be illegal under the laws governing fertilisation research. No responsible biologist would support such work, say scientists. (p. 1)

Reporting on Ian Wilmut's testimony before the science and technology select committee in Parliament, Roger Highfield, science editor of *The Daily Telegraph* quoted the Roslin team leader's opinion that 'most of the suggested applications for cloning of humans are non-sensical' and that all of the Roslin/PPL team members would find any such research 'distressing and offensive' (*The Daily Telegraph*, 7 March 1997, p. 1).

Through such statements by Wilmut, issues of feasibility were used to underscore the unlikelihood of successful human cloning – in what might be described as the 'and besides, it wouldn't be feasible anyway' argument. Similarly, the pro-cloning views of the majority of commentators culminated in a list of medical benefits on offer through cloning: new pharmaceuticals, organs, plasma, skin grafts, and research possibilities for the study of ageing.

On the basis, then, of the British press coverage of Dolly, an extensive selection of which I have collected and read, the basic Dolly position can be summarised as follows.

Dolly represents a medical-scientific breakthrough because it was thought impossible for adult cells to be returned to a state compatible with undifferentiated embryonic cells. Her birth raises the possibility that humans could be cloned, but no responsible scientist would do such a thing, and besides, even if they tried they would probably fail. Plus it is illegal. However, the Dolly technique is undoubtably a very welcome scientific advance, because it will lead to benefits for people, for animal husbandry, and even for sheep themselves, as their biodiversity can be better protected and managed.

Without intending to charicature the debate, I would argue this summary captures the gyst of the British media 'position' on Dolly. Typically, and as is characteristically the case in Britain where public opinion is generally favourable towards innovation in the life sciences, there was very little opposition to the Roslin technique. Overwhelmingly, opposition was focussed on the possibility of cloning humans, not sheep. Also typically British was the lack of any substantial, organised religious opposition to the Roslin cloning technique, and the general public acceptance of the moral legitimacy of the benefits it would bring.

Anthropological perspectives: Dolly as property

This paper is not concerned to take a position for or against cloning, and it is not my intention to enter the debate as such. In part, however, because I am sympathetic to the Habgood position, I would like to borrow some of the forms of cultural analysis specific to anthropology to examine some of the issues raised by Dolly's creation in more detail. In my own mind, it is an insufficient argument to say that animal cloning is acceptable because it brings medical benefits to humans. Simply prohibiting use of the technique on humans, while extending its use on animals also appears to me to skip over some important questions. To develop these, I propose to consider Dolly as a form of property – arguably a novel form of property. Since all forms of property are cultural inventions, my argument is based on a consideration of what it tells us to consider Dolly not only as a scientific invention, or as an ethical dilemma, but as a cultural product. One way of doing this is to consider Dolly from the perspective of what kind of property she instantiates. If, as Renee Hirschon describes it, '"property" as an analytic category can be seen to link several conceptually distinct levels of social organisation' in part 'because property relations entail social mechanisms of transmission' (1984:5), then how might Dolly be seen as an assemblage of resources, practices and values integral to a wider social order? If, moreover, as Veronica Beechey suggests (1984), it is essential to treat the interrelationship of production and reproduction as a single process, then how does Dolly's status as a form of reproductive property figure in this analysis?

Breedwealth

To develop this line of argument I take as my starting point some general observations about British sheep breeding, and the development of what I will call here 'breedwealth'. Broadly speaking sheep breeding is an agricultural industry, practiced for centuries in Britain by farmer-entrpreneurs, whose activities are focussed on the reproduction of sheep herds and the recovery of resources from them through markets and other forms of exchange. Sheep are not indigenous to the British Isles, and it is generally thought their domestication occurred in western Asia approximately ten thousand years ago (Henson 1986). It is known that by 3000 BC, flocks of small, light-coloured sheep were not uncommon within western Europe and began to be imported to Britain (Russell 1986). In Britain, it is believed that sheep were initially used primarily for milk and wool, and that they were useful for restoring areas of depleted land, where they were often put out to graze, their hardiness enabling them to prosper in conditions unfavourable for cows, pigs or horses.

The hardiness and intelligence of British sheep such as the Scottish Blackface (by whom Dolly was gestated) also favoured what has become recognised as the distinctive complexity and efficiency of the British sheep breeding system, whereby different varieties, or breeds, of sheep are raised in widely divergent ecologies – from the Scottish highlands to the lowlands of the far south. In turn, these different lines, or strains, are both inbred and cross-bred, producing a highly efficient and economical system with many benefits. Scottish Blackface ewes, such as Dolly's mother, are capable of straddling a partially 'wild' and semi-domesticated existence due to their highly valued skills of survival and social organisation. As breed historian Elizabeth Henson notes:

> [Mountain] breeds are very hardy and can withstand harsh weather conditions. They are intelligent sheep with a keen sense for survival. They carefully find shelter for themselves and their lambs and are aware of approaching storms. Female lambs which are to be kept in the flock are allowed to stay on the hill with their mothers. They live in a family group and learn the family's home range. Mountain sheep may travel many miles during a year but they have a clear knowledge of their home and are said to be hefted on to their hill. When a hill is sold, the hefted flock is sold with it. Should a new farmer try to buy ewes from his neighbour he would find them soon walking home to their own hillsides. (1986:11)

The most numerous breed of sheep in Britain is the Scottish Blackface, which makes up approximately a third of the total purebred sheep population, and epitomises the Mountain breeds in its ability to survive the harshest winters in some of the most inhospitable areas of Britain. Purebreeds such as these comprise an integral component of the stratified sheep breeding system, which is sometimes claimed to have been developed and preserved so successfully because of the number of distinct regional habitats, and island populations of sheep in Britain.

The distinctive integration of sheep breeding into agricultural development and efficient land management in Britain from the 1500s onward cannot be underestimated in its historical importance, and in particular for its role in precipitating the industrial revolution. Historian Ferdinand Braudel describes the sheep breeding as 'the key' to the 'vital transformation' in English agricultural production during the seventeenth century. Citing the increasing use of 'land previously regarded as poor, fit only for grazing sheep' he claims that 'a rapid rise in the head of livestock, especially sheep, [led in turn to] increased cereal yeilds' (1979:560). Historians who argue that a rate of agricultural production higher than population growth is the single most important precondition for successful industrialisation would agree with Braudel, who argues that the industrial revolution in Northwest England;

> came not so much from machines or wonder crops as from new methods of land use; new timetables for ploughing; new forms of crop rotation which eliminated fallow and encouraged grazing, a useful source of fertiliser and therefore a remedy for soil exhaustion; attention to new strains of crops; [and] the selective breeding of sheep and cattle . . . (1979:559)

In sum, without underestimating the complexity of the factors precipitating the unique industrial expansion in seventeenth-century Britain, it is clear that the importance of a highly specialised and densely integrated sheep breeding system was a critical factor.

Perhaps it is merely prosaic, given the amount of speculation involved, to envisage links between the unique expansion of industrialised production in Britain in the seventeenth and eighteenth centuries, and the so-called industrialisation of reproduction which has also proven a distinctly British innovation in the nineteenth and twentieth centuries. However, I suspect it is not irrelevant from a cultural standpoint that Louise Brown was born in Oldham, Lancashire or that Dolly the Sheep was born from a Scottish Blackfaced ewe near Edinburgh. In any event, and leaving such provocative leaps aside, both the mechanical animation of the Lancashire mills, and the technologically-aided conception of Scottish sheep require not only particular cultural values, but also the more familiar economic kinds of value in the form of capital.

From industrial capital to genetic capital

As machine-capital was essential to industrialised production, so is bio-capital integral to the industrialisation of reproduction, or of life itself. The form of ownership proper to both forms of wealth is the patent, understood as a form of intellectual property. The establishment of patent protection for innovation has its roots both in the formation of nation states, and the need to protect national wealth, and also in the link that connects ideas to persons as property – most notably copyright. The notion of literary property established in 16th century England is modelled on paternity, extending the analogy of a father's propriety in respect of his children to the progeny of his mind. Male procreative agency is the model borrowed to establish literary propriety, and the subsequent development of the patent as a delimited form of ownership over inventions extends from the earlier model, as the scientist or inventor is seen as the 'author' of an original idea (see further in Rose 1993).

Ownership of Dolly is thus quite complicated: to begin with, it is not so much Dolly herself, as the means of creating her, which is protected by patent. Once Dolly's patent has been granted, it will exist in the names of Ian Wilmut and his team at Roslin, but will be licensed to PPL therapeutics for their exclusive use. In turn, the form of protection afforded by a patent is essentially passive: it is only activated in the event that PPL Therapeutics decides to protect their rights in court. In this sense, the patent provides an entitlement to seek redress for infringement by a user perceived to have exploited the original invention under protection. There is thus no incentive to enforce a patent if the usurper is not also financially advantaged to provide remuneration in the case of a successful prosecution. Unlike copyright, which extends for the duration of an author's life and beyond, patent protection extends for a much shorter period, and is based on a presumed exchange: in exchange for sharing vital information that is novel, original and of utility, the patent owner is granted a privileged entitlement to any profits the invention yeilds. In turn, this right can be exchanged for remuneration through licensing agreements, somewhat akin to the royalty arrangements through which a literary estate is marketed.

Dolly's patented novelty represents a new kind of genetic capital, or breed wealth. Such shifts have occurred frequently over time, and there are now a range of strategies available to secure and protect the commodity value of distinct varieties of animals, plants and microorganisms. At the time of the industrial revolution, to which, as we have seen, selective breeding of sheep is seen to be integral, the most important changes in English breeding practices are associated with the figure of Robert Bakewell. In her astute account of Bakewell's influence, historian Harriet Ritvo argues that it was his ability to reorganise the conceptual basis of livestock ownership which accounts for his unique legacy. Specifically, she suggests, 'he assumed it was possible for the improver to redraw the conventional boundary between the sphere of nature and the sphere of agriculture' (1995:415). He accomplished this, she suggests, through successful entrepreneurial production of new property values in animals, what she denotes as their 'genetic capital'.

Previous to Bakewell's transformative influence, opinion varied among livestock breeders on the question of inherited traits. As Ritvo puts it simply 'there was no contemporary consensus about what could be inherited and how' (1995:416). Rather, she claims, 'the prevalent practices of mid-eighteenth century husbandry were based on other assumptions, particularly the predominance of such environmental factors as climate and diet' (1995:416). Bakewell, she argued, was able to increase by fourhundredfold within thirty years the value of his breeding livestock by essentially relocating the value of the animal at the level of its capacity to pass on genetic traits – to become, as Ritvo describes it, an individual template. This shift, she suggests, 'represented the entry of a whole new source of value' into the livestock market. It was 'a change in kind rather than (or as well as) a change in degree':

> Bakewell claimed that when he sold one of his carefully bred animals, or, as in the case of stud fees, when he sold the procreative powers of these animals, he was selling something much more specific, more predictable, and more efficacious than mere reproduction. In effect, he was selling a template for the continued production of animals of a special type: that is, the distinction of his rams consisted not only in their constellation of personal virtues, *but in their ability to pass this constellation down their family tree*' (1995:416, emphasis added).

The shift here could be thus be described as metonymic in the sense that the individual comes to be so closely associated with the breedline as a whole it can stand in its stead, or be substituted for it, implying they are isomorphic. More accurately, such a shift is synechdochic, in the sense that a part is used to stand in for the whole (as in *hand* for *sailor*), the specific is made to represent the general (as in *line* for *telecommunications systems*), or the substance from which it is made for an object (as in *steel* for *sword*). In the case of Bakewell's prized Dishley and Leicestershire rams, an individual specimen not only belonged to, or continued, a breedline – *particular* individuals could embody the very best traits of the breed *and this capacity could be reproduced*. What Ritvo describes as 'genetic capital' thus conjoins individual reproductive capacity (in this case paternity) with the value of the line *as a whole*.

Two additional features of this transformation deserve further note before returning to Dolly. One is that the accomplishment of the 'change in kind' argued by Ritvo to be at the heart of Bakewell's influence was achieved, like all such changes, through a set of specific practices, and in particular through the use of pedigrees. Although pedigrees of breedlines were well established among horsebreeders in the eighteenth century, they were less commonly consulted among sheep breeders. It was Bakewell who instituted a much more rigorous application of pedigree record-keeping and administration, through which he consolidated the value of his own breeds and rams.

Second, Bakewell achieved this shift to increasing reliance on pedigree without any systematic, or what might be called 'scientific' evidence, such as, for example, progeny tests. As historian Nicholas Russell points out, 'it is likely that Bakewell believed, with so many of his contemporaries, that sire line inheritance was all that really mattered'. Moreover, Russell notes, 'Bakewell's deliberate selection policy was based entirely on appearance' (1986:212-213).

From genetic capital to genetic progress

Turning to Dolly, it is possible to suggest that the nuclear transfer technology through which she was bred effects a strategic and conceptual shift that builds upon Bakewell's earlier refinements. With the twentieth-century confirmation of the mechanisms of genetic inheritance, Bakewell's assumption that the genetic capital of a breed can be narrowed to the conduit of an individual's reproductive powers is no longer either radical or controversial. If the vicissitudes of such inheritance patterns remain subject to dispute among breeders, the basic principle that certain elite individuals have greater value as breedstock is hardly contentious.

Bakewell's consolidation of a new form of breedwealth might be described as the *individualisation of value*, transforming an individual animal into a more valuable form of property or stock. Through selection of an individual animal to serve as what Ritvo describes as a 'template' for the breed, Bakewell effected a compression of genealogical time through pedigree selection. His sire lines recorded this reduction of the breed to its select few elite rams, and he eventually transferred this technique to cattle.

The Roslin technique effects a different set of transformations. Nuclear transfer also relies upon selection of prized individuals, but offers also the possibility to achieve a molecular specification to this transfer. Eliminating the genetic 'noise' of sexual reproduction, cloning narrows the conduit of genetic transfer more precisely to an exact replica of the genome of the nuclear donor. The mitochondrial genome is still provided by the egg donor, and the renucleated embryo is gestated by a surrogate – increasing the number of animals involved in the reproduction of an individual. Such a widening of genomic transfer is seen as beneficial insofar as it can be used for the transgenic production of sheep such as Polly, whose genome has been modified to include additional (human) genetic material.

According to the Roslin Insititue's own account of Dolly's importance, they state that:

> The main advantage of cloning would not be *within* selection programmes, but in the more rapid dissemination of genetic progress from elite herds to the commercial farmer. At present this is achieved through artificial insemination (which supplies only half the genes) and by limited use of embryo transfer. This process is not that efficient and recent estimates in dairy cattle suggest the performance of the average cow is some 10 years behind the best. With cloning, it would be possible to remove this difference. Farmers who could afford it would receive embryos that would be clones of the most productive cows of elite herds. In doing so, they could lift the performance of their herds to that of the very best within one generation. This would be a one-off gain, since from then on the rate of genetic progress would return to that of the elite herds. (Roslin Institute Web Pages).

This achievement is described by Roslin as 'transfer of genetic progress to the farm'. The shift in property value here is thus from 'genetic capital' to 'genetic progress' – and the added-value consists in the 'one-off gain' of a 'lift' in performance of the herd. The steps involved in the process are as follows:
a. selection of elite animals from elite herds
b. substitution of cloning for sexual reproduction
c. elimination of the genetic 'noise' of sexual reproduction
d. exact replication of desired traits.

In turn, the technologically added-value of nuclear transfer is essentially time compression: a speed-up, in the form of 'genetic progress' is achieved. The 'genetic capital' yielded by the Roslin technique is thus 'genetic progress'. It is not the genetic capital of the animal *per se* that cloning facilitates, but the ease, precision and speed with which the genetic progress the animal represents can be transferred into mass production.

Dolly thus represents three kinds of value: the 'Bakewell value' of sheep breeding in the industrial era (its genetic capital); and the 'Roslin value' of genetic progress comprised of both precise replication and time compression. As a form of breedwealth, the Dolly and Polly products thus comprise significant developments in the reproduction of biogenetic value.

From an anthropological perspective, these shifts can also be considered from the vantage point of genealogy. Dolly's coming into being represents a departure from the assumed genealogical grid of biogenetic transmission in the sense that her parentage is no longer conventionally bilateral. Either her pedigree is unilateral (as a line of maternal succession), or it is bilateral (with an udder cell nucleus and a denucleated egg cell standing in as two gametes in a dual matriline), or it is trilateral if the surrogate mother is included (in what we might call polymatrilineality). It is less clear if lineality any longer equates to genealogical descent for the more recent sheep, Polly, whose DNA is transgenic, containing human genes. This addition confers a lateral dimension to Polly's pedigree. It could be said her genealogy has been respatialised.

In sum, both Dolly and Polly belong to the new kinship universe of transgenic animals whose existence must be understood in relation to an unfamiliar genealogical system made possible through molecular genetic technology. As live-stock they both embody the technological capacities which brought them into being, and are protected by intellectual property law as forms of biowealth. Both are clearly corporate entities, the animate equivalents of industrial machinery in their production and design as manufacturing technologies. The Roslin Institute web pages describe such sheep as 'bioreactors'. They and their progeny are designed to manufacture a range of goods including pharmaceuticals, so-called neutriceuticals (such as infant formula), organs for xenotransplantation, animal models for research, embryonic stem cells and, of course, other transgenic animals like themselves.

Conclusion

I began this paper by rehearsing the emphasis on human cloning in the initial public reaction to Dolly, and by asking whether the cloning of sheep can be so readily seen as a distinct ethical question. In the discussion and examples which follow, I have tried to argue that Dolly and Polly must be seen as forms of property which are inseparable from a wider social and cultural context. In conclusion, I would suggest that it is a mistake to see new forms of reproductive property in a distinct ethical domain simply because they are not human. Such a view rests on a presumed separation between the animal and the human belied by these very animals transgenic constitution. If it is possible from the standpoint of public debate, or ethical principles, to imagine such a separation, I suggest it is less so, if not impossible, from an anthropological standpoint which presumes a number of cultural connections between Dolly and ourselves. It might seem such connections would be particularly obvious in a society such as Britain, where human reproductive models are self-consciously based on nature and biology. Yet, the reverse would seem to be true. In the very sphere of reproduction humans and other mammals are seen to share in common, biological reproduction, the question of what is done to sheep is considered an entirely distinct matter from what is permissable for humans. It is, of course, the paradoxical nature of this very proximity and disconnection which explains why Dolly's birth was immediately translated into an ethical dilemma concerning the possibility of cloning humans.

Culturally, such ricochets of connection and comparison between one domain and another can be understood as a kind of traffic in meanings, in which biology and culture, nature and nurture, humans and animals rebound off one another. As Marilyn Strathern suggests,

> Comparative awareness is also cultural awareness. A comparative excercise throws into relief the kinds of connections people make between different parts of their experiences. *How* those connections are constructed, the ways fact and opinion are brought together, reveal possible limits in forms of representation . . . [Anthropologists] would say that culture lies in the manner in which connections are made, and thus in the range of contexts through which people collect their thoughts. (1993:7)

This view of culture presumes that all human activities have a generic cultural dimension: that indeed meaningful human action is impossible without the construction of meaningful contexts of action through which it is understood – as ethical, purposeful, effectual, or pointless. This is why consideration of the ethics of cloning must attend to its cultural context, and why it is unethical for the scientific practices involved in such research to be seen as exempt from cultural scrutiny.

Note

An earlier version of this paper has been published in *Environmental Values*, 6 (1997):427-37 and is reprinted here with permission of the editors.

References

Beechey, Veronica (1979), 'On Patriarchy', *Feminist Review* 3 (3):66-82.

Braudel, Fernand (1979), *The Perspective of the World: civilization and capitalism 15th to 18th century,* volume 3. New York: Harper and Row.

Habgood, John (1997), 'Send out the clones', *The Observer*, 2 March, p. 27.

Henson, Elizabeth (1986), *British Sheep Breeds.* Princes Risborough, Buckinghamshire: Shire Publications.

Highfield, Roger (1997), 'Human clones in "two years"', *The Daily Telegraph*, 7 March, p. 1.

Hirschon, Renée (1984), 'Introduction: property, power, and gender relations', in Hirschon, Renée (ed.), *Women and Property, Women as Property*, pp. 1-22. London: Croom Helm.

McKie, Robin (1997), 'Scientists clone adult sheep', *The Observer*, 23 February, p. 1.

Ritvo, Harriet (1995), 'Possessing Mother Nature: genetic capital in eighteenth-century Britain', in Brewer, John and Staves, Susan (eds.), *Early Modern Conceptions of Property.* London: Routledge.

Rose, Mark (1993), *Authors and Owners: the invention of copyright.* Cambridge, MA: Harvard University Press.

Russell, Nicholas (1986), *Like Engend'ring Like: heredity and animal breeding in early modern England.* Cambridge: Cambridge University Press.

Strathern, Marilyn (1993), 'Introduction: a question of context,' in Edwards, Jeanette et al., *Technologies of Procreation: kinship in the age of assisted conception.* Manchester: Manchester University Press.

5 Issues surrounding preimplantation diagnosis and germline gene therapy

Alexandre Quintanilha

Biotechnological advances are making it easier to perform preimplantation diagnosis (PID) for an ever increasing number of genetic characteristics at earlier and earlier stages subsequent to fertilisation. As always occurs with any new technological advance that has clear and important implications for our society, PID is raising a plethora of views from different quarters of the social spectrum.

The key question is, as always: once the information is available, what do you do with it? Some feel that even this question should never be asked. For them, the question could perhaps be rephrased: should PID technology ever be applied? Or, since the idea of implanting a seriously defective embryo seems unreasonable, should the technology of in-vitro fertilisation ever be used (in humans)? I suspect that for these people, too, the fundamental issue is how society uses the new capabilities at its disposal. These technical capabilities become an issue, however, because they lead directly to the former question.

In the final analysis, what seems to worry and upset some concerned members of our society is the fact that the 'new' available information may eventually be used, perhaps even abused, to select our progeny. And this, of course, sounds as if the world could slide slowly (to some even quickly) into eugenics, so that instantly red lights start flashing everywhere.

Without wishing to analyse any further the 'slippery slope' arguments discussed in several previous issues of Biomedical Ethics, I submit that, in fact, we already do 'select' our progeny in several ways. Many parents insist on having genetic tests as soon as is possible and/or meaningful after the onset of pregnancy. In many societies the legal system already determines what parents can or cannot do with such information. Many instances occur when they decide to interrupt the pregnancy. Whether they can afford or have access to such technology is a different issue, one which I am not going to discuss here.

Furthermore, marriage outside the racial, religious, social or national group that one belongs to is often either frowned upon or forbidden (at the risk of being excluded permanently from such a group). Curiously, many 'developed' societies tolerate attitudes such as these, which clearly try to exclude whole populations from genetic mixing. While for many of us such a position is accepted under the umbrella of 'minority or religious rights' or as tradition, in many other societies these rules are aggressively imposed by authoritarian governments.

In most democratic societies we do not seriously question many of these precepts, despite the fact that they have clearly affected the genetic makeup of our forefathers and will continue to do so for many future generations. We also do not seem to question the societal pressures on our young when we impress and/or impose upon them our philosophical, religious or ethical principles – principles which are often not discussed but which are presented as transcendental truths transmitted to us by our forefathers and which have withstood the test of time.

How can anyone accept unquestionably the fact that we are entitled to make choices that allow us to impose upon our children – for the benefit of their mind and body, of course – so many guidelines (and restraints) in the form of education, religion, nutrition, sport and social training, all of which have indelible and unpredictable effects upon their character and health, and not accept that under specific circumstances, to be determined by the legal system, we should also be allowed to make choices regarding the genetic constitution of our offspring, whether fertilisation takes place in vivo or in vitro? And why should we not be able – also under specific circumstances and in a limited number of cases – to eliminate on a permanent basis, using germline therapy, genetic disorders that are debilitating and painful?

To answer these questions we need to analyse current developments in modern biology. Both the identification and characterisation of an increasing number of genes and the advent of genetic manipulation have had a profound impact on the manner in which we perceive and understand 'human nature'. Until the 1970s it was generally thought that the environment played a major role in the development of one's character and mind. Countless books, reviews and articles were published on how to be a good parent. One's peers mattered also, but were less important. Frequently, to my great surprise and frustration, many people of my generation (I was born in '45) still blame mostly their parents for what they have become. Freud, of course, carries a great deal of responsibility for this; in unravelling the mysteries of the mind, he placed an enormous emphasis on the interaction between the young boy or girl and his or her parents, in the determination of character or personality. Aggression, depression, homosexuality and paranoia were just a few of the personality traits that could thus be explained.

Things have changed greatly in the last three decades. Not a week goes by in which a new gene does not surface to explain some genetic disorder or at least partly explain some increased susceptibility to cancer, crime, heart disease, body weight, etc. The messages that surround and bombard us insistently are that we are determined by our DNA. And the responsibility for this state of affairs rests not only with the media; in order to secure funding for the human genome project, many scientists claimed that it would eventually help to eliminate human disease. No wonder that slowly and insidiously the equation:

(Human) DNA = Soul

has gained ground, and should today colour most of the discussions surrounding the concept of identity. Somehow DNA has become a 'sacred' constituent of living organisms. I say 'somehow', but we all know very well how this happened. If, in fact, you are what is included in your DNA, or in other words, you are determined exclusively by your DNA, then it is only a very short distance to claim that your essence is contained in that molecule.

It is claimed that while we can still overcome the social and cultural legacy of our environment, we cannot overcome the pre-determined legacy of our genes! This is clearly untrue. While some disorders are clearly related to a single gene, most characteristics and susceptibilities are multifactorial and are related to several genes. In either case, the environment we choose frequently also plays a major role. And surely I do not have to add that the choice to try to overcome our social and cultural legacy, while possible, has only been evident in a very limited number of unique individuals.

Manipulating DNA in humans and making choices based on knowledge of the characteristics of that DNA both evoke fears of irreversibility and the idea that man could use this power to generate a sort of 'Brave New World'. Again, the slippery slope argument.

Genetic engineering is still in its infancy, but so are the fields of psychotherapy, psychiatry and many others. Our societies are both fascinated and frightened by the speed at which new knowledge is being generated and applied. Western culture is filled with warnings of the dangers of knowledge. Prometheus, Adam and Eve, and Faust are just a few of the best known examples. As Victor warns Robert in Mary Shelley's Frankenstein:

Learn from me, if not by my precepts, at least by my example, how dangerous is the acquirement of knowledge, and how much happier that

211

man is who believes his native town to be the world, than he who aspires to become greater than his nature will allow.

No wonder the subtitle of this novel was 'The Modern Prometheus'.

Nevertheless, we have benefited greatly from advances in science and technology, even as we lose or risk losing valuable characteristics of our inherited patrimony. It has become a cliché to say that all new knowledge presents us with opportunities and risks. PID and germline gene therapy are no different. They provide us with unquestionable opportunities to alleviate suffering and pain. The risks that accompany these developments should be recognised and should be the starting point for discussions and debates that involve not only scientists and philosophers or medical practitioners and theologians, but also non-specialists in these domains. Parents, single or coupled, are undoubtedly one of the most important groups to involve. But others too: teachers, journalists, students, social workers, politicians, etc. would all benefit a great deal from being better informed and from being included in these discussions.

We may find that other technologies will replace these in the near future. If so, our attention will be drawn to other problems. The bottom line, however, will always be whether parents, or society, or both have the right to obtain genetic information either from an adult, a child, a fetus, an embryo or the germ cells, and what will be allowed once such information becomes available. Bioethics has attracted a great deal of added attention precisely because genetic engineering is making strong progress. Many, including scientists outside of the narrow field of genetic engineering, have a very limited idea of what is currently possible and what remains simply a desirable goal. Many more have no idea of the opportunities and risks involved. And even if they had some idea, they still would feel baffled by how this kind of information should be translated into public policy.

My own conviction is that new knowledge always requires time before it gets incorporated into our 'everyday life'. Unfortunately, we often do not have the luxury of time. So the process advances by a series of trials and errors. PID and germline gene therapy will follow a similar path.

6   Beside the point – reflections on passivity

Paul J.M. van Tongeren

This contribution will be – I am afraid – 'beside the point'. But it is so on purpose. For, what I will try to make clear (or rather: to remind the readers of, since I am sure they know already) is that there is something beside the point, and that ethics has a special responsibility to remind us of what is 'beside the point'.

In order to clarify what I mean, I should start by saying what the point, or the focus of this volume is. It has two main themes: preimplantation diagnosis and germline gene therapy; it explores many different approaches to those themes, including the medical, the ethical, the legal and the sociological approaches. Even where the interweaving of these perspectives into an interdisciplinary approach is successful, it will result in many, or at least several, points or focuses. Therefore it can only be a very rough approximation if I summarise the 'point' of the contributions to this volume as the question: What we should do (and should not do) with the possibilities given to us by recent developments in science and technology to improve our physical well-being, or – more specifically – to reduce the number of sick or handicapped human beings? In order to answer that question, we investigate what those scientific and technological possibilities are and what consequences their application would have; we list the problems this raises; we explore the desires that create the demand for the techniques being developed; we list and categorise the fears and hopes of people; we evaluate the technology by calculating its consequences and by testing them against some fundamental principles; and we try to form a consensus on this evaluation among as many people as possible.

I think that all this is very important and 'to the point'. Nevertheless I want to concentrate on what is beside the point. It seems that to the point are questions regarding our activity: what we are able to do, what we are allowed to do, and what we should do. If this is true, then it would be beside the point to concentrate on our passivity. Our activity is intended to improve our world, our natural conditions, our physical and psychological well-being. Our passivity is the other side of the fact that the effort of this activity will never be completed. However successful we will be in our attempts to make the world and ourselves the way we want them to be, there will always be a limit to these attempts, be it only because of the fact that they always re-act to, and therefore are dependent on, what is given. What I am trying to say is that it is important to also reflect ethically on this reverse side of our activity. I am not saying that we should do this instead of asking what we are allowed to and should do; I am not saying that the proper focus of the discussion should be on passivity rather than on activity. I am only saying that this passivity, although it is beside the point, is nevertheless morally important as well as our activity.

This concentration on passivity is – from a philosophical perspective – even more important at a time in which people are exclusively or primarily interested in all kinds of activity, as is apparently the case in our time. If philosophy is, as Nietzsche once called it, the bad conscience of its own age (Nietzsche 1966) it should always and in principle concentrate on what one is in danger of forgetting – even if this would mean that philosophy is almost in principle 'beside the point'.

But what should we do, if we have to concentrate on what runs the risk of being forgotten? There are many problems here, even many kinds of problems. Just to mention a few: The expression 'beside the point' indicates already one of those problems: for what is 'beside the point' is just as diverse as 'the point' is concentrated. There is always only one way to hit the bull's-eye, and an infinite number of ways to miss it. This means that I am not claiming that the problem of passivity is the only problem that runs the risk of being forgotten; I am just concentrating on this one point beside the point.

But then: reminding someone of what he is in danger of forgetting is problematic, if one conceives of conscience as a spotlight, as I am inclined to do. A spotlight always creates a lot of darkness by shedding light on one spot very strongly. To put it differently: by illuminating a dark spot, we will darken spots that were illuminated before. The only thing to do here is to acknowledge this as much as possible, and to realise that even acknowledging that every reminder will cause a forgetting and does not eliminate the forgetting. I am inclined to see this as an example of the passivity I want to focus on; and it is important to realise that even this understanding of the necessity of our passivity does not turn it into some kind of activity.

This points to a final problem I will address briefly in this contribution: for paying attention to one's passivity is, in some way or another, 'doing' something, and thus: being not passive, but active. This is only one of the ways in which thinking about passivity yields to paradoxes that cannot be solved, but have to be endured. And that is exactly what an ethics of passivity wants to make clear: it reminds us that – in the words of T.S. Eliot – 'There are two kinds of problems in life. One kind requires the question, "What are we going to do about it?" and the other calls forth different questions: "What does it mean? How does one relate to it?"' (Cole 1988).

In this contribution I can only touch upon some aspects of what this passivity is, and how we might relate to it in an adequate way. But first I want to ask the question, why we should pay attention to it at all. Above I stated that it was important to reflect ethically on our passivity, because it was an inevitable aspect of our life: all our efforts to make our life as we would like it to be remain limited in comparison with our desires (or maybe I should say that our ever transcending desires make every reality into a project of transformation). But why should ethical reflection not abstract from this characteristic, why should it not concentrate on some of the problems that the human being encounters on its way, instead of reminding him or her that this way is always longer than he or she could ever complete? What is the importance of knowing that one's efforts are ultimately limited, if within these limits there is enough to do?

The reason is that human beings in their particular actions intend more than only the performance of this action and the reaching of its particular goal. We are reminded of the opening phrase of Aristotle's *Nicomachean Ethics*, in which he says that whatever a human being does, is always aiming at some good. He goes on to explain that all those goods are hierarchically ordered, and ultimately refer to the supreme good, which is not desired for the sake of something else, but for its own sake. According to Aristotle we should try to know more about this final good, in order to learn more about what to do in each individual case.

If there is something right in this teleological framework (and I think there is), it says that also our efforts in medicine and in pre-emptive techniques, such as preimplantation diagnosis and germline gene therapy, are to be understood within a broader framework; that scientists who are involved in this kind of research and patients who are interested in the results are involved or interested, because they consider this research or this treatment or this security check to be part of how life should be, or what would be a good life.

A correct evaluation of a particular act or event should be made from the perspective of the supreme good, the ultimate good, the good of a life as a whole. If this is the case, it becomes clear that the limits of our efforts are much more important than it would be the case if I could abstract from the wider context in which my action stands. As soon as I know that whatever I do is meant to contribute to the good life as a whole, I acknowledge the interrelatedness of all the aspects of and contributions to the good life. I cannot just evaluate a particular act according to its agreement with some kind of principle, but I have to asses its value according to its contribution to the good of the life as a whole. But if it is a characteristic of our life as a whole that it has its limits and is inevitably ruled in part by chance or fortune, this should and will also have an impact on whatever I do within life. And this brings me again to my point, beside the point.

I said already that it was not my intention to suggest that we should reflect on passivity instead of asking what our activity should be. Let me add immediately that it is not my intention either to say that we should be more passive and less active, that we should let things happen more and try less to 'make things better' (of course we should treat sickness wherever we can, prevent people from falling ill, improve the conditions under which human beings are born and live, etc.; even the prevention of severe suffering through abortion and euthanasia can sometimes be a legitimised choice). The only point I am trying to make is that we should do more than we usually do, when we try to make things better: while making things better, we should at the same time learn to acknowledge that we will not ever be completely successful. I will try to elaborate on this point a little with four remarks.

Even the expression I used above – 'learn to acknowledge that we will never be completely successful' is misleading. The point is not that there will always be a remainder, or that the way to perfection is longer than anyone could go. The point is rather that all progress produces its own remainder. Speaking of our efforts never being 'completely' successful suggests that we will be more and more successful, and that the remainder of imperfection or of that which is not controlled by our own activity, will become smaller and smaller. This seems, however, not to be the case. Yes, there is progress in medicine as well as in other fields. But it is a strange kind of progress, even if we abstract from the fact that this progress is distributed in a very unfair way across the world. The progress is strange because, although we live longer and have overcome many diseases, we seem to be no less concerned about our health, and no less worried about the dangers that threaten us. The reason for this is twofold: on the one hand, every hill that I climb gives a view onto further hills that invite me to climb them. I did not want to climb the hills that I did not see, but I do want to climb them as soon as I do see them. We do not want to become as old as Methuselah, but we do want to reach at least the average age. On the other hand: our ability to endure what resists our desires seems to decrease to the

216

same extent as our ability to fulfil our desires increases. Nietzsche expresses this in a rather extreme way when he writes (Nietsche 1969):

> The curve of human susceptibility to pain seems in fact to take an extraordinary and almost sudden drop as soon as one has passed the upper ten thousand or ten million of the top stratum of culture; and for my part, I have no doubt that the combined suffering of all the animals ever subjected to the knife for scientific ends is utterly negligible compared with *one* painful night of a single hysterical bluestocking.

From this it should be clear again that I am not saying that we should limit our efforts through some kind of passivity, or that the finiteness of our activity could be translated in terms of a boundary that we would have to respect. What I am saying is not a secular version of what was ever thought of as the prohibition by God or gods. I would rather interpret the stories about a forbidding and line-drawing God as theocentric interpretations of this typical human characteristic. These stories show in a hidden way that the human being resists the acceptance of any line or limit: not only because every prohibition triggers a transgression, but also because the prohibition by God seems to translate (human) passivity into a (divine) activity. The passivity I am pointing to, however, is not an external boundary to our activity. It is not a border about which there can be a dispute as to whether or not it should be pushed back. It is rather the other side of the coin, i.e. something which will always be there. It is not so much a limit to our activity as it is like an echo of it.

Again one could ask: why should I pay (so much) attention to this aspect of human life? The answer is at least twofold. First, in order to prevent the illusion that this other side is not there or will be removed in due time. And second, in order to prevent too one-sided a development of ourselves as human beings. The first answer is tricky again. Whoever wants to avoid falling into illusions is afraid of being disappointed, and wants to ensure that nothing will happen that could ever disappoint. I am referring to the unconvincing aspect of some stoic wisdom, in which the detachment of the ideal apathia turns into apathetic unaffectedness or disinterestedness, which is in fact first and foremost an insurance against unexpected disillusions. Here, passivity is only the misleading appearance of a hidden activity, that even wants to master the unexpected and uncontrollable. But, on the other hand, this abuse of the prevention of false illusions does not take away the moral significance of a truthful life. And truthfulness is therefore one reason to pay attention to what withdraws itself from our activity.

The second reason refers to what I said before about Aristotle's teleological ethics. In order to understand it better, we should realise that with all our investments in scientific and technological research and the application of its results, we are not only extending our knowledge, refining our skills, curing patients and preventing all kinds of diseases, but in all of this we are at the same time cultivating what can be called one half of our human capacities: the active or activistic half. By 'cultivation' I mean that we train ourselves in interpreting the world and our lives in terms of what we can do with it, make out of it, etc. We have made ourselves into the activistic kind of people we are by being successful in our activities. This cultivation is implicit in the activities that were not aimed at this result, but had their own particular goals. As soon as we acknowledge this, we realise that this is like a mono-culture, that harms the other possibilities that we hold. Cultivating only our capacity to be active harms our capacity to be passive. Since our activities are at the same time, so to say, practices or training in being active, since they are at the same times, so to say, 'moral practices', we should avoid becoming morally one-sided, and not forget to cultivate and train our ability to be passive as well, and also this can only be done by practising it. But how to do that? I conclude with a brief remark on this point.

Training oneself in being passive is a paradoxical thing – I mentioned this before. Partly the paradox is only apparent, provoked by the vocabulary that we use. Being passive does not mean just doing nothing, it does not mean being lazy or indolent (something which precisely only activistic people can be). It rather means being mindful of what is happening to us, of there always being something that we do not make but receive – happily or not –, and being susceptible to the meaning of what is given, to what it has to say to us. It is not so much not doing anything, but a special kind of doing. One can look at something in a more active way (investigating something) and in a more passive way (attending to something). There is a difference between being guided by one's own interest (or by one's own interpretation of the other's interest) and being guided by what the other has to say. I find it hard to explain in a language that is not my own. But I suppose that even these few examples show that – ideally – this passivity is tied up with our activity as are the two sides of a coin. One will investigate better if one pays careful attention to what one investigates. Or, to take another example: The arrangements one makes will be more just if one does justice to the people concerned.

My suggestion is that in much of our medical activity (but not only there; it seems to be a general characteristic of our culture) we are in danger of underrating the passive side of the coin. We are much more interested in treating or preventing illnesses than we are in understanding what it is to be ill, what it is to be in pain. Is it not strange that there are not many chairs in our medical schools for pain-research? We are much more interested in cure than we are in care.

If I am right in this suspicion, then it would make sense to invest explicitly in passivity, to train ourselves in becoming more passive. And here the paradox returns, as the terminology of investment and training indicates. I do not think that this paradox can be resolved. I only think that acknowledging it and its insolubility might be a first step in our becoming more passive.

References

Cole, T. (1988), 'Aging, History and Health: Progress and Paradox', in: Schroots, J. et al. (eds), *Health and Aging,* Lisse: New York, pp. 45-63.

Nietzsche, F. (1966), *Beyond Good and Evil* § 212, (translated by W. Kaufmann), Vintage Books, New York.

Nietzsche, F. (1969), *On the Genealogy of Morals*, II, 7, (translated by W. Kaufmann and R. Hollingdale), Vintage Books, New York.

Part Five
CHOICES AND DECISION MAKING

1 What claims can be based on the desire for a healthy child? Towards an ethics of 'informed desires'

Walter Lesch

In this paper, a little extract from a work in progress, I want to suggest some more steps towards what I like to call an 'ethics of desire' (cf. Lesch 1998) which seems to be particularly appropriate to the intimate field of reproduction and parenthood where purely pragmatic and technological reasoning does not even touch the ethical problems we are going to discuss. This approach is of course no philosophical revolution that totally breaks with the tradition of ethical theory because reflection on 'ethics and emotions' has always been an important topic of research (cf. Fink-Eitel and Lohmann 1993). It is however noteworthy that the theoretical passion for the dynamics of desire is less known in German and French speaking countries (but cf. Schöpf 1987 and Audard 1998) than in the great tradition of Anglo-Saxon moral philosophy (cf. Cullity and Gaut 1997) which is one of the strongest parts of our common European heritage. The comments I want to make are not in the first place addressed to the community of philosophers, but to those who are not familiar with the technical terms of ethics. They will be offered some elements of reflection on the notion of desire which is one of the key problems in the ethical evaluation of artificial reproductive technologies.

The starting point is the following statement which is rather evident on the moral level: there is nothing special about the desire for a healthy child. On the contrary, why should we blame parents who do all they can to ensure of the health of their future child? We expect women not to smoke or to drink too much alcohol during the months of pregnancy. In this case it is considered as a moral duty to take care of the child's health and to avoid all risks of possible harm. But in spite of these obvious duties the desire for a healthy child has some new and more complicated ethical implications in the context of modern technologies of reproduction where the supposed feasibility of health becomes an integral part of the parents' desire and sometimes even the condition of the acceptance and the love they will give to the child. Without doubt health is a desirable good. The possibility of selection and enhancement of future persons is nevertheless a new dimension of reproduction.

The language of desire

Sexuality, reproduction and family relationships are nearly always linked to strong emotions and desires, hopes and fears, because they concern the sources of personal and social identity. The public image of genetics cannot be understood without this component of emotional commitment that explains to a large extent our ambivalent attitude towards the methods of genetic diagnosis and therapy. Can there be a greater hope than overcoming sterility and having not only a child of one's own, but a healthy child? In other words: being given the chance to live a happy family life, even if this sounds a little petty bourgeois nowadays. Would it not be irresponsible not to use the medical assistance that helps such wishes come true – not with an absolute certainty, but with a relatively high probability?

When we talk about the traits of a future child (as a *virtual* reality) it is always helpful to consider the parallel case of adoption (where there are already *real* children) in order to test the validity of our arguments. A couple seeking a child for adoption usually asks for a young and healthy child, if possible sharing the parents' ethnic and cultural background so that they can live like a 'natural' family. There are pragmatic reasons for such a concrete desire, but we also won't ignore the narcissist wish to create the nearly perfect illusion of procreation as a substitute for the prolongation of one's own identity. It is theoretically easy to say that the social construct of parenthood and family life is much more important than the contingent biological fact of filiation. There is still the widespread opinion that biology *does* matter, even if it is only the preference for a *healthy* adoptive child. The adoption of children with obvious disabilities is not the rule, but the expression of altruism and of a special acceptance of the child's otherness that has to be absolutely respected. This unconditionable love which public authorities demand from adoptive parents is inconsistent with the quality control that increasingly influences the definition of children who are 'acceptable' or not.

Returning to the role of genetics in reproduction I want to mention another case that illustrates the complexity of our subject. Imagine a genetic counselling situation in which parents with certain disabilities, for instance deafness, ask for assistance in having a child with the same disabilities so that the whole family will belong to the same 'cultural' minority and can act in solidarity against possible discrimination. This issue of 'deliberately producing a deaf child' (Davis, 1997, p.8) shows very well that the progress of the Human Genome Project will give rise to a number of new dilemmas for counselling and ethical reasoning. In the given case I would (together with Davis 1997) clearly plead against the parents' autonomy and for the child's right to an open future. The 'culture of deafness' seems to be a very narrow community so that nobody should be forced to become a member of it by means of genetic engineering.

> Good parenthood requires a balance between having a child for our own sakes and being open to the moral reality that the child will exist for her own sake, with her own talents and weaknesses, propensities and interests, and with her own life to make. Parental practices that close exits virtually forever are insufficiently attentive to the child as an end in herself. By closing off the child's right to an open future, they define the child as an entity who exists to fulfill parental hopes and dreams, not her own (Davis 1997, p.12).

As the examples considered so far have shown, desires are indispensable and dangerous at the same time. They express individual claims to autonomous life plans and on the other hand the undeniable influence of psychological, cultural and social factors that restrict free decisions. The history of modern ethics can be described as a constant oscillation between the two extremes of rational control and emotional creativity, symbolic order and anarchical effects.

Our language is full of words expressing the different dimensions and degrees of wishing and desiring: passion, demand, yearning, longing, seeking etc. As a desire approaches the intentional act it becomes an object of the will. According to Kant, 'good will' is the essence of morality because the will is identical with practical reason. In other philosophical theories the will is much closer to irrational powers and far from being connected with universal laws in the Kantian sense. The same diversity of meanings can be found on the level preceding the degree of desires: basic needs are sometimes regarded as the biological basis of morality because they define the necessities of organising our lives. On the other hand it is not always easy to make the distinction between basic needs that have to be satisfied (such that a failure to do so constitutes a violation of fundamental human rights) and other needs which are stimulated artificially and represent a manipulation of our free choice. The following table shows some words (without any claim to completeness) for different degrees of wishes in the English, French and German language.

Table 1. The vocabulary of desire

English	French	German
instinct, drive	instinct, pulsion	Instinkt, Trieb
need	besoin	Bedürfnis
inclination	inclination	Neigung
desire	désir	Begehren
wish	désir, souhait	Wunsch
will	volonté	Wille
demand	demande,	Forderung
claim, pretension	réclamation	Anspruch
right	prétention	Recht
	droit	

As an example, the semantics of 'pretension' reveals some aspects of our problem because the usage of 'to pretend', 'pretender', 'pretentious', 'pretentiousness' points to the mistrust of unjustified claims. As long as we are not (officially) entitled to do something (but how? and by whom?) we have to give good arguments for our pretensions. This is exactly what ethics is about.

The list from needs over claims to rights shows not only the different degrees of obligation, but also the constant shift of perspectives between individual wishes (the subjective part of morals) and socially guaranteed rights (the objective moral universe). 'The English word «desire» indicates a set of ideas that can be weak or strong, from a mild wish to a yearning or a frantic lust' (Oppenheimer 1986, p.152). There is still another problem in our evaluation of desires.

> Religious people frequently treat desire itself as inherently sinful, and especially sexual desire, so uncontrollable and often irrational. Theologians of a more positive bent have blamed Augustine's horror of 'concupiscence', mankind's fallen, distorted will, for much that is negative in Christian ethics (...) (Oppenheimer 1986, p.153).

These two opposed orientations in philosophical and religious traditions can be illustrated as follows. On the one side there is the attitude of being very demanding. In this case we consider ourselves to be entitled to the pursuit of happiness because of our basic needs and strong desires. Such a position of hedonist self-interest is often attributed to the philosophy of Epicurus although his theory of the happy life only partly corresponds to an unlimited hedonism. On the other side there would be a simple style of life with the repression of strong desires and the esteem of modesty as a virtue. This attitude is near to the stoical ideal of being undemanding without resting absolutely passive. Both models of reaching happiness by means of a cultivated art of living contain complementary aspects because pleasure is not simply the result of wild desires, but also depends on rational plans.

Obviously negative judgements on desire and delight have particularly deep roots in Christian ethics and correspond to a more or less negative view of the body and sexuality in the mainstream of this tradition. These positions are reflected in fundamental attitudes towards health, disease and handicap. If life and health are God's good gifts, they are certainly to be maintained, but not at any price because this would change the character of human beings as creatures partly depending on their creator. I suspect that in spite of secularisation and dechristianisation this tradition still has a considerable influence on our collective image of health and reproduction and leads to a firm opposition to all forms of reasoning which take place merely in terms of a cost-benefit-analysis. Can moral philosophy clearly tell us which of these two tendencies is right and which wrong? Or will all attempts at differentiation finally leave us alone in world of moral relativism? The next three sections of this paper try to give some elements of a reasonable answer.

Motivation by desire and the impact of practical reason

First of all we have to underline that our question refers to a rather old debate that was already present at the beginning of moral philosophy in ancient Greece, taken up in the positions of Hume and Kant in the eighteenth century and rather prominent in the metaethical discussions between emotivism and cognitivism in our century. I begin with this last manifestation which is not only an interesting part of the history of philosophy, but is still a sign of an acute problem of contemporary ethics. In the context of logical positivism A.J. Ayer introduced the provocative idea that there is no moral reality at all. Our moral language, as an expression of feelings, desires and beliefs, refers to nothing, so that we are just trying to convince others to share these emotions. There is no place for rational argumentation, only for the expression of attitudes and of agreement or disagreement. Such a theory will not help us to understand desires or clarify the normative status of strong desires as motivations. To a larger extent ethical theory is nearer to what we call cognitivist positions. These must not necessarily be compatible with the very severe form of Kantian ethics according to which the autonomy of the will should not depend on our natural desires. But in any case extreme emotivism is unable to give reasons for the regulation of moral practice in complex societies. In order to avoid misunderstandings it should at least be noted that emotivism is not the only form of noncognitivist ethics. R.M. Hare's prescriptivism is another, more plausible theory that works as well with the assumption that there is no universal moral reality.

The debate between cognitivists and their opponents is not only an important topic in Anglo-American moral philosophy of this century. A similar structure can already be found in the philosophy of David Hume.

> According to the standard picture of human psychology – a picture we owe to David Hume, the famous Scottish philosopher of the eighteenth century – there are two main kinds of psychological state. On the one hand there are beliefs, states that purport to represent the way the world is. Since our beliefs purport to represent the world, they are subject to rational criticism: specifically, they are assessable in terms of truth and falsehood according to whether or not they succeed in representing the world to be the way it really is. On the other hand, however, there are also desires, states that represent how the world is to be. Desires are unlike beliefs in that they do not even purport to represent the way the world is. They are therefore not assessable in terms of truth and falsehood. Indeed, according to the standard picture, our desires are at bottom not subject to any sort of rational criticism at all. (...) *in themselves*, our desires are all on a par, rationally neutral (Smith 1995, p.400).

Hume proposes an attractive model for understanding human action that has to be distinguished from the motivation to act in a desirable way. The pure motive of duty in disregard of our desires seems to be too weak to stimulate actions (cf. Schueler 1995).

Desires should thus be part of every theory of action which wants to close the gap between motivation and action. Claims have to be justified within the framework of a theory of rights, rules and mutual duties of all the persons who are concerned by a specific project. But there would be no claim without the existence of strong desires and dreams which have to be discussed and analysed in order to find out what is possible and what not. The articulation of informed desires has the advantage of crossing the border between highly individualised wishes and maxims that can be universalised. The desire for a healthy child is a good example of a wish that is not at all purely egoistic. Of course, such a wish expresses the parents' vision of a good life, but also concerns directly the chances of happiness for the child. So it is from the beginning a matter of social concern and not only of private pleasure and preference.

Nevertheless it seems to be a demand of political correctness to mistrust these sorts of desires because they could be directed against handicapped persons. But even if we do not admit it, we probably agree that it is better to live without handicaps than with them (Rippe 1997, p.7). If we accept this presupposition we are inclined to accept the possibility of prenatal diagnosis and the parents' wish to have access to it as a sufficient indication for this test (cf. the critical position of Baumann-Hölzle and Kind 1997). We would also accept the possibility of abortion in the case of a positive result of the diagnosis and welcome therapeutical interventions in order to avoid abortions. This is a logic leading to the moral approval of preimplantation diagnosis (PID) that should be dissociated from eugenics (cf. Testart 1994). The private nature of reproductive decisions is slowly transformed into a societal concern when the offer of genetic counselling helps the patients to clarify their uninformed desires. This counselling only makes sense if we have good reason to think that desires alone are no sources of value and that practical reason is not powerless when the right decision has to be found.

The psychoanalysis and psychology of desire

As some important currents of moral philosophy have neglected the field of emotions and desires, ethics can learn a lot from the interdisciplinary contact with moral psychology. There are interesting psychological theories of motivation and helpful studies on the problem of how to cope with disappointments and unfulfilled wishes. We know a lot about the dangers of wishful thinking and the psychopathology of wishes. This aspect has been thoroughly discussed in Sigmund Freud's theory of psychoanalysis where wishes are considered as illusions which find their expression in dreams (Saint Girons 1997, Boothe et al. 1998).

Another interesting contribution is Jacques Lacan's theory of the specular image. According to this approach desire is an unconscious current of our narcissist tendency to construct our own identity and our vision of the other as mirrored images (Lacan 1966). The desired child is also captured in the image the parents make against the background of their own images. As a result, individuals do not exist as independent and coherent persons, but in the complicated universe of unconsciousness structured by the symbolic order of language. Human beings constantly experience incompleteness and lack and are therefore driven by an unsatisfiable desire to be loved and to be given the impression of completeness with the help of the other's image. I cannot enter into a further discussion of these exciting ideas that should be considered more closely in the theoretical research on the desire for a child as a special case of Lacan's 'desire of the other'.

Independent from therapeutical applications a great part of recent psychological research on desire has been inspired by the philosopher Harry Frankfurt and his famous distinction of first-order and second-order desires (Frankfurt 1988). Whereas first-order desires are spontaneous wishes, impulses or needs, we are capable of adopting a cognitive attitude towards these first-order desires. On a second level we can keep our distance to spontaneous expressions and thus avoid logical contradictions, establish a chronological order and a list of priorities. This is of course not the final answer to the problem of desires from a rational point of view. We do not always have unequivocal criteria in order to know that higher order preferences are more rational than lower order desires. But this distinction shows a useful direction for the discussion of priorities and end-means-relations in genetic counselling situations.

As a provisional result we can say that psychological and philosophical criticism of wishes (cf. Kusser 1989, Wolf 1996) is indispensable to the dialogue between the emotional and the cognitive aspects of action. Without strong (and sometimes wrong) desires there would be no innovation, no change, no scientific progress. But desires alone do not direct us to good choices. We should also take a critical look at the impact of the media and their strategies of introducing genetic concepts in popular culture where DNA is sometimes seen as a new destiny or as a dangerous backdoor to eugenics (Nelkin 1994). So it is not always easy to decide which of my desires are really my own desires. Aren't they a result of my social, economic and cultural context? The specific role of ethics in the field of health in human reproduction consists in transforming hot and unreflected desires into informed (= higher order) desires. That means

to discover different degrees of desires (first- and second-order desires) and to establish a hierarchy (of course there is still the problem of evaluating such hierarchies),

to think about alternatives to a strong wish for a child,

to consider possible consequences for the child,

to balance the parents' autonomy and the child's autonomy (the child's right to an open future),

to consider the problem of justice concerning the access to diagnosis and therapy (including the legal and economic situation).

All these aspects are elements of a responsible practice of genetic counselling.

From desires to claims and from claims to rights

The last point takes us directly to the difficult transition from informed desires to justified claims. Legal regulations should not intervene too early in the process of value clarification because there is already enough work to be done on the level of ethical argumentation, especially at the intersection of individual and social ethics. From such a point of view the claim to a healthy child is more than a question of personal preferences and individual choice. A rational life plan cannot be separated from communities with shared values and moral attitudes in the case of disease and failure. In recent philosophy this type of problem can be illustrated from the debate between 'liberals' and 'communitarians'.

> Communitarian ethics as applied to health care will suggest the limits within which genetic interventions should be carried out; according to Hub Zwart, it embodies a willingness to accept, as opposed to a constant readiness to intervene. The place to start, then, in redressing the balance is by turning from questions of individualism to questions that affect the community, looking beyond the biological paradigms to the environmental causes of ill health (...). It is the response given to these questions that will determine the social context within which individual choices are made (Chadwick 1995, p.128).

Even the greatest progress of genetic control and therapy will not completely change the uncontrollable otherness of the child as an independent human being with his or her own rights. For this reason ethics should not be restricted to a case by case risk assessment, but should also take into account the cultural dynamics of genetics as an important factor in the construction of a new image of health and disease and the illusion of perfection (McGee 1997a). What about the perfect child in a world of extreme imperfection?

> (...) imagine the beautiful, intelligent, even-tempered girl developed by genetic engenering. Could she survive in an imperfect world, with bad water and fatty foods? (McGee 1997b, p.21).

In a world of rapid change we know so little about tomorrow that any kind of calculativeness could even become ridiculous. The adventure of parenthood can only partly be brought under technical control because the future is open and will again and again confront us with the necessity to decide what has to be changed and what has to be accepted. This paradox is common to medical aid and to education.

My conclusion is not an ethics of prohibition because I cannot see why PID should be considered as absolutely bad in itself. I wonder whether modesty is a virtue in the practice of biomedical ethics or only the confession of helplessness. But if clinical ethics is conceived as a contextual philosophy (Cadoré 1997) within a scientific culture of uncertainty (Malherbe 1996) I invite ethicists to adopt an attitude of scepticism regarding the long-term social effects of selection and enhancement as long as there is no legal regulation accepted by all members of the European Union and no ethical theory capable of reconciling private desires and the public interest in avoiding the abuse of genetics in reproduction and of predictive medicine in general.

References

Audard, C. (1998), 'Les désirs humains ont-ils leur place en morale?', *Magazine littéraire*, No. 361, Dossier: Les nouvelles morales, pp. 79-81.

Baumann-Hölzle, R. and Kind, Ch. (1997), *Indikationen zur pränatalen Diagnostik. Vom geburtshilflichen Notfall zum genetischen Screening* (Folia Bioethica, 20), Société Suisse d'éthique biomédicale: Lausanne.

Boothe, B., Wepfer, R. and von Wyl, A. (eds) (1998), *Über das Wünschen. Ein seelisches und poetisches Phänomen wird erkundet*, Vandenhoeck & Ruprecht: Göttingen.

Cadoré, B. (1997), *L'éthique clinique comme philosophie contextuelle*, Éditions Fides: Montréal.

Chadwick, R. (1995), 'The Gene Revolution', in Brenda, A. (ed.), *Introducing Applied Ethics*, Blackwell: Oxford, pp. 118-29.

Cullity, G. and Gaut, B. (eds) (1997), *Ethics and Practical Reason*, Clarendon: Oxford.

Davis, D.S. (1997), 'Genetic Dilemmas and the Child's Right to an Open Future', *Hastings Center Report*, Vol. 27, No. 2, pp. 7-15.

Fink-Eitel, H. and Lohmann, G. (eds) (1993), *Zur Philosophie der Gefühle*, Suhrkamp: Frankfurt a.M.

Frankfurt, H. (1988), *The Importance of What We Care about. Philosophical Essays*, University Press: Cambridge.

Kusser, A. (1989), *Dimensionen der Kritik von Wünschen*, Athenäum: Frankfurt a.M.

Lacan, J. (1966), *Écrits*, Seuil: Paris.

Lesch, W. (1998), 'Is the Desire for a Child too Strong? or Is There a Right to a Child of One's Own?', in Hildt, E. and Mieth, D. (eds), *In Vitro Fertilisation in the 1990s. Towards a Medical, Social and Ethical Evaluation*, Ashgate: Aldershot, pp. 73-9.

Malherbe, J.-F. (1996), *L'incertitude en éthique. Perspectives cliniques*, Éditions Fides: Montréal.

McGee, G. (1997a), *The Perfect Baby. A Pragmatic Approach to Genetics*, Rowman & Littlefield: Lanham.

McGee, G. (1997b), 'Parenting in an Era of Genetics', *Hastings Center Report*, Vol. 27, No. 2, pp. 16-22.

Nelkin, D. (1994), 'Genetics in the Media', in Landeshauptstadt Stuttgart, Kulturamt (ed.), *Zum Naturbegriff der Gegenwart*, Band 2, Frommann-Holzboog: Stuttgart-Bad Cannstatt, pp. 231-44.

Oppenheimer, H. (1986), 'Desire', in Childress, J.F. and Macquarrie, J. (eds), *The Westminster Dictionary of Christian Ethics*, The Westminster Press: Philadelphia, pp. 152-3.

Rippe, K.P. (1997), *Pränatale Diagnostik und 'selektive Abtreibung'* (Folia Bioethica, 19), Société Suisse d'éthique biomédicale: Lausanne.

Saint Girons, B. (1997), 'Désir & Besoin', in *Dictionnaire de la Psychanalyse*, Encyclopædia Unversalis and Albin Michel: Paris, pp. 137-44.

Schöpf, A. (ed.) (1987), *Bedürfnis, Wunsch, Begehren. Probleme einer philosophischen Sozialanthropologie*, Königshausen & Neumann: Würzburg.

Schueler, G.G. (1995), *Desire. Its Role in Practical Reason and the Explanation of Action*, MIT-Press: Cambridge, Mass.

Smith, M. (1995), 'Realism', in Singer, P. (ed.), *A Companion to Ethics*, Blackwell: Oxford, pp. 399-410.

Testart, J. (1994), *Le désir du gène*, Flammarion: Paris.

Wolf, J.-C. (1996), 'Moralischer Internalismus. Motivation durch Wünsche versus Motivation durch Überzeugungen', *Conceptus. Zeitschrift für Philosophie*, Vol. 29, No. 74, pp. 47-61.

2 The European Alliance of Genetic Support Groups

Ysbrand Poortman

The European Alliance of Genetic Support groups (EAGS) is a European umbrella organisation of patients' organisations concerned with genetic disorders. It represents European umbrella groups for specific conditions and national umbrella bodies for the whole range of genetic disorders.

The EAGS was founded in 1992 during a meeting in Elsinore (near Copenhagen) after a preliminary meeting in Leuven, Belgium (1991), and has met every year since than as a satellite of and in co-operation with the annual congress of the European Society of Human Genetics (ESHG).

42 associations from 14 countries are affiliated to the EAGS. It is estimated that the EAGS represents via its member organisations over 6 million registered families in Europe.

Objectives of the EAGS

Main objectives of the EAGS are:

to serve the common aims of individuals and families with genetic disorders
to promote the provision of services which meet the needs of these individuals
and families.

Subsidiary objectives are:

to facilitate the availability of reliable information concerning genetic disorders, their prevention and treatment
to increase public awareness concerning genetic disorders
to stimulate research into the causes, prevention, diagnosis and treatment of genetic disorders and to promote public understanding of the importance of such research
to ensure the availability of comprehensive counselling on the options available and the consequences of particular choices
to ensure the individual's right to autonomous and informed decision making
to promote the assessment of the ethical, legal, psychological and social impact of the increasing understanding of human genetics
to voice and promote the views of the members on issues of common concern
to represent the members in European and International bodies and organisations
to encourage the formation of new National and European umbrella organisations.

Bottlenecks

During the 1992 meeting of the EAGS in Copenhagen bottlenecks were listed by the representatives of the various member organisations. The complaints and problems, regardless of what country the participants came from, were the same or very similar. These statements were recently reviewed and considered still to be up to date and relevant.

The bottlenecks were summarised as follows:
primary and secondary level health care is not capable of dealing with genetics and genetic counselling; the level of awareness of health care officials and caregivers about genetics is very low or absent
relevant information reaches the people concerned (too) late or not at all
appropriate and timely decision making is often endangered by late and inaccurate diagnosis, inefficient referrals, unbalanced and unreliable information
research into the causes of congenital disorders is scarce and its importance is underestimated
the impact of genetics and congenital disorders on the people concerned is underestimated; adequate and well trained guidance is hard to find
scarce availability of reliable, well balanced and clear educational materials tailored to the various target groups such as health care workers, media, the public and the people concerned.

Priorities

Priorities determined by the EAGS:

public awareness (to make information available to the public in order to increase the general understanding about genetics and genetic disorders, in particular the new genetic technologies and their applications)
education (of e.g. medical and general practitioners, health authorities and teachers) in matters relating to genetics, genetic disorders and genetic technologies
encouragement of scientific research in (medical and community) genetics and of the free flow of information among scientists
ethics (to promote ongoing assessment and research into the ethical and social impact of the new knowledge arising form genetic research)
reproductive choice and screening (to promote access to comprehensive genetic counselling at genetic service centres, any decisions in this regard to be made on the basis of free informed choice of the individual or couple within the legal framework of each country. Such individuals or couples have the right to the understanding and full support of society for whatever decision is reached. They also have the right to complete information and confidentiality).

Threats

There has also been unanimous agreement about concerns and threats which are formulated as follows:

scope and confidentiality of genetic testing and screening
discrimination and stigmatisation
eugenic pressure
commercial exploitation of human genome data
society is not prepared for genetic progress
equity of benefits of human genetic research.
Discussion of these concerns led to the need for an ethical code. A working committee was installed which drafted a proposal – with the professional advice of the ethicist Mrs. Jeantine Lunshof. This proposal circulated among the member organisations. After many interesting discussions the sixth annual general meeting of the EAGS endorsed the proposal in London on April 12, 1996.

The EAGS' Ethical Code

In the light of recent rapid scientific advances, the EAGS has recognised the need for a basic set of statements pertaining to the ethical issues created by the increased understanding of human genetics.
The EAGS endorses the standpoint agreed by the WHO (1995):

> Genetics and biomedical technology open up vast avenues for research and can provide humankind with much needed therapeutic tools. But, where human life and dignity are at stake, technology cannot be left to govern ethics on an empirical basis.

The EAGS, therefore, expresses its basic tenets in the following statements:

Statements and guidelines

1   Medical genetics should serve the interests of the individuals who are affected or at risk from a genetic condition.
2   Needs-based access to information and facilities should be safeguarded.
3   Individuals should be free to decide for themselves whether or not to make use of the available information and facilities.
4   Genetic services are to facilitate diagnosis and provide options for and leading to informed decisions about preventative measures and/or treatment, and the consequent provision of appropriate needs-based services.
5   The continual improvement of the quality of life and of care and support of those affected by hereditary or congenital disorders is to be promoted, particularly by encouraging and supporting any necessary changes in legislation at national and at European level, to the benefit of patients with genetic disorders.
6   Persons with a disability or disease are entitled to unrestricted acceptance and solidarity from society.

The EAGS calls on behalf of families with genetic and congenital disorders for:

equal access to full information
early diagnosis at accredited centres
the maintenance of confidentiality
the freedom of choice for all within the legal framework of each country.

Commentary on the statements and guidelines

1   Genetic counselling should be undertaken by qualified personnel. It should be comprehensive in its scope. Preferably it should be available in clinical genetics centres or in affiliation with such centres. Clinical genetics centres cannot be developed in every country immediately, but the demand for them derives its legitimation from the complexity of medical genetics as such and from the need to create expertise to interpret or manage this complexity.

Genetic counselling should offer:

information about and knowledge of the hereditary aspects of conditions or diseases
referral and access to consultation with medical doctors, specialised in diagnosis and treatment of a given condition or disease.

Options should be offered:

for consultation with qualified social workers, psychologists and other relevant professionals regarding the social and familial consequences of the disease, for the meeting with representatives of patient organisations, if the counsellee wishes so.

2   Information about genetic services should be made available to all who may benefit from it. Genetic facilities should be within reach, both geographically and financially, for all who wish to make use of them.

3   Knowing one's own and/or one's partners genetic make-up creates options for action regarding genetic testing and reproductive choice. The decision concerning the preferred course of action to be taken in the light of this information rests solely with the individual or the couple, within national legal frameworks. There should be no third party coercion. This also applies to the option for prenatal diagnosis and the freedom to act upon the consequences. Utilisation of genetic services must be voluntary. Any pressure to utilise all available technology for diagnosis or risk assessment should be avoided. The principle of privacy protection and respecting a wish not to be informed may interfere with moral obligations towards relatives at risk. Within the medical and institutional setting adequate measures for data protection should be safeguarded.

4   The general goal of genetic research is treatment of genetic conditions. Genetic services are to be directed towards accurate diagnosis and treatment of genetic conditions and to provide information concerning

appropriate care and other options, if no effective treatment is possible. Genetic information can enable individuals to adopt strategies for reducing the risk of or preventing certain conditions, e.g. lifestyle changes, dietary measures or the avoidance of certain occupational hazards. This does not dismiss companies from their responsibilities for safer workplace and environmental conditions.

5   For disabled persons the limits to self-determination and the opportunities to live a fulfilled life are set by their living conditions and by the standard of care and support that is available. These depend largely upon the structure and organisation of national facilities for health and social care, and as such are amenable to being influenced by public pressure or other factors – unlike the pattern of the disabling condition. Member organisations of EAGS regard the articulation of the needs of those affected by genetic disorders and to initiation of action that will bring services into being that will respond to these needs appropriately and effectively as a major task. This will involve action at national and at European level.

6   The existing and ongoing debate on priority setting in health care reveals the possible conflict of interests between the individual and society. Discrimination against disabled persons should be excluded. Persons with a disability or disease are under all circumstances entitled to full civil and human rights and to participate fully in all aspects of the society in which they live.

Statement on prenatal diagnosis (PND)

Various members of EAGS, sometimes in close collaboration with experts or expert groups, formulated statements on topics.
The Dutch Alliance of Genetic Support groups (VSOP) issued a statement on prenatal diagnosis (PND) in 1994 with addenda on specific prenatal investigations such as pre implantation diagnosis (PID).

Summary of the statement on prenatal diagnosis

Considerations:

1. Parents are, often suddenly, confronted with very complex issues which are a consequence of progress in molecular biology and medical technology.

They are often not educated in this field and nevertheless they are supposed to be able to take the right decisions fitting in their situation.

2. There is a growing optimistic tendency in society that the new medical technologies enable parents to have babies without diseases or handicaps ("design baby", "man-made child"). Parents with a child with a genetic disease or congenital disorder face remarks like "you could have prevented it". It should be clear that prenatal genetic diagnosis can only give information on a specific disease – known in the family – which sometimes can be avoided in further offspring.

3. The increasing number of tests should not infringe the freedom of the parents whether or not to use them.

4. (Research) investment in therapies should have a higher priority than in the development of diagnostic tests.

5. Psycho-social and legal implications of genetic diagnostic tests deserve more attention and further studies are necessary.

Prerequisites for prenatal diagnosis:

1. PND must not serve any health-policy aiming at genetic improvement, but should only be used to the benefit of individuals, enabling them to make a timely and well-considered choice.

2. Utilisation of PND must be voluntary and without restrictions (e.g. that counsellees must terminate the pregnancy if a serious disorder is detected).

3. Availability of timely, well-balanced, clear, reliable, non-directive, comprehensive information and counselling.

4. Service only in certificated / recognised centres.

5. Informed consent.

6. PND should not diminish pre-conceptual policy and facilities.

Regarding pre implantation diagnosis (PID) the following additional statements were formulated:

1. The provision of PID should be restricted to a few qualified and certificated centres where technology and experience on the subject is available and which:
   - can provide psycho-social support tailored to the specific problems;
   - have available comprehensive, clear, well balanced and non directive information;
   - have facilities for data registration and long follow-up studies;
   - use recognised indications.

2. Written informed consent.

3. A normative list of diseases for which PID is allowed, is rejected.

241

The Dutch Alliance of Genetic Support groups (VSOP) advertised for arousing awareness on available genetic services in a prudent way.

References

European Platform for Patients' Organizations, Science and Industry (1996), *Biomedical Research and Patenting: Ethical, Social and Legal Aspects.*

Netherland Haemophilia Society in Cooperation with the European Haemophilia Consortium (1994), *The Ethical Aspects of Biomedical Research and the Biomedical Industry.*

WHO (1995), *Summary Statement on Ethical Issues in Medical Genetics.* Geneva, February 1995.

Zerres, K. and Rüdel, R. (1993), *Selbsthilfegruppen und Humangenetiker im Dialog: Erwartungen und Befürchtungen*, Ferdinand Enke Verlag: Stuttgart.

3 Some reflections on the use of the term 'prevention' in reproductive medicine

Elisabeth Hildt

The concept of disease prevention is widely applied to almost all fields of medicine. It is based on the assumption that it is best to avoid disease and disease-related suffering as much as possible. As the saying 'Prevention is better than cure' illustrates, the concept of disease prevention generally has a very positive touch.

In general, three levels of prevention can be distinguished: Primary prevention, which is the prevention of the initiation or occurrence of a disease; secondary prevention which refers to the prevention or amelioration of the consequences of a disease; and tertiary prevention, which is the limitation of disability going along with a disease. Other authors use the distinctions primary prevention, treatment, and rehabilitation instead of primary, secondary and tertiary prevention (Steel 1995, Bloom 1996).

The term 'prevention' has also been used in the context of reproductive medicine (e.g.: Beck-Gernsheim 1993, Euler 1984, Munthe 1996, Lieberman 1998). With the help of prenatal diagnosis followed by selective abortion, preimplantation diagnosis and – pure speculation at the moment – germline gene therapy, people aim at avoiding the occurrence of certain disorders with genetic origin. In sum, it seems that these new developments in reproductive medicine offer another level of disease prevention.

In my opinion, however, especially in the context of procedures such as prenatal diagnosis or preimplantation diagnosis it is very misleading to use the word 'prevention' since there are some important differences between the classical concept of disease prevention and the strategies implicated in these procedures.

These differences relate to issues such as (1) the status of the 'patient' involved, (2) selection, and (3) the structure of choice underlying the procedure. In what follows, I want to discuss in how far new developments in reproductive medicine can be considered to be preventive measures in the classical sense of the word.

The status of the 'patient' involved

The first difference I want to mention relates to the status of the human being involved: whereas methods of primary prevention achieve prevention of disease by removing a cause or by removing a person's susceptibility to a cause, the strategy of disease avoidance in reproductive medicine often consists in preventing the birth of an individual known to have the disease (Steel 1995, Munthe 1996). As Kathleen O. Steel puts it with regard to prenatal diagnosis (Steel 1995, p. 351):

> (In primary prevention) the disease, condition, or disability is secondary to the individual – one removes the causes, but *personhood* remains intact. Prenatal diagnosis, as it is currently used for the most part, regards the person as secondary to the disease or disabling condition. The primary aim of prenatal diagnosis is to prevent the disease, regardless of the consequences to the person.

Although I agree with Steel that in reproductive medicine the tendency to focus not on the human being involved but on the disorder is very problematic, I consider it equally problematic to extend the concept of a person to early human embryos or fetuses. Whereas preventive strategies aim at promoting the patient's well-being, procedures involving prenatal diagnosis or pre-implantation diagnosis avoid the occurrence of diseases at the price of there being no patient left in the end who has been helped by the treatment. Thus, the relation assumed between the patient involved in medical practice and his or her disease differs fundamentally between primary prevention strategies and procedures involving preimplantation diagnosis or prenatal diagnosis. Although it is obvious that most often it is the couple who is helped by these procedures and not the embryo, this argumentation assumes the embryo to be the patient and not the woman or couple who seeks to have a child. With regard to the concept of disease prevention this assumption is plausible, however, since prenatal diagnosis and preimplantation diagnosis aim at avoiding the occurence of disease in the future generation, and not in adults.

Selection

In addition to the possibilities of disease avoidance offered by prenatal diagnosis and selective abortion or by preimplantation diagnosis, there is also the possibility of avoiding some diseases by modifying the conditions leading to the existence of an individual, i.e. by changing the date of conception or by using donor insemination.

In both cases, it is not only the occurrence of a certain disease that is being avoided, but the birth of individuals with certain disorders. However, with regard to an ethical evaluation, there is an important difference here: normally, a clear distinction is made depending on whether the procedure consists in selecting between already existing embryos or fetuses according to certain criteria or in merely choosing those starting conditions that seem to be the most promising ones. The aspect of selection plays an important role in this context. In my opinion, it is very questionable to use the term 'prevention' in the context of selective procedures, since the term 'prevention' implies the attempt to avoid a disease in an already existing individual, and not to avoid the birth of this individual.

With regard to the issue of selection which has often been considered problematic in the context of prenatal diagnosis and preimplantation diagnosis (Testart 1995, Mieth 1996), germline gene therapy might have some advantages. If germline modification should ever be applied to human beings, it seems that it will be a procedure with high preventive character. Thus, it is not very astonishing that in the discussion of the pros and cons of germline gene therapy the possibility of disease prevention is considered to be an aspect which clearly speaks in favour of germline modification.

To cite Nelson A. Wivel and LeRoy Walters, for example (Wivel and Walters 1993, p. 536):

> The health professions have a moral obligation to use the best available methods in preventing or treating genetic disease (...) and at least in the case of highly prevalent genetic disorders, disease prevention through germline modification may be the most efficient approach to reducing the incidence of disease.

Notwithstanding the manifold unresolved problems linked to a possible future application of germline gene therapy to human beings, one argument in favour of germline modification clearly is that it would help to circumvent the selective procedures that are currently carried out in the context of prenatal diagnosis and preimplantation diagnosis and which in principle have to be repeated from generation to generation. One problem with germline modification is that, in principle, in all methods involving genetic transfer a procedure is necessary in order to select those cells in which the gene in question has been integrated. However, this selective procedure need not necessarily have to take place at the level of the embryo. Although at the moment not feasible, in the future it might become possible, as is currently done in mice, to introduce transgenes via embryonic stem cells, or to modify germ cells genetically (Winnacker et al. 1997, Graumann 1998). It is clear, however, that considerations like these are nothing but pure speculation for the time being.

For a critical evaluation of embryo selection, a distinction based on the developmental stage the human embryo has reached at the time of selection may have some plausibility. Especially those positions which regard the moral status of the human embryo as being highly dependent on its developmental stage may consider it adequate to adjust the moral judgement concerning selection according to the embryo's developmental stage. According to these positions, it is of great relevance from a moral point of view whether selection occurs at an earlier or later embryonic stage, or before or after implantation of the human embryo. Based on this assumption with regard to the aspect of selection, germline gene therapy and preimplantation diagnosis would have to be considered clearly less problematic than prenatal diagnosis, for example, since they are carried out at a very early developmental stage.

Although I agree that a distinction like this may have a certain plausibility, I consider it problematic that in an argumentation like this the judgement concerning selection relies mainly on the status of the human embryo that is being selected and not so much on the aspect of selection itself. In my opinion, selection and the idea of choice underlying selection can be questioned on a more fundamental level. That is why I would like to refer more directly to the concept of choice and to the structures of decision-making underlying reproductive technologies.

Same number choices versus different number choices

With respect to issues relating to people who will live in the future, another distinction between two different kinds of prevention can be made. According to this point of view, one kind of prevention consists in the avoidance of disease in an already existing individual. If a pregnant woman decides to stop smoking and drinking alcohol, this significantly reduces the health risks for her baby. Cases like these are what Derek Parfit calls 'Same People Choices', since in both cases – whether someone chooses to take preventive measures or not – the same individual will live and will be affected by the decision (Parfit 1984).

In contrast, another kind of prevention can be considered to be what Parfit calls 'Same Number Choices'. This may be the case if a pregnancy is postponed for medical reasons. For example, a couple decides to have a child not now but some months later, since the woman is forced to undergo a medical treatment that might have teratogenic effects. However, the child that will be born will be a very different child than the child that would have been born if the pregnancy had not been postponed. Thus, in Same Number Choices in both alternatives for action one child will be born, i.e. the number of future individuals will be the same, whereas the child's identity will be a different one. In contrast, in 'Different Number Choices' the number of individuals that will ever exist depends on the choice made.

With Same Number Choices a difficulty arises: Depending on the choice made, a different individual will exist in the future. That is why it is not possible to compare the two different alternatives for action by arguing on the basis of 'person-regarding' reasons. For example, it cannot be argued that for medical reasons it is better for *the* child to postpone the pregnancy since the child that will be born later will be a different one than the child that would have been born. In order to circumvent this non-identity problem, Parfit proposes to use the so-called 'Same Number Quality Claim', or claim Q (Parfit 1984, p. 360):

> If in either of two outcomes the same number of people would ever live, it would be bad if those who live are worse off, or have a lower quality of life, than those who would have lived.

With the help of claim Q it is possible to compare Same Number Choices. According to Parfit's claim Q, with regard to the example above it can be argued that it is better to postpone the pregnancy, because the individual that will then live will have a higher quality of life than the individual that would have lived if the pregnancy had not been postponed.

The Same Number Quality Claim has also been used as a basis for argumentation in the context of prenatal diagnosis and selective abortion followed by another pregnancy which serves to 'substitute' for the aborted fetus (Brock 1995, Munthe 1996). The well-known argumentation is that after having diagnosed a fetus with a genetic abnormality leading to severe disability, it is better to have an abortion followed by another pregnancy than to have the disabled child. The same strategy has also been applied to preimplantation diagnosis, it clearly can also be applied to the hypothetical possibility of germline gene therapy involving embryo selection. At first sight it seems that the procedures following prenatal diagnosis, preimplantation diagnosis or germline modification also imply Same Number Choices, since in all cases in the end *one child* will be born, although the child that will be born will be another one than the child that would have resulted without reproductive technology.

247

However, it seems to me that it is not possible to transfer Parfit's Same Number Quality Claim to procedures like these. Instead, in my opinion they involve Different Number Choices. If one assumes, and this obviously is a very modest assumption, that a human embryo deserves some respect, that from a moral point of view the fate of a human embryo matters somehow and cannot be totally neglected, then the structures of decision-making in the procedures following prenatal diagnosis or preimplantation diagnosis differ significantly from the choice to be made in a Same Number Choice.

If a couple has to decide whether or not to undergo selective abortion after prenatal diagnosis, the decision to be made clearly is a Different Number Choice, since it depends on the choice as to whether or not the embryo or fetus will continue to exist. The decision whether or not to conceive another child, to become pregnant again, clearly is another Different Number Choice, which, on the condition that prenatal diagnosis does not reveal a severe disorder, will be followed by the Same People Choice to carry the child to term. Thus, although the net effect of the procedure is quite similar to the example of postponing a pregnancy, in the overall pregnancy-abortion-pregnancy-procedure two Different Number Choices are involved.[1]

Different Number Choices are also involved in preimplantation diagnosis: After IVF-procedures in which more embryos have been created than are to be implanted, the clinicians have to make a Different Number Choice in order to decide which embryos to use for the diagnostic procedure, which embryos to discard or to cryopreserve. If a certain genetic abnormality has been diagnosed the embryo in question will not be implanted into the woman's womb. The decision whether or not to implant a certain embryo also clearly is a Different Number Choice.

Since the choice to be made in these procedures is on the level of the human embryo and not on the level of the future child, it seems to me that human embryos which already exist cannot be neglected in the overall structure of decision-making. Only a position which denies that the fate of a human embryo matters somehow can, on the basis of the overall net effect, consider these strategies as being Same Number Choices. In my opinion, procedures involving Different Number Choices (which imply the disposal of already existing human embryos) cannot be considered to be preventive measures in the classical sense.

Based on these assumptions it follows that Parfit's Same Number Quality Claim cannot be applied to procedures like prenatal diagnosis or preimplantation diagnosis which involve a Different Number Choice.

In this short contribution I have argued against a wide application of the term 'prevention' in the context of reproductive technologies. In my opinion, there are some basic differences between the classical concept of prevention and the strategies underlying most of these procedures. However, with regard to reproductive technologies a distinction like this does not necessarily lead to a position which uncritically accepts all kinds of preventive measures and absolutely condemns all other procedures. Instead, it may help to underline that apart from the concept of disease avoidance there are also other considerations which are of great relevance in this context. In aiming at the avoidance of diseases, these aspects should not be forgotten.

Note

1 For the sake of simplification this argumentation neglects the fact that each decision to have a child is in principle a Different Number Choice and that the fact of choosing a certain time for procreation is in principle a Same Number Choice.

References

Beck-Gernsheim, E. (1993), 'Zwischen Prävention und Selektion – Fortschritte und Dilemmata der Gentechnologie', in Zwierlein, E. (ed.), *Gen-Ethik*, Schulz-Kirchner Verlag: Idstein, pp. 59-78.

Bloom, M. (1996), *Primary Prevention Practices*, SAGE Publications: Thousand Oaks.

Brock, D.W. (1995), 'The Non-identity Problem and Genetic Harms – The Case of Wrongful Handicaps', *Bioethics*, Vol. 9, pp. 269-75.

Euler, H. (1984), 'Genetische Beratung und Untersuchungen als Aufgabe einer staatlichen Vorsorgemedizin', in Schloot, W. (ed.), *Möglichkeiten und Grenzen der Humangenetik*, Campus Verlag: Frankfurt, pp. 261-74.

Graumann, S. (1998), '«Präimplantationsgenetik» – Ein wünschenswertes und moralisch legitimes Ziel des Fortschritts der vorgeburtlichen Medizin?', in Düwell, M. and Mieth, D. (eds), *Ethik in der Humangenetik*, Francke: Tübingen, pp. 383-414.

Lieberman, B.A. (1998), 'Limits of Reproductive Technology', in Hildt, E. and Mieth, D. (eds), *In vitro Fertilisation in the 1990s – Towards a Medical, Social and Ethical Evaluation*, Ashgate: Aldershot, pp. 317-23.

Mieth, D. (1996), 'In vitro Fertilization: From Medical Reproduction to Genetic Diagnosis', *Biomedical Ethics*, Vol. 1, No. 1, pp. 6-8.

Munthe, C. (1996), *The Moral Roots of Prenatal Diagnosis*, Göteborg.

Parfit, D. (1984), *Reasons and Persons*, Clarendon Press: Oxford.

Steel, K.O. (1995), 'The Road that I See: Implications of New Reproductive Technologies', *Cambridge Quarterly of Healthcare Ethics*, Vol. 4, pp. 351-4.

Testart, J. (1995), 'The New Eugenics and Medicalized Reproduction', *Cambridge Quarterly of Healthcare Ethics*, Vol. 4, pp. 304-12.

Winnacker, E.-L., Rendtorff, T., Hepp, H., Hofschneider, P.H. and Korff, W. (1997), *Gentechnik: Eingriffe am Menschen – Ein Eskalationsmodell zur ethischen Bewertung*, Herbert Utz Verlag: München.

Wivel, N.A. and Walters, L. (1993), 'Germline Modification and Disease Prevention: Some Medical and Ethical Perspectives', *Science*, Vol. 262, pp. 533-8.

4   Preimplantation diagnosis – implications for genetic counselling

Ruth Chadwick

Genetic counselling: the issues

Debates about genetic counselling have tended to focus on three issues: aims, ethos and outcomes. As far as the aims are concerned, there has been discussion about the extent to which the aims are to facilitate choice on the part of clients, including reproductive choice where the counselling is concerned with reproductive issues; and the extent to which there are public health goals (Chadwick 1998). As regards ethos, debate has turned on the issues of whether non-directiveness if possible and desirable (Clarke 1991; Chadwick et al. 1993). Then there has been discussion about how the outcomes of genetic counselling are to be measured, what counts as a successful outcome (Chadwick 1993). Clearly the last issue is not unconnected with the first, as the measure of a successful outcome must have reference to the aim of the process.

The practice of genetic counselling, in espousing an ethos of non-directiveness has tried to distance itself from the charge of eugenics, with varying success, and was in fact described by Sheldon Reid as 'social work without eugenics'. This distancing has had regard to all three aspects of discussion – aims, ethos and outcomes. In addition to the non-directive ethos, the aim tends to be described as not about selection and the outcomes are *not* explained in terms of a reduction in incidence of genetic disorders.

More recently however the emphasis on individual choice in clinical genetics has been associated with eugenics by the 'back door' as the cumulative effect of individual choices leads to eugenic results (Duster 1990).

It is my aim in this article to explore the potential impact of preimplantation diagnosis on these debates. What I shall attempt to show is that preimplantation diagnosis has the potential to affect genetic counselling in the following ways:

increased vulnerability of the client which in turn has an impact on

the possibility of non-directiveness in the process and of autonomous choice on the part of the client

the closer association of genetic counselling with genetic selection.

What also has to be borne in mind, however, is the development in debates about genetic counselling generally, which seem to show a move away from non-directiveness. This provides the context in which the impact of preimplantation diagnosis has to be considered.

The context of genetic counselling

It is important first to note the different contexts in which genetic counselling may take place. Although reproductive counselling is perhaps the most central in the debate, the increase in programmes of genetic testing and screening brings with it the opportunities for counselling adults and young people about their own health status. The issues may be affected by context. The Royal College of Physicians of London says (1998, s.1.4.):

> preventing transmission of genetic disease to offspring is not a primary aim of genetic counselling. However, when the aim is to prevent the complications of genetic disease, the genetic counselling process may be more directive, with specific recommendations for surveillance, e.g. for early detection of cancer in a predisposed individual.

This quotation suggests that there may also be an issue about the particular condition about which someone is being counselled. It may be the case that the particular features of the condition in question will be thought relevant to the appropriate degree of directiveness or otherwise.

Reproductive counselling may take place both preconception and post-conception. Where what is at issue is post-conception counselling and prenatal diagnosis, the decision with regard to which counselling is offered may be whether or not to opt for a termination of pregnancy. Counselling also has a role, however, in assisting counsellees to prepare for the birth of a child with a particular condition, in the knowledge that this condition is present.

252

The intriguing question is the extent to which preimplantation diagnosis and genetic counselling differs from prenatal diagnosis and counselling about termination decisions or preparation.

Preimplantation diagnosis and genetic counselling: what is the difference?

Elsewhere I have argued (e.g. Chadwick 1998) that the ethos of non-directiveness in genetic counselling, together with the aim of facilitating choice and associated outcome measures, forms part of what I have called the 'standard view' and have examined challenges to that standard view in genetic counselling generally, including the view that non-directiveness is not possible and the view that it is not desirable. I now propose to examine the impact of preimplantation diagnosis on these debates.

The possibility of non-directiveness

There are at least three reasons why it might be argued that non-directiveness is not possible: the vulnerability of the client; the social context and the attitudes to disability therein; and the very structure of the genetic service on offer.

First, client vulnerability. We start from the fact that in professional-client relations there is typically an imbalance of power, arising at the very least out of the difference in the degree of knowledge held by the parties. There may be differences in social status as well. In the case of reproductive counselling, this may be exacerbated by the extra vulnerability of pregnancy. How might this state of affairs be affected in the context of preimplantation diagnosis? The process is surrounded by the procedures of IVF, with the extra strains this places on the couple, especially the woman. Let us think of an example of a case in which preimplantation diagnosis might be indicated. A couple in which both partners are carriers of cystic fibrosis are trying to have a child. They have had two pregnancies in which prenatal diagnosis was carried out. In both cases the fetus was found to have cystic fibrosis, and in both cases the couple opted for a termination. They cannot face the prospect of another termination but are still desperate for a child and so they are referred for preimplantation diagnosis. It seems clear that the stress and anxiety for such a couple are likely to increase their vulnerability. While preimplantation diagnosis is offered only comparatively rarely, it is also couples who are in this type of situation who are prime candidates for referral.

Second, attitudes to disability. There has been much discussion about the potential for developments in genetics to affect social attitudes to disability. The issues here are complex and it is beyond the scope of this paper to deal with them adequately. What should be mentioned, however, is the argument that in a society which does display intolerance of disability the possibility of non-directiveness in genetic counselling is undermined. Deborah Lynne Steinberg has suggested that this intolerance has played a part in supporting the view of the move towards the practice of preimplantation diagnosis as both necessary and desirable and a form of 'progress' over prenatal diagnosis with the option of termination (Steinberg 1997).

The significance of this point here is that if social attitudes are anti-disability, they will play a part in producing a perception of preimplantation diagnosis as an improvement on prenatal diagnosis and this will affect the practice of genetic counselling in this context.

Thirdly, the nature of the service. The fact that genetic counselling is offered for certain conditions, with the possibility of termination of affected pregnancies, it has been argued, in some way suggests that these conditions are undesirable (see e.g. Clarke 1991). So in addition to being affected by social attitudes, genetic counselling reinforces those attitudes and in some way, however, minimal, suggests to clients that there are certain decisions that ought to be taken. Although there is explicit adherence to the ideal of choice, implicitly certain decisions are expected.

Whatever view we take of this account in relation to prenatal diagnosis and counselling, it seems that the logic of preimplantation diagnosis is such that it becomes more intimately associated with selection. It is important to note, however, that *in principle* it could facilitate a choice of embryo with, for example, the potential to become a child with restricted growth, if that was what parents wanted. It has been argued, however, that although preimplantation diagnosis is portrayed as an improvement for women, in particular, because it relieves them of the trauma of termination of pregnancy, it in fact takes power out of their hands and puts it firmly into the hands of clinicians (see Steinberg 1997; Draper and Chadwick 1998). A woman may decline to have a termination of an affected fetus but is dependent on the co-operation of the clinician to choose to have a particular embryo implanted.

Non-directiveness is not desirable

The prevailing ethos of non-directiveness has been criticised on the grounds that (a) it may not be what clients want, being cold and unhelpful (Nuffield Council on Bioethics 1993); and at a deeper level (b) that the principle of autonomy which provides its theoretical underpinning may not be the most appropriate principle in this field (cf. Royal College of Physicians 1991). It has been argued that there is a right, if not a duty, to make reproductive decisions in the light of much information as possible. The suggestion of a duty marks a move away from autonomous decision-making about reproduction to the suggestion that there are certain constraints on what decisions we ought to make. It is not clear what the grounds of this duty are meant to be e.g. whether they are considerations of the welfare of future people or whether some other factor is thought relevant (Chadwick et al. 1993).

The 1998 report of the Royal College of Physicians of London, however, marks another move away from the standard view in relation to genetic counselling. It is worth quoting some sections of the report in detail.

> It is generally held that the desired outcomes of genetic counselling for those who face threats presented by a genetic disorder are to be assessed not only in terms of patients' knowledge of the disorder, its significance for them and of the preventive and therapeutic actions open to them but, more importantly, in terms of their adjustment to this knowledge. These are psychological outcomes (4.1.).

Section 4.2. makes clear that the report continues to recognise the element of personal choice and non-directiveness: choice is enabled but not directed by the counselling process. For some families the outcome may include the birth of children with, or at risk of developing a genetic disorder. Although there is evidence that one consequence of the informed reproductive decisions that couples make will be a reduced prevalence of certain serious genetic disorders, this is not a primary purpose of genetic counselling and its use as a measure of the outcomes of genetic counselling is mistaken.

So as regards the aims, they subscribe to the view that reduction in incidence of genetic disorders is not a 'primary' purpose and also reject such a reduction as an outcome measure. In section 5.10, however, it is admitted that "[s]ignificant reductions in morbidity and mortality may become outcome measures in time but at present they remain within the remit of research". As regards the ethos, they subscribe to non-directiveness, with a caveat about context. What is interesting however is the emphasis on 'adjustment' rather than choice as the final aim.

What counts as healthy adjustment and is a commitment to healthy adjustment as the outcome aimed at consistent with the ethos of non-directiveness? The fact that adjustment is the aim might be taken to imply that prior to counselling the counsellee was not 'adjusted', which has implications for the extent to which the counsellee is regarded as having a capacity for autonomy. The question also arises as to how the 'adjustment' is to be understood. The Royal College considers various possible measure of psychological outcome:
 − recall of information
 − changed perception of risk
 − perception of risk and [relationship with] reproductive decisions
 − patient satisfaction
 − better understanding
 − restoration of confidence in making reproductive decisions.

All of these are found to be problematic in the report, as measures of psychological outcome. In considering testing recall of information the range of types of information (e.g. family implications, medical genetics) has to be taken into account. Changed perception of risk is not likely to be satisfactory as an outcome measure because of the variation in individuals' perception of risk. There is no clear relationship between perception of risk and reproductive decision-making. Patient satisfaction is not a good outcome measure because patients might be satisfied with bad advice and vice versa. Restoration of confidence in decision-making is difficult to assess because, for example, there is insufficient data on those clients who do not return after counselling. So what of better understanding? The report claims (para. 4.10) that for some clients this is the main benefit, and also that "reassurance and peace of mind is a health gain". Without further discussion of this last point, however, the Royal College concludes that none of these is suitable as an outcome measure for service use and that multidisciplinary research is needed to develop measures that would be suitable.

The report under discussion does not explicitly consider genetic counselling in the context of preimplantation, as opposed to prenatal, diagnosis, but it is worth trying to tease out the implications. What could count as 'healthy adjustment' in the context of preimplantation diagnosis? As the list of possible measures of psychological outcomes shows, adjustment might be interpreted in different ways – in terms of change to the decisions that people make, or in terms of state of mind. The impact on reproductive decisions is an example of the first; the reference to patient satisfaction is an example of the second. It is far from clear, however, what could count as an example of healthy adjustment to matters such as the status of the embryo, a key feature in preimplantation diagnosis, and to the issues surrounding making a choice between embryos.

What *is* clear is that the implications of an emphasis on healthy adjustment mark a move away from the autonomy end of the spectrum towards the paternalism end, despite the professed continuation of adherence to non-directiveness. When combined with the other factors at work in preimplantation diagnosis, there is potential here for a marked change to hitherto predominant ways of viewing the process of genetic counselling.

Preimplantation diagnosis and genetic selection

As stated above, the practice of genetic counselling has been vulnerable to charges of eugenics and has attempted to distance itself from this with varying success. The question arises as to whether in the context of preimplantation diagnosis this becomes a more difficult task. The reasons for this are partly connected with the greater influence of clinicians over decision-making, but lie partly elsewhere, namely in the fact that in the case of preimplantation diagnosis, as opposed to prenatal diagnosis, an embryo might be more likely to be rejected on the basis of a carrier state. Thus in the case of genetic disorders where what is being tested for is a recessive condition such as cystic fibrosis or thalassemia, the focus of attention in prenatal diagnosis of a fetus would be the homozygous state. In preimplantation diagnosis, however, it might seem to be the case that the rational choice is to implant not only heterozygotes rather than homozygotes, but embryos that are not even heterozygous for a particular condition. This line of thought supports Steinberg's view of the inevitable trajectory towards greater control in the move from prenatal diagnosis to preimplantation diagnosis.

This possibility raises interesting questions about the associated counselling. In the case mentioned above, of the couple who want to avoid another pregnancy in which the fetus is affected by cystic fibrosis, should the issue of carrier status even be raised? If they simply want to avoid an affected fetus, is it relevant whether an embryo is a carrier or not? Or should they have regard to the possibility that their child when grown may have to make the same choice that they are now wrestling with? It is in relation to this type of question that preimplantation diagnosis may raise issues about the aims of counselling of a more far-reaching kind. Even if it is thought, however, that this choice ought to be put before the counselled couple, it is still not clear to what extent the aim is to facilitate *their* choice (i.e. not only whether or not to have an affected child, but whether or not to have a carrier child) and to what extent it is offered with an eye to the reproductive choice of the next generation or further reaching effects on the incidence of the disorder.

It is not the role of this paper to discuss whether and to what extent it is morally desirable to engage in some kind of genetic selection – I have discussed these matters elsewhere (cf. Chadwick 1992; 1998). All that I am trying to show is the way in which preimplantation diagnosis has implications for genetic counselling, and it does seem to be the case that it has the potential for increasing the vulnerability of the client, with consequential results for the possibility of non-directiveness and the greater degree of genetic control. But what has to be borne in mind is that there are also other trends away from what I have called the standard view, namely towards outcome measures in terms of psychological adjustment. Hence any consideration of the impact of preimplantation diagnosis on genetic counselling must have regard to other challenges to what I have called the standard view of this practice.

References

Chadwick, R. (1993), 'What counts as success in genetic counselling?', *Journal of Medical Ethics* 19 (1) 43-6.

Chadwick, R. (1998), *"Can genetic counselling avoid the charge of eugenics?" forthcoming in Science in Context.*

Chadwick, R., Coli, D., ten Have, H., Husted, J., Ngwena, C., Nørby, S., Pogliano, C., Shickle, D. (1993), *Ethical Implications of Human Genome Analysis for Clinical Practice in Medical Genetics with special reference to Genetic Counselling: a report to the Commission of the European Communities,* Cardiff: Centre for Applied Ethics.

Chadwick, R.F. (ed.) (1992), Ethics, *Reproduction and Genetic Control,* Revised edition, Routledge: London.

Clarke, A. (1991), "Is non-directive genetic counselling possible?", *Lancet* 338: 998-1001.

Draper, H. and Chadwick, R. (1998), *"Beware! Preimplantation genetic diagnosis may answer some old problems but it also raises new ones",* Forthcoming in Journal of Medical Ethics.

Duster, T. (1990), Backdoor to Eugenics, London: Routledge.

Nuffield Council on Bioethics (1993), *Genetic Screening Ethical Issues,* Nuffield Council on Bioethics: London.

Royal College of Physicians (1991), *Ethical Issues in Clinical Genetics,* Royal College of Physicians: London.

Royal College of Physicians of London (1998), *Clinical Genetic Services: Activity, Outcome, Effectiveness and Quality: a report from the Clinical genetics Committee of the Royal College of Physicians of London,* Royal College of Physicians: London.

Steinberg, Deborah Lynn (1997), *Bodies in Glass: Genetics, Eugenics, Embryo Ethics,* University Press: Manchester.

Part Six
HEALTH CARE, JUSTICE AND REGULATION

1 Legal regulations concerning preimplantation diagnosis

Jennifer Gunning

Preimplantation diagnosis (PID) allows genetically defective embryos to be detected and weeded out before implantation. This allows couples, who are at risk of transmitting a serious genetic disease to their offspring, to enter a pregnancy with greater confidence that the resulting child will be normal. Generally one or both partners will have been genetically screened and found to be a carrier before PID is offered.

PID was developed in 1989 at the Hammersmith Hospital in London exploiting the then novel technique of polymerase chain reaction (PCR). Now PID is possible for some two dozen genetic diseases but some 200 disorders would be amenable. New analytical techniques, such as fluorescence in situ hybridisation (FISH), are also being applied to PID but they are not yet entirely reliable. It is clear that, if PID is to continue, embryo research has to continue in parallel to ensure that, for each particular disease, the test is not applied clinically until it is properly validated.

The aim of this paper is to give a flavour of the current inconsistencies and anomalies which exist in Europe in the regulations affecting PID. Positions range from upholding absolutely the sanctity of human life, through permitting restricted access to human reproduction techniques to a fairly permissive legislative approach; and then there are those countries which have no legislation at all. One or two examples will be given to illustrate each approach. The impact of the European Convention on Human Rights and Biomedicine will also be examined.

The absolutist approach

In 1994 Pope John Paul II established *motu proprio* the Pontifical Academy for Life whose vice-president is also chairman of the board of directors of the Centre of Bioethics at the Catholic University of the Sacred Heart in Rome. In 1997 the Centre published a statement, which is effectively a statement from the Holy See, against experimentation on human embryos (*Bulletin of Medical Ethics* 1996). The statement is critical of artificial fertilisation techniques, in particular in vitro fertilisation (IVF), because apart from providing a method of manipulating human procreation, it also provides the chance to exploit or eliminate human individuals. The statement asserts that human embryos

> are human beings from the first moment they are formed, with a fully personal individuality, and are able to develop completely even if they are temporarily frozen.

It concludes that

> The creation of human embryos to be used in experimentation is to be considered ethically unacceptable, as is any form of experimentation on spare human embryos in a 'state of abandonment' or on those judged unsuitable for transfer to the woman's genital tract.

Two strongly Catholic countries provide an example of upholding absolutely the sanctity of human life, in line with statements from Rome. In the Republic of Ireland the human embryo is specifically protected by the Eighth Amendment in the Irish Constitution. This includes the statement

> The State acknowledges the right to life of the unborn and, with due regard to the equal right to life of the mother, guarantees in its laws to respect, and, as far as practicable, by its laws to defend and vindicate that right.

Abortion is illegal in Ireland; there is currently no research being undertaken on human embryos; PID would not be acceptable under the law.

In 1993 in Poland a significant change was made to the legal status of the human embryo/fetus with the introduction of a new anti-abortion law (E. Zielinska, personal communication, 1994). Article 1 of the Act declares 'every human being shall have an inherent right to life as from the time of its conception' and 'The life and health of the child shall be placed under the protection of the law, as from the time of its conception'. The Penal Code was also amended by a new article (23a) under which 'the conceived child may not be subject to any procedures other than those invented to protect its life and health, or its mother's life or health'.

A subsection to this article limits prenatal examinations to those that do not significantly increase the risk of abortion. That is, prenatal diagnosis followed by a termination is not possible. Prenatal testing is only authorised where
- the conceived child belongs to a family manifesting a genetic burden;
- it is assumed that the genetic condition may be cured or that it may be possible to remedy the condition or to limit its effect at the fetal stage;
- a presumption exists that the fetus presents a serious defect.

All non-therapeutic experimentation on human fetuses is prohibited in Poland. Moreover, the Polish citizen who participates abroad, where it is lawful, in research causing death or injury of the conceived child may be subject to criminal responsibility in Poland (articles 114 and 116 of the Penal Code). However, what is meant by 'the conceived child' and 'moment of conception' is not defined. Two interpretations exist; one that the law applies to embryos in vitro and in vivo; the other that legal protection only applies after implantation in the womb. Needless to say, the net effect of this legislation has been to decrease the availability of assisted reproduction. The withdrawal of cover for such services from national insurance has caused some public hospitals to cease performing IVF altogether. PID is not an option.

The inconsistent approach

Most other countries in Europe allow the termination of a pregnancy where the fetus is discovered to be suffering from a serious genetic defect. Prenatal screening and testing programmes are widespread. But in those countries where strict laws addressing IVF and embryo research have been passed one finds the anomaly that prenatal diagnosis followed by termination is permitted but that PID which would avoid the trauma of abortion is not.

In Germany PID and the selection of healthy embryos before beginning a pregnancy is forbidden yet an abortion some weeks later of a fetus diagnosed as affected by genetic disease is allowed. The Embryo Protection Act 1990 prohibits fertilisation other than for the purposes of pregnancy and the fertilisation of a human egg cell for any purpose other than to start a pregnancy in the woman who produced the egg (Gunning and English 1993). An embryo is defined as a fertilised developing egg from the time of karyogamy (fusion of the two pronuclei) and also any totipotential cell which is able to divide and develop into an individual. Research is therefore forbidden and, by implication, PID. It might be suggested that biopsy of late stage embryos, i.e. when cells are no longer totipotent, might be permissible under the law as it stands. However, an application to conduct a trial of PID in Lübeck was turned down in 1996 by the local ethics committee on legal rather than ethical grounds (Mueller 1997).

The conduct and use of IVF in Germany is covered by the guidelines of the Federal Physicians Chamber. These allow IVF only for the treatment of infertility but not genetic selection by means of PID. On the other hand the Abortion and Family Planning Act of 1995 decriminalises abortion for medical indications which include hereditary diseases which can be genetically tested by DNA or chromosome analysis. Genetic counselling and prenatal diagnosis are controlled by professional self-regulation rather than by law. Over one hundred centres offer genetic counselling in Germany.

A similar situation obtains in Austria. Section 9 (1) of the Austrian Act on Procreative Medicine (Official Gazette, 1992, No. 275) states,

> Pre-embryos may only be used for medically assisted reproduction. They may only be medically examined and treated as far as it is deemed necessary according to medical science and experience for establishing a pregnancy. The same applies to semen and ova which are to be used in medically assisted reproduction.

This would imply that while interventions for the benefit of the embryo itself would be permissible, PID is forbidden because affected embryos would be discarded.

In its Bioethics Law of 1994 France has taken a comprehensive approach to reproductive medicine including PID and prenatal diagnosis. PID is allowed exceptionally under the Public Health Code, articles L162-16 and L162-17. It is permitted only where couples have a high probability of giving birth to a child likely to be affected by a life-threatening, serious genetic defect. The risk has to be confirmed by a doctor working in a recognised genetics centre. Both members of the couple have to give consent in writing. The PID has to be undertaken in a centre authorised for this purpose by the National Commission for Reproductive Medicine and Biology and Prenatal Diagnosis. This Commission is also established under the Public Health Code (article L184-3). It would seem that PID is only allowed for prevention and treatment and for research into the particular problem of the individual couple (Auby 1994, Vigneau 1994).

Although the law would seem to allow research in the context of PID it is in fact unclear. Article L152-8 of the Public Health Code forbids the creation of embryos for research and all embryo research except in special cases where research is for a medical end and causes no harm to the embryo. This would seem to eliminate invasive procedures but PID through the removal of cells from an embryo, which may be seen as invasive procedure, is allowed in article L162-17. Despite the fact that the law makes provision for PID it seems that there remains some unease about the effects and consequences of embryo biopsy among clinicians and the technique is not yet applied in France (Auroux 1995, Laplane and David 1996).

Legislative recognition of PID

Two countries have produced comprehensive legislation on assisted reproduction which both allows PID and related research. The Spanish Act 35 of November 1988 in article 1 states that the techniques of assisted reproduction may be used in the prevention and treatment of illnesses of a genetic or hereditary origin. Diagnosis and treatment is addressed in articles 12 and 13 and extends implicitly to both PID and prenatal diagnosis. Article 12.1 states,

> Every intervention on the pre-embryo, alive, in vitro, with diagnostic purposes, will have no other aim but the assessment of its viability or non-viability, or the detection of hereditary diseases, in order to treat them, if possible, or to advise against its transfer for purposes of procreation.

Article 13 sets out the conditions under which interventions are allowed. There must be informed consent for the couple, or woman - the law makes provision for single women to have access to assisted reproduction - and genetic selection for or against non-pathological characteristics is forbidden.

Research and experimentation is allowed under the Act and articles 14 - 16 set the conditions. Research must be carried out in authorised centres and the parties concerned must have given written consent. Research beyond 14 days after fertilisation is not permitted. Research is generally restricted to non-viable embryos but research on viable in vitro pre-embryos will be authorised if

- it is applied research of a diagnostic character or if it has a therapeutic or prophylactic purpose;
- the non-pathological genetic patrimony is not modified.

This may be interpreted as meaning that research relating to PID is permissible but research on germline gene therapy is not. Embryos which have been the subject of research may not be returned to the womb.

The Act made provision for the establishment of a National Committee of Assisted Reproduction to regulate assisted reproduction services in Spain. However, the law was challenged immediately upon enactment as being unconstitutional and referred to the Constitutional Court. It has therefore not been implemented. Assisted reproduction is governed by professional self regulation and statistics are collected by the Spanish Fertility Society (Gunning and English 1993, p. 164).

In the United Kingdom the Human Fertilisation and Embryology Act 1990 made provision for the establishment of a statutory authority, now the Human Fertilisation and Embryology Authority (HFEA), which would licence centres for the provision of clinical services and to undertake research (Gunning and English 1993, p. 133-42). The authority was required to publish a code of practice to regulate the activities of centres. Schedule 2 of the Act sets out the activities for which licences may be granted. Research licences may specifically be granted for research which has the purpose of 'developing methods for detecting the presence of gene or chromosome abnormalities in embryos before implantation'.

Other than reiterating the purposes for which the HFEA may grant a research licence and those activities prohibited by law, the Code of Practice does not specifically address PID. However, the Code of Practice does require research projects to be approved by a properly constituted ethics committee. This often will be the local hospital research ethics committee although clinics are permitted to establish their own ethics committees and the Code of Practice provides advice on their constitution. Like the Spanish legislation, embryos which have been the subject of research may not be returned to the womb.

Currently four centres in the UK are licensed to undertake PID and its associated research. Recently the HFEA has become aware that this technology is reaching maturity and, with the rapid increase in knowledge about genetics, that demand for it will grow; yet there are no guidelines regulating its conduct. Jointly with the UK Advisory Committee on Genetic Testing, the HFEA has established a working group to decide what criteria should be used in deciding when PID is, and is not acceptable. In the interim the HFEA is drawing up its own guidelines. The HFEA has also considered the issue of sex selection in assisted reproduction and has announced that this should not be undertaken for social reasons (HFEA 1997).

The European Convention on Human Rights and Biomedicine and its implications

The European Convention on Human Rights and Biomedicine (ETS164) was laid open for signature in Oviedo in April 1997 (Council of Europe 1997). Twenty-one countries signed on that occasion followed by a further signature by Moldova in May 1997. Table 1 details the countries which have signed the Convention. So far the only country to ratify the Convention is Slovenia (15 January 1998). The Convention contains three articles relevant to PID:
Article 12 on predictive genetic tests states that

> Tests which are predictive of genetic diseases or which serve either to identify the subject as a carrier of a gene responsible for a disease or to

detect a genetic predisposition or susceptibility to a disease may be performed only for health purposes or for scientific research linked to health purposes, and subject to appropriate genetic counselling.

Article 14 addresses sex selection and states that

The use of techniques of medically assisted procreation shall not be allowed for the purpose of choosing a child's future sex, except where serious hereditary sex-related disease is to be avoided.

Finally, article 18 addresses research on embryos and states that

1. Where the law allows research on embryos *in vitro*, it shall ensure adequate protection of the embryo.
2. The creation of human embryos for research purposes is prohibited.

How is the Convention to be interpreted? Predictive genetic tests are allowed for health purposes only and subject to genetic counselling. Sex selection is allowed only for the avoidance of serious hereditary sex-related disease and it is only in this context that assisted procreation is mentioned. But articles 12 and 14 are conditioned by article 18. As has been mentioned earlier, predictive genetic tests are only available for a handful of the diseases which could be detected and new approaches and refinements to the detection of genetic diseases are needed. This means that there is an ongoing need for embryo research in the field of PID. But article 18 effectively prohibits embryo research. What is meant by 'adequate protection of the embryo' is not defined. Presumably this will be addressed by the protocol to the Convention but, where embryo destruction is inevitable for analysis or the embryo is not reimplanted, it is difficult to see how this condition can be met. Some countries, such as the United Kingdom, do not allow the replacement in the womb of embryos which have been the subject of research.

The creation of embryos for research is specifically prohibited but while diagnostic tests remain unreliable embryos will need to be created for research if PID is to be a viable option for affected couples. As it stands, the Convention would seem to restrict PID to sex selection in the context of X-linked diseases or allow PID if it is to be followed by an attempt at gene therapy.

Those countries which have already passed legislation allowing embryo research can avoid the implications of article 18 by making a reservation with respect to that article, citing the relevant law. Some countries may choose not to ratify the Convention at all. But what is the outlook for those countries which currently have no legislation on assisted reproduction? Portugal is one of the April 1997 signatories to the Convention. It has no law regulating assisted reproduction although a comprehensive draft (which refers to PID) was sent to the Parliament in the autumn of 1997. This was prepared by the Ministry of Health and evaluated by the National Council of Ethics for Life Sciences. No centres currently offer or undertake research on PID. This seems unlikely to change since, once Portugal ratifies the Convention, the law will have to respect article 18. On the other hand, prenatal diagnosis is routinely offered in general hospitals with standards set and overseen by the Portuguese Medical Association. Prenatal tests are reimbursable through the National Health Service (Dispatch 9108/87, 13 October 1997). This will put Portugal in the same class as Germany and Austria, that is, allowing prenatal diagnosis followed by abortion but forbidding PID. Interestingly, Austria and Germany have not yet signed the Convention.

Italy and Greece are also signatories to the Convention. Neither of these countries has passed legislation regulating assisted reproduction but both have a strong tradition in the prenatal diagnosis of genetic disease. In Greece PID is being offered to patients carrying thalassaemia and cystic fibrosis but it is not clear how much research, if any, is being undertaken. Prenatal diagnosis is regulated by health legislation but PID is not included and is therefore controlled by professional self regulation. In Italy access to genetic testing is regulated by law and pregnant women are expected to be offered the opportunity to be tested by the National Health Service, though the specific criteria for being offered tests is determined by individual centres or, in a very few cases, by the Regional Government. Very recently a task force, set up by the Instituto Superiore della Sanità, has prepared guidelines for genetic testing for the Ministry of Health and National Government. No public centre has, so far, undertaken PID but a private centre in Bologna has been performing chromosomal investigations by FISH to achieve better implantation in IVF. This implies that PID may well be available in the private sector. There will inevitably be some conflict of approach in these two countries if PID is to be available and to progress. As signatories to the Convention they will be expected, on ratification, to respect article 18.

Belgium has an active programme of IVF and embryo research but has no legislation on assisted reproduction. It has not signed the Convention. There is a distinction, in Belgium, between the Catholic and the Free university hospitals in their approach to assisted reproduction. In the Catholic infertility centres IVF is only offered for the purpose of establishing a pregnancy for a 'married' couple and only using the husband's sperm; PID will shortly become available, having received recent ethical approval. At the Free Universities, which are secular, treatment is less restricted although only one or two centres have a strong programme of embryo research and PID. Since 1984 the Belgian College of Physicians has required ethical approval for research projects and doctors can be disciplined if they are found conducting experiments without ethical approval.

Other recommendations

Given that PID has been feasible for nearly a decade its regulation has been given remarkably little consideration. However, with the rapid advances in human genetics and the increasing availability of commercial tests and testing services, it would seem that some action needs to be taken particularly in those countries where PID is available and unregulated. There has been some activity, however, in the general area of genetic testing where some recommendations should be equally applicable to PID. The EC Group of Advisers on the Ethical Implications of Biotechnology published an *Opinion on Ethical Aspects of Prenatal Diagnosis* in February 1996. In the UK the issues have been addressed by the Nuffield Council on Bioethics (December 1993) and the Advisory Committee on Genetic Testing (ACGT), which reports to the Department of Health (ACGT 1997). One aspect on which all are agreed in relation to genetic testing is that there must be adequate genetic counselling. Assisted reproduction centres may provide infertility counselling but, unless they are associated with a hospital with a genetics centre, they cannot routinely provide genetics counselling. This could be important as commercial testing becomes readily available. Couples would have access to genetic tests without referral from a genetics centre and present themselves at an IVF clinic requesting PID. Where the clinic is part of the National Health Service patients would undoubtedly be referred back to an appropriate genetics centre but in the private sector, if the demand becomes sufficient, there may be the temptation to offer a commercial service but PID implies more than applying a test. Another area of consensus is the need for fully informed consent by the woman or couple. This can only be given following adequate counselling.

The ACGT in its Consultation on Genetic Testing for Late Onset Disorders (November 1997) also addresses the scientific and clinical valididity of tests and the quality of the laboratory service available. It emphasises that scientific and clinical validity should be clearly established before any test is used in clinical practice stating:

> It must be clear that the genetic change found is causally related to the disorder, before it is used as the basis for a genetic test. Validity should be based on published, peer reviewed evidence.

> The extent and limitation of the association between the test result and the disorder (false positive and false negative rates) should be accurately known.

The error rate and failure rate should be known to those requesting the test...

I suggest that these recommendations apply equally strongly to PID and support the need for continuing research. Tests validated for prenatal diagnosis on the fetus will need to be revalidated on the embryo.

With regard to laboratory services the ACGT considers the following issues to be important and they apply equally to PID.

All laboratories providing a genetic testing service should be appropriately accredited for this as well as taking part in internal and external quality control schemes.

Research laboratories should not normally be the basis for a genetic testing service; where they are, because of the rarity of the disorder or other factors it is essential that the service delivered conforms to the same standards expected in an approved service laboratory.

Genetic testing should be undertaken only by laboratories closely linked with other genetics services.

Conclusion

In ethical terms, PID raises no new questions. The same arguments for and against the sanctity of human embryonic or fetal life pertain. In those countries with an absolutist approach to the sanctity of human life PID is not currently an option and prenatal diagnosis of genetic disease is only permissible in so far as it may allow better management of an affected pregnancy and the resultant offspring. The legislative and regulatory approach is consistent. Looking ahead, PID might become acceptable in these countries if it enabled treatment of an affected embryo, perhaps by gene therapy. But any treatment of this kind must be validated by embryo research. A country forbidding such research but permitting the treatment of embryos, based on the research of others, would lay itself open to accusations of hypocrisy.

Elsewhere inconsistencies need to be addressed so that patients have access to PID as well as prenatal diagnosis since patients requesting PID are most likely to be those who have already had an affected child and will, quite likely, already have undergone the trauma of prenatal diagnosis and abortion of subsequent affected children. These services should be available through national health services. If PID is only available in one or two countries, patients in those countries without PID services will have to travel abroad for tests and some may not be able to afford to do so.

On the regulation of PID, the UK seems now to be taking the lead with the current collaboration between the HFEA and the ACGT to produce recommendations. When published, the resultant report may provide a model on which regulations throughout Europe could be based. It will need to set out criteria for access to PID, and for the distribution and monitoring of services provided. Should PID be undertaken by IVF or genetics centres? Informed consent, genetic counselling and confidentiality will need to be addressed. It will also need to address issues such as whether PID should be limited to the diagnosis of a specific list of diseases (the Spanish law seems to think so) and, if so, with the increasing availability of new genetic probes, what criteria should be used to add diseases to the list? Should conditions for which there are currently prenatal and neonatal genetic screening programmes be considered for inclusion in such a list? Finally, the method of patient referral will be important if inappropriate commercialisation is to be avoided.

Acknowledgements

I would like to ackowledge the help of Professor Walter Osswald, Professor Panagiota Dalla-Vorgia, Professor Erwin Bernat and Professor Bruno Brambati in bringing me up to date with regulation in their countries.

Table 1: Signatories to the European Convention on Human Rights and Biomedicine

Member States	Date of Signature	Date of Ratification
Denmark	04.04.1997	
Estonia	04.04.1997	
Finland	04.04.1997	
France	04.04.1997	
Greece	04.04.1997	
Iceland	04.04.1997	
Italy	04.04.1997	
Latvia	04.04.1997	
Lithuania	04.04.1997	
Luxembourg	04.04.1997	
Moldova	04.04.1997	
Netherlands	04.04.1997	
Norway	04.04.1997	
Portugal	04.04.1997	
Romania	04.04.1997	
San Marino	04.04.1997	

Slovakia	04.04.1998	
Slovenia	04.04.1997	15.01.1998
Spain	04.04.1997	
Tfyrmacedonia	04.04.1997	
Turkey	04.04.1997	

The Convention will enter into force when it has been ratified by 5 countries including 4 member states

References

Advisory Committee on Genetic Testing (1997), *Consultation on Genetic Testing for Late Onset Disorders*, Health Department of the United Kingdom: London.

Auby, J-M. (1994), *Les Petites Affiches,* No. 149, pp.14-24.

Auroux M. (1995), *Bulletin de l'Académie nationale de médecine*, Vol. 179, pp.1729-41.

Bulletin of Medical Ethics (1996), October bulletin, pp. 9-11.

Council of Europe (1997), *Convention on Human Rights and Biomedicine*, Council of Europe, Strasbourg.

Group of Advisers on the Ethical Implications of Biotechnology (1996), Opinion No.6, *Ethical Aspects of Pre-natal Diagnosis*, European Commission: Brussels.

Gunning, J. and English, V. (1993), *Human in vitro Fertilization*, Dartmouth Publishing: Aldershot.

Human Fertilisation and Embryology Authority (1990), *Code of Practice*, HFEA: London.

Human Fertilisation and Embryology Authority (1997), *Annual Report*, HFEA: London.

Laplane, R. and David, G. (1996), *Bulletin de l'Académie nationale de la médecine*, Vol. 180 No. 2.

Mueller, S. (1997), *Eubios Journal of Asian and International Bioethics*, Vol. 7, pp. 5-6.

Nuffield Council on Bioethics (1993), *Genetic Screening*, Nuffield Council on Bioethics: London.

Vigneau, D. (1994), *Les Petites Affiches*, No. 149, pp. 62-9.

2 Reproductive technology and the slippery slope argument: A message in Blood

Tony McGleenan

Introduction

Slippery slope arguments are a recurrent feature of the discourse relating to reproductive technology (Schauer 1985, van der Burgh 1992, Holtug 1993, Whitman 1994, McGleenan 1995). Literary and cultural analogies, from Mary Shelley's *Frankenstein* to Spielberg's *Jurassic Park*, offer constant reminders of the dangers of failing to check the technological imperative. Historical parallels, from state sterilisation policies to Nazi experimentation, also fuel public and political concerns about the development of reproductive technology. Structural factors within reproductive technology ensure that this debate is particularly prone to the suggestion that liberal practices will ultimately lead to a calamitous outcome. Over the past twenty years we have witnessed the genesis of a technology which, while offering tremendous potential benefits, threatens significant harms. This is the classic formula for the emergence of 'horrible results' style slippery slope arguments. New revelations as to the possibilities presented by technology such as cloning appear in the various media on an almost daily basis and demonstrate why such arguments can carry great rhetorical force.

The slippery slope argument is often dismissed as little more than rhetorical scaremongering. Critics claim that the empirical realities demonstrate that actual slippery slopes are rare. One common counter argument is that even on a slippery slope there will always be 'handholds' and that even though we may slide some way down the slope we will not necessarily descend directly to the bottom and the dreaded horrible result. The 'handholds' objection to the slippery slope argument refers directly to the possibilities offered by legislation and regulation to place viable and durable impediments across any treacherous moral incline. A second counterargument rejects the presumption that there will always be a downward pressure towards the horrible result. In many instances, the counterargument goes, this downward pressure will be entirely absent. In the Netherlands, for example, it is pointed out that there is no need to fear a slippery slope in relation to euthanasia because there will be no downwards momentum; there simply will not be large numbers of people who wish to see their relatives killed. Similarly, there will be little demand for human cloning because few people would be willing to contemplate the risks involved. The argument presented in this paper is that the recent history of the regulation of reproductive technologies in the United Kingdom may demonstrate the weaknesses of some of these counterarguments. In the first instance I shall, by way of a brief outline of the history of reproductive regulation in the United Kingdom, seek to demonstrate that the 'handholds' provided by a procedural system of regulation may offer only a temporary and illusory respite on the descent. Secondly, and more specifically I shall argue that the ruling of the English Court of Appeal in the recent and remarkable *ex parte Blood* case demonstrates that there are certain structural features within European Community law which actually generate a downward regulatory pressure. Consequently, I suggest that regulation which applies across the European Union, in medico-moral as well as economic issues, will ultimately reach the lowest common denominator in that the law which will be applied in the event of a dispute will be that of the most liberal state.

The Human Fertilisation and Embryology Authority (HFEA), Procedural Regulation and the Handholds Argument

July 25, 1998 was an important day for Louise Brown. It was her 20th birthday. However, unlike the many others born on that day in 1978, Louise Brown's birth carries a special significance. As the world's first test tube baby her very existence provoked a widespread public debate about the future of reproductive technology (Steptoe and Edwards 1978). In response to this concern the United Kingdom government established a committee under Dame Mary Warnock which finally reported in 1984 (Warnock 1985). The committee recommended that the law be changed and in 1990 a legislative framework was built around the central principles of the Warnock report. It was finally passed in the form of the Human Fertilisation and Embryology Act.

The legislation established a novel system of regulation. Alongside a relatively sparse legislative framework the law provides for a system of procedural regulation. This procedural regulation operates through a licensing authority known as the Human Fertilisation and Embryology Authority

(HEFA).[1] The central feature of the legislation is contained in section 3 of the Act which states:

'No person shall:-

(a) bring about the creation of an embryo, or

(b) keep or use an embryo,

except in pursuance of a licence'.

This method of regulation has obvious attractions in the medico-moral field. It enables the government to distance itself significantly from any political fallout which might be generated by controversial issues. The Code of Practice under which the Authority operates can be altered at any time and so enables a large degree of flexibility to be retained within what is, ostensibly, a statutory system. Quangos such as the HFEA are also vulnerable to more general criticism. The Authority does not meet in public, does not usually publicise its deliberations, does not grant an automatic right of appeal against a decision and does not contain a single member known to be opposed to the practice and development of the new reproductive technologies. A further difficulty with this mode of regulation is that it lends itself particularly well to consequentialist reasoning. There are few moral absolutes contained within the 1990 Act apart from the prohibition on embryo experimentation after the emergence of the 'primitive streak'. However, a close reading of the Warnock Report will reveal that even this was informed by a practical utilitarian ethic. It is submitted here that slippery slope type practices are more likely to develop in a soft or procedural regulatory climate based on a consequentialist ethic than in a substantive legislative framework which clearly defines the boundaries of acceptability. Is this supported by the actions and practices of the HFEA in the 1990s?

HFEA: Soft regulation and slippery slopes

The first major controversy to require the intervention of the HFEA after the legislation came into force in 1991 was prompted by the opening of the London Gender Clinic in 1992. This was a commercial enterprise which offered couples the chance to select the sex of their children through the use of the Ericsson sperm sorting technique (Ericsson et al. 1993). In response to adverse public reaction the HFEA embarked upon a six month consultation exercise (HFEA 1993), at the end of which the authority issued a press release to the effect that while sex selection for social reasons would not be permitted, sex selection for medical purposes would be allowed. (HFEA 1993).[2] Even before the issue of sex selection had been fully resolved the HFEA had been forced to begin another consultation exercise in response to widespread public disquiet over suggestions that fetal ovarian tissue transplantation might be used to treat infertile women (HFEA 1994). The consultation document asked for views on whether it was acceptable to use eggs or ovarian tissue from fetuses or cadavers in research or infertility treatment.[3] Once again a six month consultation period elapsed after which the authority advised that it would be unacceptable to use fetal ovarian tissue in the treatment of infertile women. (Caplan 1987, Cefalo and Engelhardt 1989, Strong 1991, Bopp and Burchtael 1989, Gelfand and Levin 1993). In both these instances significant policy matters had been decided upon by the Authority without any parliamentary debate, having been subject only to a public consultation exercise. The discussion in both instances was significantly shaped by the consultation documents themselves which seemed to focus heavily on the potential consequences of the proposed treatments.

The next controversy to strike the HFEA and the system of regulating reproductive technology in the United Kingdom related to the vexed question of frozen embryos. This matter had only been partly addressed in the legislation. The legislation stated that unused embryos could be stored under licence for a 'statutory storage period'(HFEA 1990). Schedule 3 paragraph 8 of the legislation set out the conditions under which embryos could be stored:

> An embryo the creation of which was brought about *in vitro* must not be kept in storage unless there is an effective consent, by each person whose gametes were used to bring about the creation of the embryo, to the storage of the embryo.

As the legislation had come into force in the United Kingdom on August 1 1991 the statutory storage period expired on August 1 1996. The majority of couples who had cryopreserved their embryos were contacted and were able to express their views as to the fate of the embryos. However, the 'parents' of 3300 embryos could not be contacted. Consequently, all the unclaimed embryos were destroyed in the period immediately following the expiry of the statutory storage period (Young 1996). This episode again provoked a significant adverse reaction from the public and the media. An Italian research organisation, Artemisia, offered to transport the frozen embryos to Italy to implant them in volunteers (Utley 1996). The government responded to the dilemmas posed by the destruction of the frozen 'orphan' embryos simply by raising the statutory storage period from five years to ten.[4] Shortly after the frozen embryo crisis had been resolved a fresh challenge to the authority of the Authority was posed by the case of a young woman who sought to utilise the techniques of posthumous insemination in order to have a child. This matter brought the HFEA before the courts and placed the spotlight firmly on questions of reproductive technology.

Diane Blood had been married to her husband Stephen for four years. On 26 February 1995 he contracted meningitis and passed into a coma. Two days later Mrs Blood spoke to the doctors caring for her husband and raised with them the possibility of obtaining a sample of sperm by electro-ejaculation. Two samples of sperm were taken and shortly afterwards Mr Blood was certified dead. Mrs Blood applied to the HFEA for permission to use the gametes for artificial insemination. She stressed that she and her husband had intended to have children. At the hearing she laid emphasis on the fact that they had been married according to the 1662 Anglican Book of Common Prayer service which focussed on the role of procreation in marriage. The HFEA refused to allow the use of the stored gametes based on the fact that the law required a written informed consent from both parties before treatment services could be provided and that Mr Blood had not given any such consent. With significant public and media support Mrs Blood began a protracted legal battle in pursuit of what she saw as her right to reproduce. The matter was first heard in the Family Division of the High Court where Sir Stephen Brown ruled that the law on the matter was clear insofar as written, informed consent was required in advance of any treatment and since such consent had not been obtained the HFEA was correct in law in refusing to authorise the treatment. (Morgan 1997).

Downward pressure: Articles 59 and 60

Following the decision of Stephen Brown in the High Court, Diane Blood brought an appeal to the Court of Appeal. In this instance she buttressed her legal argument with the provisions of the Treaty of Rome, in particular, Articles 59 and 60 which provide for freedom of movement within the European Community in order to provide or receive services (Weatherill and Beaumont 1993). The essence of Article 59 is a rule against discrimination based on nationality. In *Van Binsbergen* the European Court of Justice described Article 59 as a means of preventing 'any discrimination against a person providing a service by reason of his nationality or of the fact that he resides in a state other than that in which the service is in fact to be provided'. In *Blood* the applicant sought not to provide a service but rather to receive a service. Nevertheless, European Community Law had already established the principle of freedom of movement to *receive* services. In *Luigi and Carbone* v *Ministero del Tesoro* (1984) two Italian nationals argued that restrictions on the export of Italian currency curtailed their freedom to receive the service of tourism outside Italy. The European Court of Justice (ECJ) ruled that:

the freedom to provide services includes the freedom, for the recipients of services, to go to another member state in order to receive a service there, without being obstructed by restrictions, even in relation to payments, and that tourists, persons *receiving medical services* and persons travelling for the purpose of education or business, are to be regarded as recipients of services.

The question of whether the receipt of medical services would include controversial issues such as abortion and the new reproductive technologies had already been emphatically answered by the ECJ in *SPUC* v *Grogan* (1991) where it held that:

the termination of pregnancy, as lawfully practiced in several Member States, is a medical activity which is normally provided for remuneration, and may be carried out as part of a professional activity.[5]

From these raw materials Lord Lester, the lawyer acting for Mrs Blood, constructed the argument that just as the Italian nationals in *Luigi and Carbone* were entitled to supercede national legislation restricting the use of a commodity necessary to receive services (currency) in another member states so Mrs Blood was entitled to overcome the provisions of the HFE Act 1990 because they similarly impeded her ability to receive services (by denying her the right to export her dead husbands gametes). This argument was rejected in the High Court where Sir Stephen Brown expressed surprise that European Community law could require a Member State to permit an activity which the national Parliament had enacted legislation to explicitly prohibit.

In the Court of Appeal Lord Woolf took a different view of the situation. He found that there were three issues to be resolved. First, there was the question of whether it would be lawful to store and use sperm in the United Kingdom. Secondly, the court had to consider the law which applied to the export of sperm from the United Kingdom to another European state. Thirdly, since the court was actually engaged in judicial review proceedings, they would have to determine whether the decision of the HFEA was a reasonable one.

On the first issue Lord Woolf reviewed the relevant legislation. The 1990 Act stated that gametes could only be stored under licence. The conditions for such a licence were contained in Schedule 3 of the Act which stated that a consent to the storage or use of gametes must be given in writing, specify the maximum period of storage and state what must be done with the gametes in the event of the consenting parties death. In addition paragraph 3 of the Schedule states that an individual giving consent must be given relevant information and counselling. The Court of Appeal found that since the adequate consent had not been obtained for the storage of the sperm 'technically ... an offence was committed by the licence holder'.

The Court also considered whether the taking of the sperm from the unconscious Mr. Blood was in itself unlawful. This issue is governed by the widely held common law principle that any touching without consent amounts in law to an assault. The Court found that the taking of sperm from Mr. Blood without consent was not a lawful action. Consequently, Lord Woolf affirmed the High Court ruling that the use of the sperm for treatment in the United Kingdom was prohibited.

The second matter the Court considered was the law in relation to the export of the sperm. The HFEA had a power under the 1990 Act to authorise a licence for the export of sperm.[6] Lord Woolf clearly stated that even though the case was being heard under a United Kingdom statute the relevant law on this matter included European law and the Treaty of Rome which was now to be regarded as national law. The Court followed the decisions of the ECJ in *Grogan, Alpine* and *Gaston Schul Douane* noting that the jurisprudence generated a two stage test in relation to cases involving disputes under Article 59. Firstly, the court must determine whether the challenged action or decision was an infringement of the citizens' right to free movement. If it finds such an infringement the court must then go on to consider whether the restrictions are justified according to the legitimate requirements of the state. Lord Woolf found that there had clearly been an infringement in this case in that Mrs Blood was prevented from receiving services in another Member State because she was being denied a commodity essential to the procurement of those services. The court ruled that the infringement of Article 59 could only be justified where it was:

  non-discriminatory
  justified by an imperative requirement in the general interest
  suitable for securing the attainment of the objects which it pursues
  proportionate

The Court of Appeal applied this two stage test and found that the Authority had given inadequate consideration to the effect of Article 59 on the right of Mrs Blood to freedom of movement in order to obtain services. In reaching the original decision the Authority had not taken into account the fact that the applicant was entitled to receive posthumous insemination treatment in Belgium. In light of this the Court ordered the HFEA to reconsider their decision not to permit the export of the gametes. This the HFEA duly did and the conclusion was reached that Mrs Blood ought to be permitted to export the gametes to another Member State.

Conclusion

The significance of the decision in *Blood* lies in the fact that the national appeal court of a Member State felt that it must permit an activity prohibited by national legislation because an individual citizen sought to avail of a service which was permitted by a more liberal regulatory system in another member state.

Even if the United Kingdom, or any other European state, had the most rigorous legislation possible in relation to in vitro fertilisation or gene therapy, if a commercial company from a state where such practices were not prohibited wished to set up there and offer treatment services there would be nothing that could be done to stop the practice even if it conflicted with national legislation because of the protections afforded by the provisions of Article 59. The burden of the argument presented here is that the jurisprudence developed by the ECJ in relation to Article 59 generates a structural downward pressure so that ultimately any regulation in Europe in relation to reproductive technology will gravitate towards the most liberal laws available. What broader lessons can be drawn from this for the development of European policy on reproductive technology and bioethical issues? First, it appears from the recent history of the HFE Act in the United Kingdom that the protections offered by a procedural or 'soft' system of regulation can be somewhat illusory because any controversial issue tends to be resolved according to consequentialist reasoning. Secondly, the rules of freedom of movement to receive services clearly both supercede national boundaries and apply to reproductive technology. This must lead to the conclusion that there should be a Community wide policy on reproductive technology. A coordinated approach is necessary with agreement on a minimum policy standard because, as the *Blood* case so clearly illustrates, individual citizens with the means to travel will always be able to circumvent any national prohibition.

Notes

1   For a more general critique of this method of regulation see generally, McGleenan 1997.

2   For a general survey of the issues surrounding selection of fetal sex see Young 1991.

3   For the background to this issue see McGleenan 1994. For a report on the science of this technique see Cha 1991.

4   For discussions of the ethical and legal dilemmas surrounding the cryopreservation of human embryos see generally Perry and Schneider 1992, Katz 1994, Davis 1990. For a discussion of the *Davis v Davis* litigation on the ownership of frozen embryos see Robertson 1994.

5   For a general discussion of the development of this jurisprudence see Phlelan 1992 and O'Leary 1992.

6   Section 24(4) 'Directions may authorise any person to whom a licence applies ... to send gametes or embryos outside the United Kingdom in such

circumstances and subject to such conditions as may be specified in the directions'.

References

Alpine Investments BV v *Minister van Financien* (1995) ECR I-1141.

Bopp, J., Burchtael, J.T. (1989), 'Fetal Tissue Transplantation: The Fetus as Commodity', *This World*, Vol. 26, p. 54.

Caplan, A. (1987), 'Should Fetuses or Infants Be Utilized as Organ Donors?', *Bioethics*, Vol. 1, p. 119.

Cefalo, R.C., Engelhardt, H.T. (1989), *Journal of Medicine & Philosophy*, Vol. 14, p. 25.

Cha, K.Y., Koo, J.J., Choi, D.H., San, S.Y. and Yoon, T.K. (1991), 'Pregnancy after in vitro Fertilisation of Human Follicular Oocyte Collected from Non-stimulated Cycles', *Fertility & Sterility,* Vol. 55, pp. 109-13.

Davis, T.L. (1990), 'Protecting the Cryopreserved Embryo', *Tennessee Law Review*, Vol. 57, p. 507.

Ericsson, R.J., Beernink, F.J. and Dmowski, W.P. (1993), 'Sex Preselection Through Albumin Separation of Sperm', *Fertility & Sterility*, Vol. 59, p. 382.

Gaston Schul Douane Expediteur BV v *Inspecteur der Invoerrechten en Accijnzen Rosendaal* (1982), ECR, p. 1409.

Gelfand, G. and Levin, T.R. (1993), 'Fetal Tissue Research: Legal Regulation of Human Fetal Tissue Transplantation', *Washington and Lee Law Review*, Vol. 50, p. 631.

HFEA Press Release, (20 July 1993), 'HFEA Publishes Second Annual Report and Announces Outcome of Sex Selection Consultation'.

Holtug, N. (1993), 'Human Gene Therapy: Down the Slippery Slope?', *Bioethics*, Vol. 7, p. 402.

Human Fertilisation and Embryology Authority (January 1993), *Sex Selection: Public Consultation Document*.

Human Fertilisation and Embryology Authority (January 1994), *Donated Ovarian Tissue in Embryo Research and Assisted Conception: Public Consultation Document*.

Katz, K.D. (1994), 'Ghost Mothers: Human Egg Donation and the Legacy of the Past', *Albany Law Review*, Vol. 57, pp. 733 –80.

Luisi and Carbone v *Ministero del Tesoro* (1984), ECR 26/83, p. 377.

McGleenan, T. (1994), 'Back to Basics on Fetal Ovarian Tissue', *Bulletin of Medical Ethics*, Vol. 99, p. 12.

McGleenan, T. (1995), 'Human Gene Therapy and Slippery Slope Arguments' *Journal of Medical Ethics*, Vol. 21, pp. 350-5.

McGleenan, T. (1997), 'The Regulation of Gene Therapy in the United Kingdom: Hard or Soft Options?' in Muller, S., Simon, J. and Westing, J.W. (eds), *Interdisciplinary Approaches to Gene Therapy: Legal, Ethical and Scientific Aspects,* Springer: Hamburg.

Morgan, D. and Lee, R.G. (1997), 'In the Name of the Father? *Ex parte Blood*: Dealing with Novelty and Anomaly' *Modern Law Review*, Vol. 60, p. 840.

O'Leary, S. (1992), 'The Court of Justice as a Reluctant Constitutional Adjudicator: an Examination of the Abortion Information Case', *European Law Review*, Vol. 17, p. 138.

Perry, C. and Schneider, L.K. (1992), 'Cryopreserved Embryos: Who Shall Decide Their Fate?', *Journal of Legal Medicine*, Vol. 13, pp. 463-500.

Phelan, D.R. (1992) 'Right to Life of the Unborn v Promotion of Trade in Service: The European Court of Justice and the Normative Shaping of the European Union', *Modern Law Review*, Vol. 55, p.670.

R v Human Fertilisation and Embryology Authority ex parte *Blood* (1997) 2 All ER 687 (Court of Appeal); 35 BMLR 1 (High Court).

R v Secretary of State for Transport ex parte Factortame (1990), CMLR, Vol. 3, p. 1.

Re T (adult:refusal of treatment) (1992), Schloendorff v New York Hospital 211 N.Y. 125 (1914); All ER, Vol. 4, p. 649.

Robertson, J. (1994), '*Davis v Davis*: An Inconsistent Exception to an Otherwise Sound Rule Advancing Procreative Freedom and Reproductive Technology', *De Paul Law Review*, Vol. 43, pp. 523-75.

Schauer, F. (1985), 'Slippery Slopes', *Harvard Law Review*, Vol. 99, pp. 361-83.

Society of the Protection of the Unborn Child v *Grogan* (1991), ECR I-4685 .

SPUC v *Grogan* 159/90 [1991] 3 CMLR 849.

Steptoe, P.C. and Edwards, R.G. (1978), 'Birth After the Reimplantation of a Human Embryo', *Lancet*, Vol. 2, p. 336.

Strong, C. (1991), 'Fetal Tissue Transplantation: Can It Be Morally Isolated From Abortion?' *Journal of Medical Ethics*, Vol. 17, p. 70.

Utley, T. (1. August 1996), 'Time Runs Out for 3000 Embryos as Last Appeals Fail', *Daily Telegraph*.

Van Binsbergen v *Bestuur van de Bedrijsvereniging voor de Metaalnijverheid* (1974), ECR, 33/74, p. 1299.

Van der Burgh, W. (1992), 'The Slippery Slope Argument' *Journal of Clinical Ethics*, Vol. 3, pp. 256-68.

Warnock, M. (1985), *A Question of Life: Report of the Committee of Inquiry into Human Fertilisation and Embryology*, HMSO.

Weatherill, S. and Beaumont, P. (1993), *European Community Law*. Penguin: London. Chapter 19.

Whitman, J. (1994), 'The Many Guises of the Slippery Slope Argument', *Social Theory and Practice*, Vol. 20, No. 1, p. 85.

Young, H. (1. August 1996), 'Science That Produces More Life Than Death', *The Guardian*.

Young, R. (1991), 'The Ethics of Selecting for Fetal Sex', *Baillière's Clinical Obstetrics & Gynaecology*, Vol. 5, pp. 575-90.

3 Measuring the benefits of IVF

Emma McIntosh and Mandy Ryan

Introduction

The phrase 'people should have access to an adequate level of health care' is commonly quoted and it rests on what people think is *important*. In this paper relating to the assessment of the benefits of in vitro fertilisation (IVF) and other related technologies this statement gives rise to the fundamental question 'How *important* do we think reproduction and having healthy children is?' In economics, this is translated to 'Are the benefits of IVF and other related technologies *worth* the cost?', and the issue of importance is tied up with the definition of benefit. Health economists address this issue of *worth* by comparing the costs and benefits of health care programmes within an economic evaluation framework. In order to do this, information is required on the resources used by IVF and related technologies and the associated benefits that would be obtained from such resource use. Only when this information is available, can a decision be made as to which combination (if any) of IVF and related technologies will maximise *benefit* from a given budget.

The following section introduces the concepts of scarcity, choice and opportunity cost. The paper then outlines the use of economic evaluation tools in determining the issue of *worth* before proceeding to examine specific challenges in the economic evaluation of IVF and related technologies with specific reference to the measurement of *benefit*.

Opportunity cost

Resources are scarce, this means that choices have to be made about which health care activities should be undertaken and which activities should not be undertaken. Therefore it is inevitable that opportunities to use resources in some activities will be given up or forgone. The benefit or *utility*, which would have accrued from such forgone opportunities, are opportunity costs (Donaldson and Shackley 1997). Therefore, in economics, the cost of a programme is defined as its opportunity cost. The opportunity cost of the use of resources in a health care programme is equivalent to the benefits forgone in the best alternative use of these resources (Donaldson and Shackeley 1997).

Economic evaluation

The aim of economic evaluation in the health care field is to ensure that the benefits of a programme are greater than the opportunity costs of such a programme. Benefit is often referred to as *utility*, where utility is a measure of preference or satisfaction for a commodity. Thus, returning to the concept of scarcity and choices, it can be seen that choices must be made in order to maximise utility in the provision of assisted reproductive services. The question 'Should infertile couples at high risk for a genetic disorder be allowed to benefit from assisted reproductive technology (ART)?' has been identified as an area of potential ethical conflict and controversy (Meschede 1997). From an economist's perspective, this can be translated into 'What is the *opportunity cost* of providing ART to infertile couples at high risk for a genetic disorder?' If the opportunity cost or *benefit forgone* by investing in one programme and not another is greater, this implies an inefficient use of resources, suggesting that more benefit could be achieved by investing the resources elsewhere. Economic evaluation in health care uses three techniques (Donaldson and Shackley 1997): cost-effectiveness analysis (CEA); cost-utility analysis (CUA) and cost-benefit analysis (CBA) to compare the costs and benefits of alternative programmes. These techniques differ only in the way they measure and value the benefits of a health care intervention. The resource costs of technologies can normally be readily identified, measured and valued in a standard fashion. Resources involved in the provision of ART include the following: drug treatment; tubal surgery; artificial insemination and IVF, all of which incur costs of staffing, administrative costs, hospital stay, tests and medications, freezing and thawing and so on (see Ryan and Donahson 1996, Neumann et a. 1994).

286

Benefit assessment

The paper has so far defined opportunity cost in relation to the allocation of resources to infertile couples at high risk for genetic disorders. However, before the opportunity cost of a programme can be established, the definition of *benefit* must be clear in order that it can be compared to *benefit forgone*. This is where the challenge lies in the economic evaluation of IVF and related technologies, namely, defining and measuring *benefit*. The remainder of this paper will concentrate on the area of benefit assessment in the area of IVF and related technologies as this is where many of the unresolved issues lie.

Traditionally, economic evaluations which have attempted to inform the debate about the provision of IVF and related technologies have implicitly assumed that the only factor important to users is whether they leave the service with a child. The dominant technique used by health economists has been CEA. This technique permits one, uni-dimensional measure of success to be incorporated into the economic evaluation. Thus, previous evaluations in this area have estimated a cost per *live birth*, cost per *maternity* or cost per some other narrow medical definition of *benefit* (Ryan 1996a). Such a narrow approach ignores the following factors: the importance of outcomes beyond some narrow medical definition of success; the majority of users who leave the service childless and the importance of the actual process of treatment (Ryan 1996a). The problem with 'the CEA' approach is that it takes no account of other potential benefits from having gone through with infertility treatment i.e. coming to terms with infertility or knowing you have done everything possible to have a child. If we take into account these potential benefits, then we can no longer assume that those women who leave the service childless obtain no *benefit*. Thus, this paper argues that any benefit assessment of IVF and related technologies must consider all factors of *importance* i.e. all factors which influence the utility or satisfaction of users. An evaluation which considers all factors that may influence utility would ideally include health, non-health and process benefits. The non-health benefits important to people using the service may include information, reassurance and psychological outcomes such as regret and disappointment. Process attributes of importance may include waiting times, choice, continuity of staff and location. Health economists are currently using two techniques in an attempt to include all the important attributes in the assessment of benefit. They are willingness-to-pay and conjoint analysis. Each of these techniques and their application to IVF and related technologies will be outlined in the following section.

Willingness-to-pay

Willingness-to-pay (WTP) is a method of measuring the benefits of health care interventions in monetary terms within CBA. The principle of WTP is very simple – the utility that an individual gains from something is valued by the maximum amount that he or she would be willing to pay for that something (Donaldson and Shackley 1997). Unlike the restrictive CEA approach, which only permits the inclusion of one outcome, WTP has the advantage that it allows individuals to take account of *all* factors that are important to them in the provision of a service. The application of WTP in health care has been limited due to the fact that, in some countries, people do not have to pay for health care at the point of consumption and it is therefore considered unacceptable to ask people their WTP for health care. In addition, people may have difficulty in assigning monetary values to things which are considered to be incommensurate with monetary valuation. However, a study by Ryan (1996a) used WTP to assess the benefits of assisted reproductive techniques since it has the advantage that it allows individuals to value all factors of importance to them. The aim of this study was to establish the importance of factors beyond some medical definition of success in the provision of assisted reproductive techniques, using WTP. The study showed that the average WTP for an attempt at assisted reproduction was $2,506. The results also suggested that there is some value in going through the service, even if the couple leaves it childless. Another study used WTP to establish the value which infertile couples place on IVF in Scotland (Ryan 1997a). The objective of the paper was to inform the debate on the public provision of IVF. The results of the study suggested that users of the service had a mean WTP of over £5,000 for an attempt at IVF. When this benefit *valuation* is compared with the average government expenditure of £2,700 the results suggest that the benefits outweigh the cost and that, where possible, public provision of IVF should be encouraged. The importance of psychological outcomes in the provision of IVF was established in another WTP study of ART (Ryan 1998). The results suggested that there was some perceived utility from undertaking treatment, even if the individual leaves the service childless. Of the total respondents, 89% agreed with the statement *One of the reasons we are trying (or tried) IVF is so that in later life I will know that we have tried everything possible to have a child*. Further, 93 % agreed that even if they left the service childless, they would still be glad they tried it. This study obtained WTP estimates separately for individuals providing an *ex-ante* and *ex-post* evaluation. Psychological outcomes were found to be significant predictors of WTP for both these groups, with evidence being presented that the psychological feelings of *regret* and *disappointment* may be major motivators for individuals seeking ARTs. Of the 78 individuals who gave an ex-post valuation, 65 had left the service childless. Whilst those who had a child from IVF gave significantly higher valuation than those who left it childless, the childless still provided a positive valuation for the service. Thus, it would be inappropriate to ignore the childless when examining user values in the economic evaluation of ARTs, as CEA does.

Conjoint analysis

Conjoint analysis (CA) is a technique for establishing the relative importance of different attributes in the provision of a good or service. It assumes that any service can be defined as a combination of levels of a given set of attributes. The total benefit or *utility* that an individual derives from a good is thereby determined by the utility to the individual of each of the attributes. The aim of CA is to estimate the relative importance of the individual attributes and the total benefit or utility score for different combinations of attributes (Ryan 1996b). This technique allows estimation of a broad range of benefits as the attributes can be health, non-health or process attributes. To date, the application of CA in the area of health economics has been relatively limited. In the UK, CA has been used by health economists to establish the monetary value of time spent on the National Health Service (NHS) waiting lists (Propper 1990); to examine the trade-offs that individuals make between the location of clinic and waiting time in the provision of orthodontic services (Ryan and Farra 1994); to assess women's preferences for surgical versus medical management of miscarriage (Ryan and Hughes 1997); to assess patient preferences in the doctor-patient relationship (Vick and Scott 1998); to assess the importance of a patient health card in the provision of general practice services (Ryan et al. 1998) and to assess the relative importance of different attributes in the treatment of menorrhagia (San Miguel et al. 1998).

One study used CA to estimate the relative importance of various attributes in the provision of IVF services (Ryan 1997b). Previous economic evaluations of IVF had assumed that the only important factor to users is whether they leave the service with a child. This study challenged this view by attempting to look at how individuals traded-off the *chance of having a child* with other, potentially important factors in the provision of IVF services. Based on literature reviews and previous studies, six attributes were identified as being *important* to users: chance of taking home a baby; follow-up support; time on the waiting list; continuity of staff; cost; and attitudes of staff. These attributes were interesting for a number of reasons. Only one of these attributes was a health outcome (chance of taking home a baby). There were also non-health outcomes (follow-up support) and process type attributes (waiting time, continuity of staff and attitudes of staff). The results showed that all the attributes included were significant i.e. they were all 'important' to individuals in the provision of IVF services. This study provided evidence that, within IVF, there are other attributes of *value* beyond leaving the service with a child.

This finding, along with the results from the WTP studies above has important implications for future evaluations of IVF and related technologies.

Discussion

The main challenge in the economic evaluation of IVF and related technologies lies in the definition, measurement and valuation of benefit. The studies outlined have shown that within the area of IVF and related technologies, there is more to the definition of *benefit* than traditionally assumed. Benefit includes not only health outcomes but non-health and process outcomes. Thus, in order for a fully comprehensive and informative economic evaluation of IVF and related technologies to be carried out, it is crucial that these other forms of benefit be included. The techniques of WTP and CA offer potential solutions to the problems of the traditional *narrow* measures of benefit assessment in economic evaluation.

References

Donaldson, C. and Shackley, P. (1997), 'Economic Evaluation', in Detels, R., Holland, W., McEwen, J. and Omenn, G. (eds), *Oxford Textbook of Public Health Third Edition*, Vol. 2, Oxford University Press, pp. 849-71.

Meschede, D. (1997), 'Assisted Reproduction for Infertile Couples at High Genetic Risk: An Ethical Consideration', in *Biomedical Ethics*, Vol. 2, No.1, pp. 4-6.

Neumann, P.J., Gharib, S.D. and Weinstein, M.C. (1994), 'The Cost of a Successful Delivery With In Vitro Fertilisation', *The New England Journal of Medicine*, Vol. 331, No. 4, pp. 239-43.

Propper, C. (1990), 'Contingent Valuation of Time Spent on NHS Waiting Lists', *The Economic Journal*, Vol. 100, pp. 193-9.

Ryan, M. (1996a), 'Using Willingness to Pay to Assess the Benefits of Assisted Reproductive Techniques', *Health Economics*, Vol. 5, pp. 543-58.

Ryan, M. (1996b), 'Using Consumer Preferences in Health Care Decision Making. The Application of Conjoint Analysis', *Office of Health Economics*.

Ryan, M. (1997a), 'Should Government Fund Assisted Reproductive Techniques? A Study Using Willingness to Pay', *Applied Economics*, Vol. 29, pp. 841-9.

Ryan, M. (1997b), 'Assessing the Benefits of Health Interventions: A Role for Conjoint Analysis?' Paper Presented for the Labelle Lectureship in Health Service Research, McMaster University, Hamilton, Ontario.

Ryan, M. (1998), 'Valuing Psychological Factors in the Provision of Assisted Reproductive Techniques Using the Economic Instrument of Willingness to Pay', Forthcoming, *Journal of Economic Psychology.*.

Ryan, M. and Donaldson, C. (1996), 'Assessing the Costs of Assisted Reproductive Techniques', *British Journal of Obstetrics and Gynaecology*, Vol. 103, pp.198-201.

Ryan, M. and Farrar, S. (1994), 'Conjoint Analysis: A New Tool for Eliciting Patients' Preferences', *Briefing Paper for the NHS in Scotland No.6, Health Economics Research Unit*, University of Aberdeen.

Ryan, M. and Hughes, J. (1997), 'Using Conjoint Analysis to Assess Women's Preferences for Miscarriage Management', *Health Economics*, Vol. 6, pp. 261-73.

Ryan, M., McIntosh, E. and Shackley, P. (1998), 'Methodological Issues in the Application of Conjoint Analysis in Health Care', Forthcoming, *Health Economics Letters.*

San Miguel, F., Ryan, M. and McIntosh, E. (1998), 'Some Methodological Issues in Applying Conjoint Analysis in Health Economics: An Application to Menorrhagia', Paper presented at the *Health Economists Study Group meeting*, Sheffield.

Vick, S. and Scott, A. (1998), 'Agency in Health Care. Examining Patients' Preferences for Attributes of the Doctor-patient Relationship', Forthcoming, *Journal of Health Economics*, p. 571.

4   Justice and preimplantation diagnosis

Joke de Witte

From a perspective of resource allocation in health care preimplantation diagnosis (PID) is just one more technology waiting to be financed. Or is it? Preimplantation diagnosis is a newly developed technology in the field of genetic screening. Since we are confronted as a society with the limits of the health care budget, we have to make some decisions with regard to this technology. Should we spend money on further research and development? Should this technology become a part of the health care services? Should everybody who needs it have access to it?

We do not want our answer to these questions to be arbitrary, so we need to try to find a just way of deciding what should be accessible and to whom within the health care services. This question of justice in health care, however, is a very difficult topic.

Justice in health care

Justice in health care is a topic that has received considerable philosophical attention. Probably the most influential work is the book *Just Health Care* by Norman Daniels (1985). According to Daniels a right to health care is only possible if it can be deduced from a general theory of distributive justice, or more specifically, from a theory of justice in health care. To bring health care within the domain of distributive justice (on the macro-level) it must be shown that health care is a social good comparable to other social goods that are distributed by society in accordance with particular principles of justice. To distinguish health care needs from all the other things we need, Daniels opts for the following definition: health care needs are the needs that are necessary to achieve or maintain species-typical normal functioning. Impairments of species-typical normal functioning reduce the range of opportunities available to an individual to realise his own plan of life. This definition of the importance of health care needs makes it possible to connect health care with a theory of justice that has as its central aim the promotion of fair equality of opportunity. If a theory of justice demands fair equality of opportunity, and if health care services contribute to this principle by maintaining or restoring species-typical normal functioning as much as possible, then health care is one of the social goods that should be distributed by society.

Another example is an article by Allan Buchanan concerning philosophical perspectives on access to health care (Buchanan 1997). Buchanan summarises several criteria for justice in health care. There is a moral right to health care, because health care serves particular fundamental interests of people (in preventing death, relieving suffering and offering information to plan our futures) and because it is unreasonable to expect people to pay for these services themselves. Distributive justice not only demands access to health care, but access without undue burdens. Serious barriers to obtaining services should be removed. The next question is what exactly distributive justice demands with regard to access to health care: access to all there is? This is impossible, because we cannot spend all our money on health care. There are other important social goods, such as education. It would also put too much stress on our solidarity with each other. The right to health care is the right to an adequate level of care. In addition to these criteria Buchanan mentions three other criteria for distributive justice in health care. The realisation of universal access to an adequate level of care without undue burdens should be realised through a fair distribution of costs and through a fair distribution of rationing. The last criterium is that the fruits of publicly funded medical research should be distributed fairly. If research is publicly funded, the public should benefit from it.

In short, from a perspective of distributive justice in health care, everybody should have equal access to an adequate level of health care, without undue financial, geographical or other burdens.

These are just two examples from the literature, but from my point of view this is the most reasonable account of justice in health care and matches more or less the principles which underly the organisation of health care services in (most) Westeuropean countries. For example, one article of the Dutch Constitution specifies that the government take measures to promote public health (Article 22, Dutch Constitution). The interpretation of this article is that the government has the obligation to ensure the quality and financial and geographical accessibility of health care services.

Justice and PID

But has this attention to justice in health care gotten us any further with respect to a decision about PID? We have arrived at the position that everybody should have equal access to an adequate level of care without undue burdens. If rationing is necessary because of limits to the health care budget, this rationing should be fair. This, however, is the most difficult part. Assuming that we cannot provide access to all that health care can offer, how do we go about setting priorities or rationing within the health care system?

Here we are facing a number of problems. One of the practical problems is the immensely difficult financial structure of the health care system (at least in the Netherlands). As a consequence, rationing between services that are relevant with regard to one health problem is not always easy, because they are regulated and financed in a different way. Another problem is that we do not start from scratch. Health care services are already in existence. This means that it will be difficult to change existing mechanisms of development and introduction of new medical technologies. Reality can make the implementation of ethical principles difficult.

The most important problem from the perspective of justice, however, is that justice is probably too general a concept to solve rationing problems between services. Daniels and Buchanan both make remarks to this extent (Daniels 1996, Buchanan 1997). I think this shortcoming is reflected in the difficulty governments have, or the Dutch government has, in reforming the health care system. It is easy enough to say that all citizens should have equal access to an adequate level of care, but to decide what should be included in this adequate level and how to weigh different services against each other is not just a matter of justice.

Some thoughts about PID

Whether resources should be reallocated to finance the further development of PID, whether PID should be part of the health care services and whether everybody in need should have access to PID, depends on what we, as a society, think is important. Justice plays its part, but it is not enough to make decisions about PID. To make a decision with regard to PID, it is important to analyse the way PID is looked at and find the problem it is supposed to solve. However, before presenting two possible ways of looking at PID, I want to make some preliminary remarks.

If PID is morally unacceptable, for example because the selection and destruction of embryos is thought to be morally unacceptable, or because the risks involved are too high, PID should not be part of the health care services.

If it is possible to base a claim on the desire for a healthy child, or if it is possible to formulate any rights at all with regard to PID, this would influence the decisions concerning priorities and rationing in health care. At this point I am assuming that it is not possible to formulate a claim or a right with regard to PID.

In the examples I have seen of adequate levels of care and of priorities within health care services (philosophical and government documents), the basic health care services that have to be offered to all are all forms of care meant to help existing individuals. PID would not be part of the core of the health care services. From this perspective it would be difficult to justify financial cuts on the core services for the sake of PID. If we were to use Daniel's concept of species-typical normal functioning, for example, infertility would probably count as a disease. PID, however, would not, because the problem is not an impairment of species-typical normal functioning.

Ways of looking at PID

PID as just an extension of the methods available within the field of genetic screening technologies. PID is a form of early prenatal diagnosis. Since we have accepted prenatal diagnosis, we can also accept PID.

What does PID offer? It offers a possibility to screen embryos in vitro for the presence of genetic disease. The affected embryos are discarded and only 'good' embryos are implanted in the womb of the future mother. A couple with a high risk of having a child with a genetic disease can start the pregnancy without fear and does not face the traumatic experience of prenatal diagnosis and abortion in case the fetus has the disease. Maybe offering PID can also reduce the amount of abortions. This would be good, because although abortion may be accepted, it remains morally problematic. These are some of the positive aspects of PID.

The disadvantage is that PID is coupled to in vitro fertilisation (IVF) and the succes rate of IVF is not high. A further consideration is that PID is still a rather expensive technology. If the succes rate of IVF does not improve, it could be more cost-effective to apply prenatal diagnosis to existing pregnancies.

From this perspective the decision with regard to PID depends ultimately on how much importance is attached to the positive aspects of PID in comparison to the costs.

How about access to PID? If a society wants a completely egalitarian health care system, the decision about PID will depend on whether this society can afford to offer PID to all who need this treatment, without doing an injustice to legitimate claims to other health care services. If this society cannot offer PID to all, they should decide not to include PID within the health care services.

PID is not just another technology for genetic diagnosis. Prenatal genetic diagnosis is justified, at least in the Netherlands, with the arguments that it helps to prevent human suffering and that it enables people to make a free, informed decision with regard to reproduction. It enables them to decide whether or not to continue a pregnancy in the case that the fetus has a genetic disease. But what about PID? PID also helps to prevent human suffering (especially for the parents). However, does it also contribute to free, informed reproductive decision making? Or does PID rather extend the possibilities for reproduction?

Is not the fundamental question of this whole discussion about genetics and reproduction how we think as a society about the importance of reproduction and having children? And more specifically: how we think as a society about the importance of having healthy children that are genetically our own. People with a high risk of having a child with a severe genetic disease do have other options. Apart from deciding to give up any further attempts at becoming pregnant, they could opt for adoption or for donor insemination or for IVF with the use of donor material. From this perspective what PID offers is the possibility of having a healthy child, that is genetically their own. It is possible that these alternatives offer no solution or that the future parents won't want to use them. But does that mean that society should offer them the possibility to have their own healthy child?

As a society we need a discussion about the importance of reproduction. With every new reproductive or genetic technology, we express our worries with regard to the effect all these technologies are supposed to have on our way of thinking about having children. We repeat over and over again that people do not have a right to a healthy child. We continue, however, to finance and accept these new technologies. The implicit assumption seems to be that reproduction and helping people to have a healthy child is very important. We should, however, make our assumptions explicitly. There are several possibilities:

For example, if we do not think that it is the task of society, especially when faced with limits to the budget, to help people realising their desire for a healthy child, we should not develop and offer new technologies, such as PID. People should realise that they cannot have all they want. They should learn to accept their unfortunate situation.

Or, if we recognise that it is important for people to be able to reproduce and to have a healthy child, we could reallocate money for the development of these technologies. In addition we could ask people to contribute financially to this treatment (include it in an additional insurance package).

Or if reproduction and the ability to have your own healthy child is, however, considered to be of the utmost importance, we should spend at least some money on the development of all sorts of technologies and include these technologies in the basic level of health care services.

At this moment, however, there is a gap between theory and practice. The health care system already offers all sorts of reproductive technologies and money has already been spent on the development of PID. In other words, was a decision about the availability of PID not made at the moment it was decided to finance PID or to accept PID as an experimental treatment? If we, as a society, do not think that it is a task of society to help people realise their deepest desire to have a healthy child and we are faced with limits in the health care budget, we should not have promoted the development of PID. Now that PID is being developed it will be extremely difficult not to use the technology, because it offers the possibility to relieve suffering and help people.

References

Buchanan, A. (1997), 'Philosophical Perspectives on Access to Health Care: Distributive Justice in Health Care', *The Mount Sinai Journal of Medicine*, Vol. 64, No. 2, pp. 90-5.

Daniels, N. (1985), *Just Health Care*, Cambridge University Press: Cambridge.

Daniels, N. (1996), 'Justice, Fair Procedures, and the Goals of Medicine', *The Hastings Center Report*, Vol. 26, No. 6, pp. 10-2.

5 The role of ethics codes in medicine – how can they be helpful in making decisions?

Stella Reiter-Theil

Introduction

Ethics codes and the codification of ethics have become a well recognised and widespread phenomenon since the Nuremberg Code was formulated in 1947 as a result of the Nuremberg Doctors' Trial against Nazi physicians. International documentation shows an exponential increase of upcoming new codes in the health sector in general and for the professions and subspecialties involved in particular (Reich 1995, Reiter-Theil 1998/in press a, Tröhler and Reiter-Theil 1998). But the significance and legitimacy of such codes are not clear. Despite the political impact and the professional or public awareness of codes, profound understanding and knowledge about the working of codes is lacking, due to a lack of specific research.

In this paper a tentative analysis will be presented for discussion about codifying ethics in medicine in general, and in reproductive medicine and preimplantation diagnosis (PID) in particular. The considerations offered go back to a broad interdisciplinary and international project of investigating the implications and the impact of ethics codes in medicine and biotechnology in depth since 1947, which has been recently undertaken in Freiburg at the Center for Ethics and Law in Medicine.[1] The goal of this paper is to show some of the possibilities as well as the difficulties connected with codifying ethics in the health sector and to stimulate debate and further research. One premise of the paper is that reflection about codes and codification is a challenge to reconsider the role of medical ethics in the whole of medicine and biomedical research as compared to law. The author hopes to contribute to a profile of medical ethics as mediating between the sphere of legal norms, which are all too often remote from medical practice, and the sphere of practical and clinical medicine, which is frequently uninformed or reluctant to deal with requirements of the law respectively.

What are medical ethics codes supposed to achieve?

In the following the term 'ethics codes' will be used in a broad sense including declarations, conventions, guidelines or recommendations concerning ethical issues in the health sector. Among these, professional (ethical) guidelines of medicine play an important role.

Quite often ethics codes are characterised as 'soft law' in the sense of being 'less' legitimate, valid or important than real laws. Therefore it seems necessary to clarify the relation between these two kinds of instruments for implementing ethical principles or rules. As a point of departure, the pejorative aspect of the label 'soft law' should be rejected. This view should open up the possibility to study what codes are expected or supposed to achieve. From the practical point of view, codes may provide better responses to present-day problems than laws. One reason for this is that they may be modified and optimised more easily than laws, i.e. that they allow for more flexibility in judgement, decision-making and action. Thus, they seem rather to be complementary to and more specific than the more general laws. And they can prepare the ground for national and international legal initiatives, which means that they can even contribute to competent legislation.

In comparing the role of the law as opposed to codes as a means for implementing medical ethics, it is interesting to consider the words of a clinician in reproductive medicine who advocates professional self control in the case of IVF:

> They [the General Medical Council] are highly knowledgeable of the facts and procedures of IVF and other medical procedures. They have the immense advantage of practising medical ethics, as opposed to the imposition of law by politicians, administrators, and lawyers. Ethics is not necessarily prohibitive; it is more constructive and responsive to a given situation, and medical ethics is practised by professionals ... (Edwards 1998, p. 13).

This view may help understand the significance of ethics codes up to the point, where guidelines are involved as instruments of professional self control. But a code seems to have a more general meaning and to demand a higher level of legitimacy than the criteria of a profession alone. The ethics underlying a code should not be the kind of medical ethics restricted to the particularities of the professional perspective. So, the internal means of safeguarding ethical standards within the medical profession as such would not qualify as a basis of an ethics code in a special medical domain such as reproductive medicine. There must be something more. We will come back to this.

How can ethics codes be helpful in the health sector?

We can distinguish at least six fields, where codes may be of use or even helpful for practical purposes:
– in jurisdiction;
– in policy making;
– as guidelines for medical decision-making and action;
– as an orientation for patients or clients;
– as an instrument of legitimation;
– as a set of criteria for 'ethical' quality control.
These fields will be illustrated and discussed by examples.

Jurisdiction

Example: The 'Nuremberg Code' (formulated in 1947 in the course of the Nuremberg Doctors' Trial):
The Nuremberg Code with its emphasis on free consent on the basis of specific information given to the research subject in medicine is the most prominent example of an effort to protect people from getting involved in precarious research which may not be in their best interests. At the same time the Nuremberg Code serves the purpose of excluding non-competent persons or patients from research to which they could neither consent nor dissent. As Krause and Winslade have shown for the US, the Nuremberg Code proved to be a useful source of ethical arguments against risky research with non-consenting subjects at court, but they also showed that it took decades for the impact of the Code was to be appreciated and respected in American jurisdiction (Krause and Winslade, in press).

Example: The 'Guidelines for Medical Aid in Dying' (issued by the German Federal Association of Physicians, 1993, 1997 rev.):
The Guidelines for Medical Aid in Dying are an attempt to answer the many questions which arise in the context of letting patients die under circumstances of terminal illness and pain. In the formulation of 1993 the guidelines do not address the option of a will to live and the consequences for medical decision-making. But this is done in the revised form suggested for discussion in 1997, where wills to live are appreciated as valuable indicators of the patient's will

that should be respected under certain circumstances. Several German court decisions about withdrawal of treatment or letting a patient die in recent years have referred to the 1993 guidelines and in some cases the judge commented that the judgment would have been easier, had there existed a will to live of the patient concerned (Koch 1997).

The relevance of codes can be objectified by showing that they are valuable sources for ethical argumentation at court. Lawsuits are seen as the 'via regia' of gaining jurisprudential knowledge, of clarifying new legal conflicts and uncertainties basically and comprehensively at the first instance. But problems remain: codes are merely 'soft law', which means that there is great uncertainty about the outcome of appealing to them. For the people involved, lawsuits are exhausting, burdensome and expensive. And for severely ill persons even a successful outcome does not always mean that necessary help or prevention is possible anymore.

Excursion about preimplantation diagnosis

Another way in which ethics codes can gain impact in the legal sphere is when they serve as preparation for the process of legislation. In the context of reproductive medicine, PID is a good example of possible interactions between the law and codes. In Germany PID is prohibited on the grounds of the Embryo Protection Act (see also Bundesärztekammer, 1991). But at some German Medical Faculties there have been discussions about the possibility to offer PID to a strictly defined group of couples with a high genetic risk of conceiving severely handicapped children, e.g. in Lübeck (Hildt 1996, Ludwig 1996). Until now, PID has not been offered in Germany due to the legal restriction in the country, although some argue that the possibility to avoid embryopathic abortion should ethically override the prohibition of the technique (Kommission für Öffentlichkeitsarbeit und ethische Fragen der Gesellschaft für Humangenetik 1995, Müller 1996, Schreiber 1996). Along with this line og thought one can also hear the argument that the Embryo Protection Act would have been formulated differently, had its drafters anticipated the possibility of PID and its potential benefits (Eser 1996). Before a change of the law becomes possible, it seems much more feasible to formulate guidelines considering and evaluating the empirical needs and clinical indications for PID. Such guidelines might allow for limited use of the technique within particular centres and under specific monitoring (as has been suggested by the Kommission für Öffentlichkeitsarbeit und ethische Fragen der Gesellschaft für Humangenetik). But all efforts to formulate preliminary rules for ethically justifiable application of PID have in any case to face the necessity of formulating limits of the practice as well. Like many other biotechnologies, PID opens up a wide spectrum of possible applications, which might be accompanied by the instrumentalisation of human beings, e.g., when a child is brought to term in order to become a bone marrow donor for another family member (Green, Fibison and Hughes 1997). After a period of time in which the practice will have been evaluated, the law might be reconsidered in the light of new experiences and data. As one form of codifying ethical principles for practice, guidelines could thus play an important role in furthering forward informed and competent legislation.

Policy making

Example: 'Convention for the Protection of Human Rights and Dignity of the Human Being with Regard to the Application of Biology and Medicine: Convention on Human Rights and Biomedicine' (ETS no. 164, Orvieto):
The Convention on Human Rights and Biomedicine is a recent initiative to harmonise the ethical grounds for human biomedical research in Europe. Although welcomed by many as an instrument for setting reasonable minimum standards for research practice still unknown in a number of European countries, the Convention has been criticised for neglecting the protection of non-competent patients from research. In the light of the Nuremberg tradition, which arose from condemning the inhumane abuse of imprisoned persons and patients for 'research' purposes, ethical criteria such as voluntary and informed consent have been given the highest priority. For non-competent persons, however, a legal substitute may give proxy consent to research, if the Convention becomes reality.

Thus, this attempt to codify ethical standards for research comes into conflict with the most prominent Nuremberg Code, a conflict which cannot be easily reconciled. The provision of medical help for those groups of patients, who by definition cannot give informed consent, often requires them to enrole in studies. This is the case in research with demented patients, in emergency research or in neonatal research. The enrolment of embryos or fetuses in experimental practices such as PID is a complicated problem because of the controversial views about the moral status of embryos or fetuses.

The consideration of these difficulties for the codification of ethics in medicine provokes questions such as: to what extent are codes, interculturally and historically universal? How can we handle difficulties with the legitimacy of codes and conflicts between codes, both nationally and internationally? The comparative analysis and evaluation of ethics codes is still in its infancy and has produced only preliminary findings. It will require great effort to draw systematic conclusions from the experiences with codes in the last decades, but it seems that it will be inevitable to proceed with the exponential production of codes even before we have gained adequate insight into the phenomenon.

In many fields of practical and clinical medicine difficult decisions have to be made about the continuation or withdrawal of treatment. This is particularly serious where prognosis is uncertain and where the individual involved is only at the beginning of his or her life. There are two medical fields of extreme difficulty, for which specific guidelines have been formulated by professional groups, assisted by interdisciplinary colleagues: neo- or perinatology and fetocide in reproductive medicine.

First Example: 'Einbecker Empfehlung' – 'Limits of doctors' duties to treat newborns with severe handicaps' (formulated by the German Society for Medical Law, revised 1992) and
Second Example: 'Guidelines for Fetocide' issued by the German Federal Association of Physicians (1989):
Doctors often have problems with making decisions about the continuation or withdrawal of treatment of severely handicapped newborns. The parents of these children are under extreme pressure in such situations and may ask desperately for heroic efforts to save the child's life. On the other hand, parents are sometimes afraid to face living with a child who would never become able to take care for him- or herself because of severe handicaps, or who would suffer enormous pain before dying due to the illness. The Einbecker Empfehlung was initiated to provide doctors and other health care professionals involved with ethical orientation, and revised after a period of experience. Doctors can use these guidelines as a starting point for reflection and discussion. This may facilitate rational and balanced reasoning and argumentation. One advantage of the Einbecker Empfehlung is that it includes other professionals such as nurses involved in caring for the child as well as the parents.

Multiple pregnancies with up to five embryos may be a result of hormone stimulation in women who have had problems becoming pregnant. Although it is in principle now possible to control the conditions of this treatment and so avoid multiple pregnancies, the problem has not yet disappeared, not even in medical centers with high standards: the long desired pregnancy occurs, but with the high risk that none of the children will survive. Irrespective of the moral problems with abortion in cases where the woman decides to carry the child to term, killing a number of embryos in order to facilitate the survival of the remaining ones poses a moral dilemma (Reiter-Theil and Kahlke 1995). The guidelines for fetocide were formulated in order to make this dilemma easier for the doctor and to help him or her to act in favour of maintaining the pregnancy – at least in the 'reduced' form.

In order to make use of the guidelines, the professional involved must have knowledge of them, understand them correctly and put their spirit into practice. But despite the advantages of the guidelines, some difficulties will remain. Doctors or others engaged in the decision-making process have to interpret the guidelines as in the light of their personal convictions as well as of the specfic conflict involved. This is a difficult task when it comes to existential issues of life and death, of uncertain prognosis, lifelong suffering, fear and guilt.

Both guidelines have stimulated professional controversies and provoked protest: the Einbecker Empfehlung was criticised from the perspective of handicapped persons, who expressed fear that letting handicapped newborns die might become easier and more acceptable because of these guidelines than protecting their lives and living with them; the guidelines for fetocide were criticised on the grounds that reproductive medicine created moral problems – multiple pregnancies – which should then be solved by immoral interventions – namely by terminating the lives of some of the embryos.

Orientation for patients or clients

Codes or guidelines can also help patients or clients to become more aware of their rights and duties in the health context. They can thus be valuable tools for the enhancement of self-determination, good care and protection from harm. Despite the official discussion of ethics in medicine, patients continue to have significant internal and external difficulties with realising their potential self-determination, be it in decisions about treatment choices (Reiter-Theil 1998/in press b) or in formulating and putting forward the wills to live (Reiter-Theil 1998/in press c), not to mention decisions in intensive or terminal care, where patients per definitionem are rarely able to participate actively (Herych and Reiter-Theil, 1998, Hiddemann 1997). In conferences with patients as well as health care professionals about ethical issues such as informed consent or withdrawal of therapy, evidence was found that there is a great need for information and participation, and, even more importantly: there is considerable competence among patients to engage in dialogue with the doctors about the underlying ethics of treatment relevant to them, if they are addressed in a fair way (Reiter-Theil 1998 a, Zerres and Rüdel 1993).

Among the problems with codes or guidelines for patients involved are the following:

– How many patients or clients really know about codes dealing with their rights and the complementary duties of health care professionals in medicine?

- How do they gain information – if at all – about codes?
- To what extent are they able to make use of concepts such as the right to be informed about the risks of a treatment or the responsibility to take the interests of an unborn child into account?
- Do we ask patients, clients or future parents to be moral agents in their personal decision-making – as we do with doctors or other health care professionals?
- What are the limits of personal (moral) preferences?
- Who is entitled to judge morally about peoples' life decisions?

Example: Ethical Code (endorsed by the European Alliance of Genetic Support Groups, 1996):
In the statements and guidelines of the ethical code formulated by this European patient organisation six major ethical issues are addressed:
- medical genetics should serve the interests of the individuals affected or at risk from genetic disease,
- services should be oriented to needs,
- freedom of choice to make use of the services,
- services should facilitate informed decisions,
- the quality of life of those affected should be improved by national or European legislation,
- persons with disabilities or diseases should be entitled to unrestricted acceptance and solidarity from society.

All of these statements reflect fears and doubts about the situation of genetically affected patients both in medicine as well as in society as a whole. However, the ethical principles referred to are the same universal concepts dominant in the general discussion of medical ethics – reflected and formulated from the perspective of the persons in need of help and protection. Even as the ethics codes of the medical profession or other academic groups rarely reach the patients directly, this patients' code will be less known among geneticists. This fact makes obvious the need for dialogue between the groups involved in medical genetics – the providers of professional help and those who are in need of it.

Legitimation

To understand the impact of codes in the realm of legitimising ethical positions, it is necessary to look at the epistemological status of codes and guidelines. A code may provide us with new reasons for legitimation. It may help us as a frame of reference, corresponding to our own preferences. Agreement between the decision taken and a relevant code may provide political or legal protection for the professional. A code may also provide a simple directive imposed by a professional association which can be followed.

Therefore, a code may induce or reinforce heteronomous morality. Conflict between a relevant code and one's own judgement may lead to disorientation. Uncertainty is one of the consequences of difficulties in applying codes to practice. Contradictions between codes and professional rules create dilemmas. As a result, we have to accept that codes or guidelines do not solve the moral problems arising from the pluralism of values in complex societies. Universalism, being one of the corner stones of ethical theory, is rather a normative and methodological concept than an empirical fact. As Baker has pointed out, it is most often not principles, rules or values which are interculturally or universally valid. It is rather a commonality of problems, conflicts and needs for solutions, which brings groups, countries or cultures together (Baker 1998). Codes play in this way the particular role in pluralism of defining and defending one dominant position preferred by the relevant professional body or societal group, but not once and for all. We have also learned that there is no absolute ethical 'neutrality' possible in the treatment and counselling of people in need of help and that it is instead necessary to reflect and to follow explicit ethical principles rather than trying to practice 'value free' medicine (Reiter-Theil 1998). What is most important is to continue the international dialogue about cultural and religious essentials and to further a universal human ethics as far as possible.

'Ethical' Quality control

Finally, guidelines and codes may be used as instruments to assess the ethical quality of health services. Possible criteria are:
– adequate patient/client information and advice
– respecting patients' preferences or choices
– minimising harm
– providing help
– confidentiality
– empathy
– organising social support

It is obvious that medical services cannot take responsibility for societal solidarity towards patients directly. Solidarity is one of the six major points in the ethics code of the European patients' organisation mentioned above. But the attitude of professional organisations, statements in ethics codes of medicine and the official medical ethics discourse are important factors in shaping the ways in which society responds to patients with certain diseases or disorders. In medicine the efforts for quality assessment and assurance have gained high priority recently. It seems reasonable to include explicit ethical criteria in the criteria catalogues and to link these two branches of self-referential reflection in medicine – quality assurance and ethical discourse – in one approach.

Conclusion

A unified Europe needs clear and valid ethical guidelines and codes for the advancement of medicine and biotechnology, if the present and future practice is to be consistent with universal ethical ideas arising from the traditions of the countries involved. But such ethics codes and guidelines must go beyond the traditionalist moral grounds of particular groups such as ethnic populations or professions in order to develop an integrative unifying value. To cope with the ever increasing new possibilities created by medicine and biotechnology, ethics codes and guidelines have to be formulated as flexible instruments which allow for specific and immediate reaction to innovations challenging the familiar limits of our thinking and doing.

The Europe wide debate about the 'Convention on Human Rights and Biomedicine' has taught us the lesson that consensus is all but easy to achieve, particularly when it comes to issues concerning the beginning and the end of life, or when the rights of vulnerable groups are drawn into question. But there seems to be no alternative to codification as a means of preparing supranational legislation in fields where empirical evidence, research data and technical potential are changing so rapidly as in medicine and biotechnology today. It is all the more important to develop methodological strategies to analyse and to compare codes with the objective of evaluating their impact on the ethical quality in applying our most ambitious innovations in humans.

Note

1   We are grateful for the generous grant from the German Ministry for Education, Science, Research and Technology permitting us to realise the project 'Ethics Codes in Medicine and Biotechnology' (1995-1998).

References

Baker, R. (1998/in press), 'Transcultural Medical Ethics and Human Rights', in Tröhler, U. and Reiter-Theil, S. (eds) (in collaboration with E. Herych), *Ethics Codes in Medicine. Foundations and Achievements since 1947,* Ashgate: Aldershot, pp. 310- 29.

Bundesärztekammer (1989), 'Mehrlingsreduktion mittels Fetozid', *Deutsches Ärzteblatt*, Vol. 86: B, pp. 1575-7.

Bundesärztekammer (1991), 'Zentrale Kommission zur Wahrung ethischer Grundsätze in der Reproduktionsmedizin, Forschung an menschlichen Embryonen und Gentherapie: Richtlinien zur Verwendung fetaler Zellen und fetaler Gewebe', *Deutsches Ärzteblatt*, Vol. 88, pp. 2360-3.

Bundesärztekammer (1993), 'Richtlinien der Bundesärztekammer für die ärztliche Sterbebegleitung', *Deutsches Ärzteblatt*, Vol. 90, No. 37:C, pp. 1628-29 (Guidelines for Medical Aid in Dying 1993, 1997).

Bundesärztekammer (1997), 'Entwurf der Richtlinie der BÄK zur ärztlichen Sterbebegleitung und den Grenzen zumutbarer Behandlung (Stand: 25.4.1997)', *Deutsches Ärzteblatt*, Vol. 94, No. 20: C, pp. 988-9.

Edwards, R.G. (1998), 'Introduction and Development of IVF and its Ethical Regulation', in: Hildt, E. and Mieth, D. (eds), *In Vitro Fertilisation in the 1990s. Towards a Medical, Social and Ethical Evaluation*, Ashgate: Aldershot, pp. 3-18.

Einbecker Empfehlungen (1992, rev), 'Grenzen ärztlicher Behandlungspflicht bei schwerstgeschädigten Neugeborenen', *MedR*, Vol. 4, p. 206.

Eser, A. (1996) 'Statement', in: *Biomedical Ethics*, Vol. 1, No. 2, pp. 33-5.

European Alliance of Genetic Support Groups (EAGS) (1996), *Ethical Code*, London: Soestdijk.

Green, R.M., Fibison, W.J. and Hughs, M.R. (1997), '«Planned Parenthood»: Case Commentary, *Cambridge Quarterly of Health Care Ethics,* Vol. 6. pp. 101-5.

Herych, E. and Reiter-Theil, S. (1998), 'Entscheidungen am Lebensende: Innere und äußere Grenzen der Selbstbestimmung', in Blonski, H. (ed.), *Ethik in Gerontologie und Altenpflege*, Kunz: Hagen, pp. 75-91.

Hiddemann, W. (1997), 'Das Thema Sterben und Tod im Unterricht: Beispiel einer Vorlesung', in Reiter-Theil, S. (ed.), *Vermittlung Medizinischer Ethik. Theorie und Praxis in Europa*, Nomos: Baden-Baden, pp. 120-30.

Hildt, E. (1996), 'Preimplantation Diagnosis in Germany? A Report from a Press Conference', *Biomedical Ethics*, Vol. 1, No. 2, pp. 28-9.

Convention for the Protection of Human Rights and Dignity of the Human Being with Regard to the Application of Biology and Medicine: Convention on Human Rights and Biomedicine, Council of Europe, ETS No. 164. Orvieto, 04.IV.1997.

Koch, H.G. (1997), 'Self-Determination, Privacy, and the Right to Die. A Comparative Law Analysis (Germany, United States of America, Japan)', *European Journal of Health Law*, Vol. 4, pp. 9-25.

Kommission für Öffentlichkeitsarbeit und ethische Fragen der Deutschen Gesellschaft für Humangenetik e.V. (1995), 'Stellungnahme zur Präimplantationsdiagnostik', *Med Genetik*, Vol. 7, p. 420.

Krause, T. and Winslade, W. (1998/in press), 'The Nuremberg Code Turns Fifty', in Tröhler, U. and Reiter-Theil, S. (eds) (in collaboration with E. Herych), *Ethics Codes in Medicine. Foundations and Achievements since 1947*, Ashgate: Aldershot, p. 140-62.

Ludwig, M. (1996), 'Statement', in *Biomedical Ethics*, Vol. 1, No. 2, pp. 30-1.

Müller, H. (1996), 'Statement', in *Biomedical Ethics*, Vol. 1, No. 2, pp. 31-2.

'The Nuremberg Code (1947)', in Reich, W.T. (ed.) (1995), *Encyclopedia of Bioethics*, Vol. 5, Appendix. Simon and Schuster Macmillan, pp. 2763-4.

Reich, W.T. (ed.) (1995), 'Encyclopedia of Bioethics'.

Reiter-Theil, S. (1998 a), 'Voice of the patient', *The Patients' Forum Medical Ethics. Bull Med Ethics.*

Reiter-Theil, S. (1998), 'Ethical Neutrality in Counselling? The Challenge of Infertility', in: Hildt, E. and Mieth, D. (eds), *In Vitro Fertilisation in the 1990s – Towards a Medical, Social and Ethical Evaluation*, Ashgate: Aldershot, pp. 257-68.

Reiter-Theil, S. (1998/in press a), 'Answers to Change: The Problem of Paradigm Shift in Medical Ethics from the German Perspective', in Tröhler, U. and Reiter-Theil, S. (eds) (in collaboration with E. Herych), *Ethics Codes in Medicine. Foundations and Achievements since 1947*, Ashgate: Aldershot, pp. 257-68.

Reiter-Theil, S. (1998/in press b), 'Therapiebegrenzung und Sterben im Gespräch zwischen Arzt und Patient. Ein integratives Modell für ein vernachlässigtes Problem', *Ethik Med.*

Reiter-Theil, S. (1998/in press c), 'Ethische Aspekte der Patienten-Verfügung. Eine Chance zur Gestaltung des Sterbens', *Forum DKG.*

Reiter-Theil, S. and Kahlke, W. (1995), 'Fortpflanzungsmedizin', in Kahlke, W. and Reiter-Theil, S. (eds), *Ethik in der Medizin*, Enke: Stuttgart, pp. 34-45.

Schreiber, H.P. (1996), 'Embryonenforschung und Präimplantationsdiagnostik im Spannungsfeld von Ethik und Recht', in Holzhey, H. and Schaber, P. (eds), *Ethik in der Schweiz*, Pano Verlag: Zürich, pp. 199-205.

Tröhler, U. and Reiter-Theil, S. (eds) (in collaboration with E. Herych) (1998/in press), 'Ethics Codes in Medicine. Foundations and Achievements since 1947', Ashgate: Aldershot.

Zerres, K. and Rüdel, R. (eds) (1993), *Selbsthilfegruppen und Humangenetiker im Dialog. Erwartungen und Befürchtungen*, Enke: Stuttgart.

Index

315

Printed and bound by CPI Group (UK) Ltd, Croydon, CR0 4YY

21/10/2024

01777088-0002